2008
YEAR BOOK OF
DERMATOLOGY
AND
DERMATOLOGIC
SURGERY™

The 2008 Year Book Series

Year Book of Anesthesiology and Pain Management™: Drs Chestnut, Abram, Black, Gravlee, Lee, Mathru, and Roizen

Year Book of Cardiology®: Drs Gersh, Cheitlin, Elliott, Graham, Sundt, and Waldo

Year Book of Critical Care Medicine®: Drs Dellinger, Parrillo, Balk, Bekes, Dorman, and Dries

Year Book of Dentistry®: Drs Olin, Belvedere, Davis, Henderson, Johnson, Ohrbach, Scott, Spencer, and Zakariasen

Year Book of Dermatology and Dermatologic Surgery™: Drs Thiers and Lang

Year Book of Diagnostic Radiology®: Drs Birdwell, Elster, Gardiner, Levy, Manaster, Oestreich, and Rosado de Christenson

Year Book of Emergency Medicine®: Drs Hamilton, Handly, Quintana, Werner, and Bruno

Year Book of Endocrinology®: Drs Mazzaferri, Bessesen, Clarke, Howard, Kennedy, Leahy, Meikle, Molitch, Rogol, and Schteingart

Year Book of Gastroenterology™: Drs Lichtenstein, Dempsey, Drebin, Jaffe, Katzka, Kochman, Makar, Morris, Osterman, Rombeau, and Shah

Year Book of Hand and Upper Limb Surgery®: Drs Chang and Steinmann

Year Book of Medicine®: Drs Barkin, Berney, Frishman, Garrick, Loehrer, Phillips, and Khardori

Year Book of Neonatal and Perinatal Medicine®: Drs Fanaroff, Ehrenkranz, and Stevenson

Year Book of Neurology and Neurosurgery®: Drs Kim and Verma

Year Book of Obstetrics, Gynecology, and Women's Health®: Dr Shulman

Year Book of Oncology®: Drs Loehrer, Arceci, Glatstein, Gordon, Hanna, Morrow, and Thigpen

Year Book of Ophthalmology®: Drs Rapuano, Cohen, Eagle, Flanders, Hammersmith, Myers, Nelson, Penne, Sergott, Shields, Tipperman, and Vander

Year Book of Orthopedics®: Drs Morrey, Beauchamp, Huddleston, Peterson, Swiontkowski, and Trigg

Year Book of Otolaryngology-Head and Neck Surgery®: Drs Gapany, Keefe, and Sindwani

Year Book of Pathology and Laboratory Medicine®: Drs Raab, Parwani, Bejarano, and Bissell

Year Book of Pediatrics®: Dr Stockman

Year Book of Plastic and Aesthetic Surgery™: Drs Miller, Bartlett, Garner, McKinney, Ruberg, Salisbury, and Smith

Year Book of Psychiatry and Applied Mental Health®: Drs Talbott, Ballenger, Buckley, Frances, Markowitz, and Sarles

Year Book of Pulmonary Disease®: Drs Phillips, Barker, Lewis, Maurer, Tanoue, and Willsie

Year Book of Sports Medicine®: Drs Shephard, Cantu, Feldman, Jankowski, McCrory, Nieman, Pierrynowski, Rowland, and Shrier

Year Book of Surgery®: Drs Copeland, Bland, Daly, Eberlein, Fahey, Jones, Mozingo, Pruett, and Seeger

Year Book of Urology®: Drs Andriole and Coplen

Year Book of Vascular Surgery®: Dr Moneta

2008

The Year Book of DERMATOLOGY AND DERMATOLOGIC SURGERY™

Editor-in-Chief

Bruce H. Thiers, MD

Professor and Chair, Department of Dermatology, Medical University of South Carolina, Charleston, South Carolina

Associate Editor

Pearon G. Lang, Jr, MD

Professor of Dermatology, Pathology, Otolaryngology, and Communicative Sciences, Medical University of South Carolina, Charleston, South Carolina

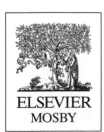

ELSEVIER
MOSBY

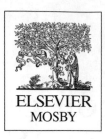

ELSEVIER
MOSBY

Vice President, Continuity: John A. Schrefer
Developmental Editor: Ali Gavenda
Supervisor, Electronic Year Books: Donna M. Adamson
Electronic Article Manager: Jennifer C. Pitts
Illustrations and Permissions Coordinator: Linda S. Jones

2008 EDITION

Printed in the United States of America
Composition by Thomas Technology Solutions, Inc.
Printing/binding by Sheridan Books, Inc.

Editorial Office:
Elsevier
Suite 1800
1600 John F. Kennedy Blvd
Philadelphia, PA 19103-2899

International Standard Serial Number: 0093-3619
International Standard Book Number: 978-1-4160-5151-0

Contributors

Margaret M. Boyle, BS
Research Associate, Dermatoepidemiology Unit, Brown University, Providence, Rhode Island

Gillian M. P. Galbraith, MD
Professor of Biomedical Science, University of Las Vegas School of Dental Medicine, Las Vegas, Nevada

Michael H. Gold, MD
Medical Director, Gold Skin Care Center and Tennessee Clinical Research Center, Nashville; Clinical Assistant Professor, Division of Dermatology, Department of Medicine, Vanderbilt University Medical School and Vanderbilt University Nursing School, Nashville, Tennessee; Visiting Professor of Dermatology, Huashan Hospital, Fudan University, Shanghai, China

Sharon Raimer, MD
Professor of Dermatology and Pediatrics; Chair, Department of Dermatology, University of Texas Medical Branch, Galveston, Texas

Martin A. Weinstock, MD, PhD
Professor of Dermatology and Community Health, Brown University; Chief of Dermatology, VA Medical Center; Director, Pigmented Lesion Unit and Photomedicine, Rhode Island Hospital, Providence, Rhode Island

Table of Contents

Journals Represented

Journals represented in this YEAR BOOK are listed below.

Acta Dermato-Venereologica
Aesthetic Plastic Surgery
Allergy
American Journal of Clinical Nutrition
American Journal of Epidemiology
American Journal of Human Genetics
American Journal of Managed Care
American Journal of Medicine
American Journal of Pathology
American Journal of Roentgenology
American Journal of Sports Medicine
American Journal of Surgery
American Journal of Surgical Pathology
Annals of Epidemiology
Annals of Internal Medicine
Annals of Plastic Surgery
Annals of Surgical Oncology
Antiviral Research
Archives of Dermatological Research
Archives of Dermatology
Archives of Internal Medicine
Arthritis and Rheumatism
Australian Journal of Dermatology
BMC Health Services Research
Blood
British Journal of Cancer
British Journal of Dermatology
British Medical Journal
CA: A Cancer Journal for Clinicians
Cancer Epidemiology, Biomarkers and Prevention
Cell
Clinical Cancer Research
Clinical Infectious Diseases
Cochrane Database for Systematic Reviews
Dermatologic Surgery
Dermatology
Digestive Diseases and Sciences
Drugs & Aging
European Journal of Cancer
European Journal of Nuclear Medicine and Molecular Imaging
European Journal of Plastic Surgery
European Journal of Surgical Oncology
Experimental Dermatology
Giornale Italiano di Dermatologia e Venereologia
Gynecologic Oncology
Health Education & Behavior
International Journal of Gynecology & Obstetrics
Journal of Allergy and Clinical Immunology
Journal of Bone and Joint Surgery (American Volume)

Journal of Clinical Investigation
Journal of Clinical Microbiology
Journal of Clinical Oncology
Journal of Cutaneous Pathology
Journal of Dermatology
Journal of Drugs in Dermatology
Journal of General Internal Medicine
Journal of Hepatology
Journal of Immunology
Journal of Infectious Diseases
Journal of Investigative Dermatology
Journal of Nutritional Biochemistry
Journal of Pediatric Surgery
Journal of Pediatrics
Journal of Plastic, Reconstructive & Aesthetic Surgery
Journal of Reproductive Medicine
Journal of Rheumatology
Journal of Surgical Oncology
Journal of Urology
Journal of the American Academy of Dermatology
Journal of the American College of Surgeons
Journal of the American Geriatrics Society
Journal of the American Medical Association
Journal of the European Academy of Dermatology and Venereology
Lancet
Mayo Clinic Proceedings
Modern Pathology
Molecular Medicine
Nature
Nature Medicine
New England Journal of Medicine
Oncogene
PLoS Medicine
PLoS Pathogens
Photodermatology Photoimmunology and Photomedicine
Plastic and Reconstructive Surgery
Proceedings of the National Academy of Sciences
Radiology
Respiratory Medicine
Science
Surgery

STANDARD ABBREVIATIONS

The following terms are abbreviated in this edition: acquired immunodeficiency syndrome (AIDS), cardiopulmonary resuscitation (CPR), central nervous system (CNS), cerebrospinal fluid (CSF), computed tomography (CT), deoxyribonucleic acid (DNA), electrocardiography (ECG), health maintenance organization (HMO), human immunodeficiency virus (HIV), intensive care unit (ICU), intramuscular (IM), intravenous (IV), magnetic resonance (MR) imaging (MRI), ribonucleic acid (RNA), ultrasound (US), and ultraviolet (UV).

NOTE

The YEAR BOOK OF DERMATOLOGY AND DERMATOLOGIC SURGERY™ is a literature survey service providing abstracts of articles published in the professional literature. Every effort is made to assure the accuracy of the information presented in these pages. Neither the editors nor the publisher of the YEAR BOOK OF DERMATOLOGY AND DERMATOLOGIC SURGERY™ can be responsible for errors in the original materials. The editors' comments are their own opinions. Mention of specific products within this publication does not constitute endorsement.

To facilitate the use of the YEAR BOOK OF DERMATOLOGY AND DERMATOLOGIC SURGERY™ as a reference tool, all illustrations and tables included in this publication are now identified as they appear in the original article. This change is meant to help the reader recognize that any illustration or table appearing in the YEAR BOOK OF DERMATOLOGY AND DERMATOLOGIC SURGERY™ may be only one of many in the original article. For this reason, figure and table numbers will often appear to be out of sequence within the YEAR BOOK OF DERMATOLOGY AND DERMATOLOGIC SURGERY™.

COLOR PLATE I

Gold Fig 1

COLOR PLATE II

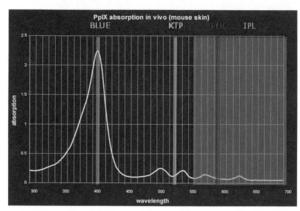

Gold Fig 2

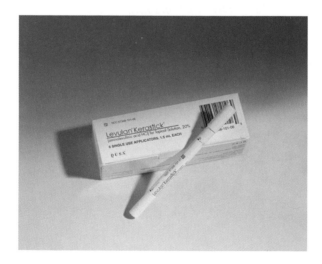

Gold Fig 3

COLOR PLATE III

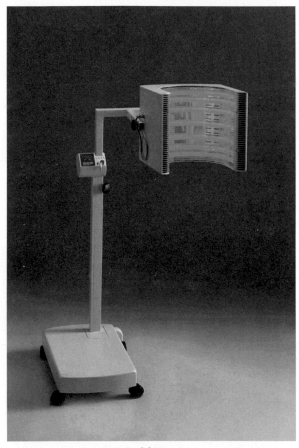

Gold Fig 4

COLOR PLATE IV

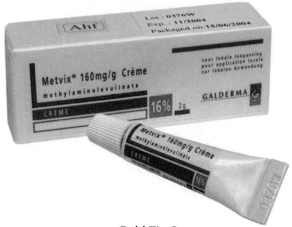

Gold Fig 5

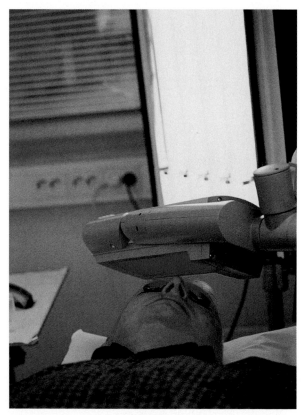

Gold Fig 6

COLOR PLATE V

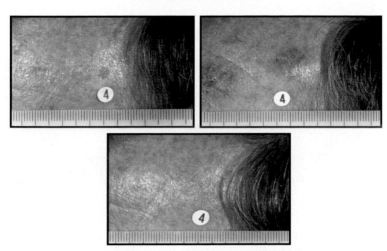

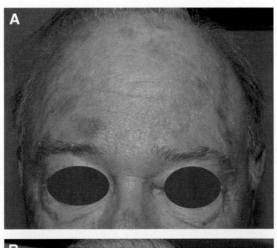

Gold Fig 7

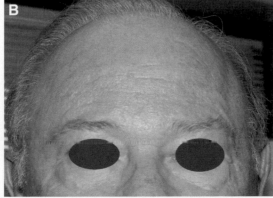

Gold Fig 8, A-B

COLOR PLATE VI

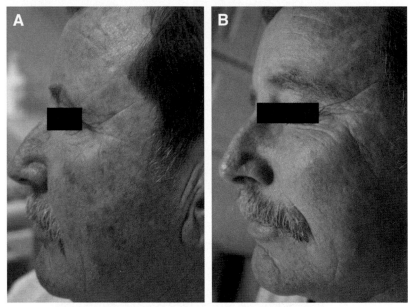

Gold Fig 9, A-B

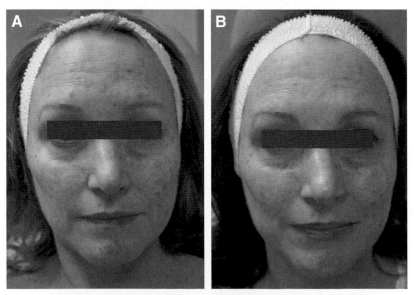

Gold Fig 10, A-B

COLOR PLATE VII

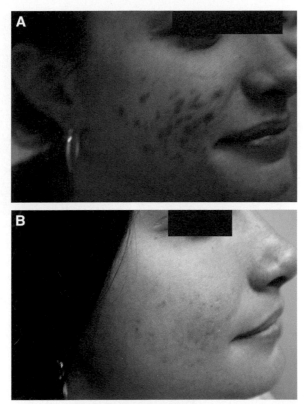

Gold Fig 11, A-B

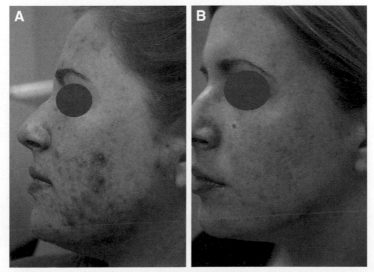

Gold Fig 12, A-B

COLOR PLATE VIII

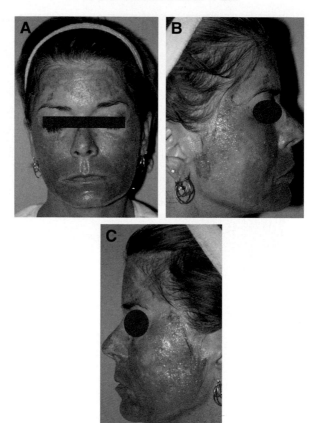

Gold Fig 13, A-C

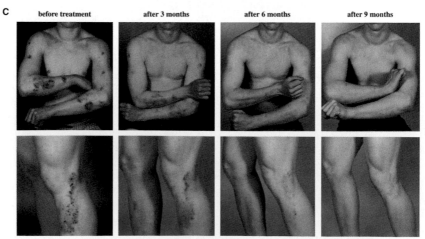

Fig 1C, page 64

COLOR PLATE IX

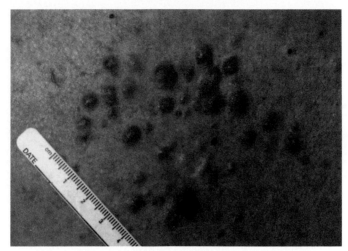

Fig 1, page 243

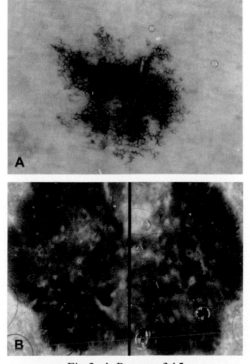

Fig 2, A-B, page 345

COLOR PLATE X

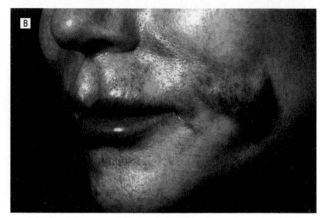

Fig 1B, page 418

Case 5

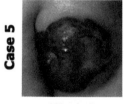

Week 0

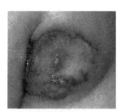

Week 5

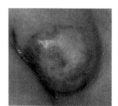

Week 11

Fig 1, Case 5, page 430

ALA-PDT: State of the Art in the United States, 2008

MICHAEL H. GOLD, MD*

Medical Director, Gold Skin Care Center, Tennessee Clinical Research Center; Clinical Assistant Professor, Division of Dermatology, Department of Medicine, Vanderbilt University Medical School, Vanderbilt University Nursing School, Nashville, Tennessee; Visiting Professor of Dermatology, Huashan Hospital, Fudan University Shanghai, China

INTRODUCTION

The state of the art for aminolevulinic acid (ALA) photodynamic therapy (PDT) is very strong. Both in the United States and in many parts of the world, the utilization of ALA-PDT has shown a steady increase in the number of conditions being treated with this form of therapy and in the number of physicians who now routinely use this therapy in their clinical, medical, and surgical dermatological practices. ALA-PDT has become available to our colleagues in Latin and South America as well as in Asia. ALA-PDT is still, at the time of this writing, not available in a commercial form in Europe and Australia, but this may change in the near future. In these countries, the methyl ester form of ALA is available and will also be reviewed in this article. Also to be reviewed in this article is ALA-PDT in detail, from its history to its current uses and indications. This report will also focus on the proper use of ALA-PDT and its proper aftercare necessary to minimize any potential adverse events and to make ALA-PDT treatments the most useful and effective for our patients.

HISTORY OF PDT

PDT is not new. In fact, it has been around since the turn of the last century, having been described in both the medical and dermatological literature. Raab,[1] back in 1900, was the first to report in the literature that when paramecia cells (*Paramecium caudatum*) were first exposed to either acridine orange or light, there was no effect on the cells but that cell death was quick, within 2 hours after exposure to both acridine orange and light at the same time. In 1904, Von Tappeiner and Jodblauer[2] described the term "photodynamic effect" when they showed the oxygen-consuming reaction in protozoa after the application of aniline dyes and fluorescence. In 1905, Jesionek and Von Tappeiner[3] reported their experiences with a topical 5 percent eosin. The topical 5 percent eosin was used as a photosensitizer; when utilized with an artificial light source, they were able to successfully treat several dermatological entities in human beings. These included nonmelanoma skin cancers, lupus vulgaris, and condylomata lata. They postulated that the eosin, once incorporated into the cells and in the presence of oxygen, would produce a cytotoxic reaction when exposed to an appropriate light source. These were the first reported cases of the use of PDT in patients and paved the way for future research into the use of PDT.

The use of porphyrins as potential photosensitizing agents became the focus of PDT research. In 1911, Hausman[4] described experiences with the use of hematoporphyrin as a photosensitizer. He demonstrated that light-

1

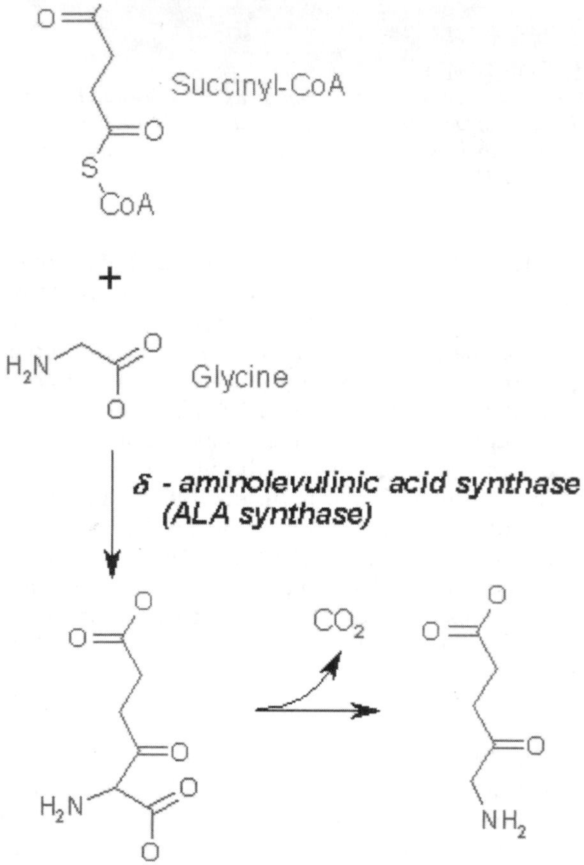

FIGURE 1.—Heme biosynthetic pathway.

activated hematoporphyrin could photosensitize both guinea pigs and mice. In 1913, Meyer-Betz[5] injected himself with hematoporphyrin. He found that when these injected areas were exposed to light, the sites became swollen and painful. Unfortunately, for the practical use of PDT, the phototoxic reaction in Meyer-Betz lasted for over 2 months. Significant clinical research on the use of PDT in dermatology was not performed for the next 30 years following this disheartening practical information.

In 1942, Auler and Butler[6] showed that hematoporphyrin, given systemically, concentrated more in certain dermatological tumors than in their surrounding tissues and that, when fluoresced, the tumors became necrotic. Figge et al[7] later reported that hematoporphyrin was also selectively absorbed into other cells, including embryonic cells, traumatized skin, and neoplastic cells.

In 1978, Dougherty et al[8] described a new systemic photosensitizer known as hematoporphyrin purified derivative (HPD). HPD was a complex mix-

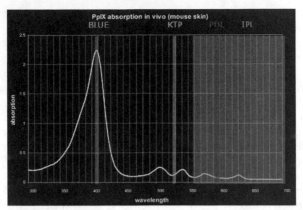

FIGURE 2.—PpIX absorption spectrum.

ture of porphyrin subunits and byproducts. This group showed that HPD could be used successfully to treat cutaneous nonmelanoma malignancies with red light. Systemic use of HPD became the standard tool for PDT, and a variety of medical uses emerged for PDT, both oncologic and nononcologic.

The skin, being so easily accessible to researchers, became the prime focus for much of the PDT research which was to follow. HPD, the only photosensitizer available during this time period, however, remained phototoxic in the skin several months after its systemic uptake, making its practical use in dermatology difficult. In 1990, the most important breakthrough of modern PDT research came when Kennedy et al[9] introduced the first topical porphyrin derivative, ALA. This photosensitizer, in the form of a prodrug, has the ability to penetrate the stratum corneum, be absorbed not only by actinically

TABLE 1.—Uses of Photodynamic Therapy in Dermatology

AKs

Photodamage and associated AKs*
Bowen's disease
Superficial basal cell carcinoma
Superficial squamous cell carcinoma
Cutaneous T-cell lymphoma
Kaposi's sarcoma
Malignant melanoma
Actinic chelitis
Keratoacanthoma
Psoriasis vulgaris
Human papillomavirus
Molluscum contagiosum
Alopecia areata
Hirsutism
Acne vulgaris*

*Common indications for 5-ALA-PDT in the United States.

damaged skin cells, but also by nonmelanoma skin cancer cells and the pilosebaceous units. Kennedy and his group described the PDT reaction of topically applied ALA; once ALA is incorporated into a cell, it is converted to its active form for a PDT reaction to occur. This active form is known as protoporphyrin IX (PpIX). The heme pathway is shown in Fig 1. ALA is seen in this biochemical loop, as has PpIX, which has been shown to be activated by a variety of lasers and light sources. Fig 2 shows the absorption spectrum of PpIX, with peak absorption bands in both the blue light (known as the Soret band) and red light spectrums. Smaller peaks of energy are also seen, and this has become important as ALA-PDT moves into this new century. A variety of different lasers and light sources are being utilized with PDT in today's world, all based on the varied peaks in the absorption spectrum of PpIX.[10]

Many dermatological entities have been successfully treated with ALA-PDT, and much research into other diseases is actively being studied by PDT researchers (Table 1).

Of note, and critical to the topical use of ALA-PDT, is that the heme biosynthetic pathway (Fig 1) is maintained under a very close feedback loop, not allowing for buildup of heme or its precursors in tissues. Exogenous ALA forming PpIX is cleared from the body much more rapidly than its predecessor, HPD. Thus, the potential for phototoxicity from ALA-induced PpIX is reduced to days instead of several months.

LEVULAN PDT

PDT seems to have undergone 2 unique paths as scientists and clinicians have begun to utilize this unique therapy over the past 10 to 15 years. In the United States research has centered on the 20 percent 5-ALA solution (Levulan Kerastick, DUSA Pharmaceuticals, Wilmington, Mass) and its ability to treat actinic keratoses (AKs), photorejuvenation, moderate to se-

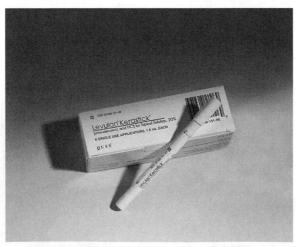

FIGURE 3.—Levulan® Kerastick (DUSA Pharmaceuticals, Wilmington, MA). (Permission to use images granted by DUSA Pharmaceuticals.)

vere inflammatory acne vulgaris, sebaceous gland hyperplasia (SGH), and hidradenitis suppurativa (HS). The Levulan Kerastick is shown in Fig 3, and the original blue light source, the BluU (DUSA Pharmaceuticals), described for its use is shown in Fig 4. As previously mentioned, this form of ALA-PDT is available in the United States, Latin and South America, and Asia. This commercial form of ALA-PDT is not available at this time in Europe or Australia; work toward that end is progressing.

In contrast, European and Australian research has focused on the methyl ester derivative of 5-ALA (Metvix, PhotoCure ASA, Norway; Metvixia, Galderma, Fort Worth, Tex) in treating nonmelanoma skin cancers, Bowen's disease (squamous cell carcinoma in situ), and AKs. Interest in the treatment of photorejuvenation and inflammatory acne vulgaris is just beginning with methyl-ALA.[10] Metvix is shown in Fig 5, and the red light

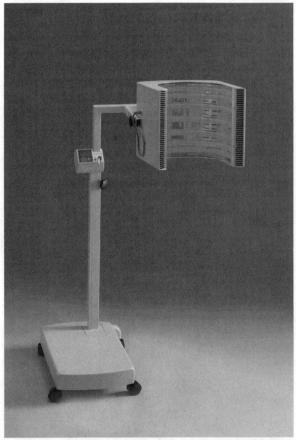

FIGURE 4.—BluU® (DUSA Pharmaceuticals, Wilmington, MA). (Permission to use images granted by DUSA Pharmaceuticals.)

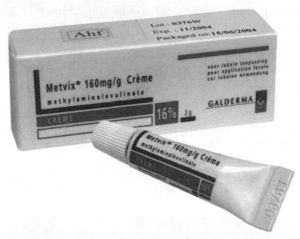

FIGURE 5.—Metvix® (PhotoCure ASA, Norway; Galderma, Ft. Worth, TX). (Permission to use images granted by Photocure, ASA, Norway.)

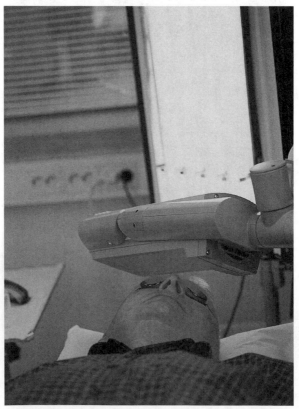

FIGURE 6.—Red Light Source, Aktilite(r) (PhotoCure ASA, Norway; Galderma, Ft. Worth, TX). (Permission to use images granted by Photocure, ASA, Norway.)

source used with it, known as Aktilite (PhotoCure ASA; Galderma), is shown in Fig 6.

Levulan PDT is Food and Drug Administration (FDA) approved in the United States for the treatment of nonhyperkeratotic AKs of the face and scalp utilizing a 14- to 18-hour drug incubation period and subjecting the treatment site to 16 minutes and 40 seconds of blue light. All other indications studied with Levulan PDT and being used currently are considered off-label uses of the product and must be thoroughly explained to patients receiving this therapy, which is very common in today's PDT world.

This report reviews the pivotal United States clinical trials that led to the FDA approval, various intriguing open-label clinical trials that confirm the effectiveness of the off-label use of Levulan PDT, as well as the split-face clinical trials that helped solidify its use in today's medical environment. Also, several new clinical studies and reports are cited to add an even further cause for the use of Levulan PDT in today's medical environment.

PIVOTAL LEVULAN PDT CLINICAL TRIALS FOR AKs

The Phase II Levulan PDT pivotal clinical trials were reported by Jeffes[11] in 2001. A total of 39 patients were enrolled in the clinical trial. The patients were required to have numerous nonhyperkeratotic AKs of the face and scalp, and each patient received 16 minutes and 40 seconds of blue light after a 14- to 18-hour ALA drug incubation period. The AKs were individually treated in this protocol. Pain was a common occurrence during the therapy as well as after the treatment, and posttreatment erythema and edema, which often led to crust formation, lasted upwards of 1 week. Eight weeks after the ALA-PDT treatment, 66 percent of the individually treated AKs resolved. For those lesions not completely cleared, a second treatment was

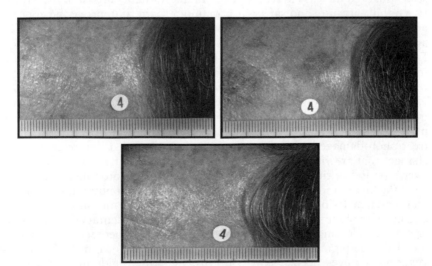

FIGURE 7.—Clinical example from Levulan Phase III trial (Courtesy of Gold MH. Photodynamic therapy with lasers and intense pulsed light. *Facial Plast Surg Clin North Am.* 2007;15:145-160. Copyright Elsevier, 2007.)

given. Results at 16 weeks showed 85 percent individual complete clearance of the AKs.[11]

Results from the successful Phase II clinical trials led to a larger Phase III multicenter clinical trial. In this clinical trial, 243 patients were included for AK treatment following the same protocol as described in the Phase II clinical trials. Once again, individualized AKs were treated; the ALA incubation time was 14 to 18 hours and the lesions were exposed to 16 minutes and 40 seconds of blue light. Results from this pivotal clinical trial showed that there was a greater than 70 percent complete clearance of the individual AKs at 12 weeks. Once again, those not completely cleared were retreated for a second time using the same clinical parameters. At 24 weeks, 88 percent of the individuals in the clinical trial had a 75 percent or greater clearance of their AKs compared with 20 percent in the placebo arm.[12] An example of an AK treated during this Phase III clinical trial is shown in Fig 7. Downtime with healing, described in both the Phase II and in this Phase III clinical trial, described by this author as the "PDT effect" and pain, was again evident in the majority of individuals participating in this clinical trial. A secondary but equally important and exciting clinical end point from this trial was that 94 percent of the individuals (and 92 percent of the physicians) rated the cosmetic appearance following the Levulan PDT treatment as either excellent or good. This finding, an improved cosmetic appearance, intrigued a number of investigators, including this author, and research initiatives on the use of ALA for several dermatological disorders began to take shape.

PHOTOREJUVENATION WITH LASERS/LIGHT SOURCES

Aesthetic cosmetic dermatological surgery has expanded greatly over the past several years. Noninvasive aesthetic dermatological surgery has also seen a marked increase in recent years, unquestionably linked to the explosive popularity, use, and safety of botulinum toxin to improve the appearance of fine lines and wrinkles on the face. Better and longer lasting filler agents have emerged as well, including the hyaluronic acid filling agents. Furthermore, noninvasive lasers and light source procedures are increasing in record numbers, as our procedures are producing better and better clinical results with less and less downtime, which is key to these treatments.

Lasers and light sources have always played a prominent role in the treatment of photodamaged skin. The term photorejuvenation appeared as a marketing term several years ago as lasers and light sources were utilized to treat photodamaged or photoaged skin. Photodamaged skin refers to skin changes that are visible on the skin surface from the effects of visible light over a period of time. Nestor et al[13] helped define photorejuvenation and were the first to introduce the concepts of type I photorejuvenation (for benign vascular lesions, including telangiectasias, the symptoms of rosacea, and flushing of the skin; also dyschromias or other pigmentary skin changes, erythema following laser resurfacing procedures, pigmentary sun damage, mottled hyperpigmentation, photoaging, and lentigines). Type II photorejuvenation involves deeper skin concerns, including epidermal or dermal structural changes, rhytids, elastotic changes in the skin, collagenous and connective tissue changes, and the appearance of large pores.

Conventional lasers and light sources, especially with the use of either the intense pulsed light (IPL) source or the pulsed-dye laser (PDL), can successfully treat both types 1 and 2 photorejuvenation and have been reported on in the medical literature many times over the past several years. The IPLs have had a great deal of experience in the treatment of photorejuvenation since their original descriptions by Goldman and Eckhouse[14] in 1966. The IPLs use a broadband wave of light conforming to the principle of selective photothermolysis, as first described by Anderson and Parish.[15] The theory states that light can be selectively absorbed by a specific chromophore within the skin, destroy the targeted chromophore, and leave the surrounding skin and structures unaffected. IPLs are by far the most common of the light sources available to clinicians worldwide.

In 2000, Biter[16] was the first to describe the use of an IPL for photorejuvenation. In his 49 patients, more than 90 percent experienced a greater than 75 percent improvement in rosacea symptoms (facial erythema and flushing), 84 percent improvement in wrinkles, 78 percent improvement in facial pigment, and 49 percent improvement in pore size after a series of 5 IPL ses-

TABLE 2.—Commonly Available Intense Pulsed Light Sources

Manufacturer	Brand Name
Aesthera	Spectra Pulse
	McCue Ultra Variable Pulsed Light
Adept Medical Concepts	SpectraPulse
	McCue Ultra Variable Pulsed Light
American Medical Bio Care	Omnilight FPL
	Novalight FPL
Candela	V-Beam
Cutera	CoolGlide XEO
	XEO SA
	Genesis Plus
Cynosure	Cynergy PL
	Cynergy III
	PhotoSilk Plus
Danish Dermatologic Development	Ellipse I2PL
DermaMed USA	Quadra Q4 Platinum Series
Laserscope	Solis
Lumenis	IPL Quantum SR
	VascuLight Elite
	Lumenis One
McCue	Ultra VPL
MedSurge Advances	Prolite II
Novalis	Clareon SR
	Solarus SR
Palomar	StarLux System
	MediLux System
	EsteLux System
Radiancy	SkinStation
	S P R
Sciton	Profile-MP
	Profile-S BBl
Syneron	Aurora SR
	Galaxy

sions performed. Further works by Goldberg and Cutler[17] and Zelickson and Kist (personal communication) have shown that through the use of IPLs improvement in collagen and elastic tissue at the treatment sites is seen. Others have also shown positive experiences with IPLs, including Weiss et al,[18] who in a 5-year retrospective review, showed that patients were able to maintain improvement in skin texture (83 percent), telangiectasias (82 percent), and skin dyschromias (79 percent); Negishi et al[19] and Hernandez-Perez[20] have shown that IPLs can be successfully used on a variety of ethnic skin types, again making this type of therapy popular all over the world.

Recent advances in IPLs have made things even better for clinicians. Squaring of the IPL pulse and more reliable computerized software have made IPLs much more predictable and more reliable than their early precursors. This concept, described eloquently by Town et al,[21] is a must read for all those who are in the market to purchase an IPL. A list of commonly available IPLs is shown in Table 2.

In 2006, Nestor et al[22] reported on what is commonly referred to as type 3 photodamage—those changes associated with chronic actinic damage, actinic keratoses, and superficial skin cancers. This is where the use of ALA-PDT with either blue light or other lasers/light sources plays a significant role.

LEVULAN PDT CLINICAL TRIALS: OPEN LABEL FOR AKS

A variety of open-label clinical trials have been performed to show that ALA-PDT is useful for the treatment of photorejuvenation and AKs with a variety of lasers and light sources.

Alexiades-Armenakas and Geronemus[23] first demonstrated the safety and efficacy of the use of a long PDL in the treatment of AKs of the face and scalp with ALA. They were also able to demonstrate that those who received short-contact ALA (3 hours) responded similarly to those who received the longer contact drug incubation (14 to 18 hours).

In 2002, Gold[24] reported on early experiences with ALA-PDT on photorejuvenation and associated AKs with ALA-PDT and a blue light source. From these observations, not only was there successful resolution of the treated AKs but, surprisingly, a response was also seen in contiguous areas to those being treated, resulting in a "rejuvenation" effect, as shown in Fig 8. A PDT effect, which was described as downtime with healing, was also evident in this series of patients who received long drug incubation periods.

To further address this PDT effect and make the therapy more acceptable to patients and physicians, a number of clinical researchers began to focus their energies on (1) shorter drug incubation times and (2) treatment of the entire face so that both clinical and subclinical AKs would be treated, giving a full photorejuvenation effect. Two significant studies appeared that were very significant in modern usage of ALA-PDT. The first, by Touma et al,[25] showed that a 1-hour drug incubation time was as efficacious as a 14- to 18-hour drug incubation time in improving AKs and the parameters of photodamage. This group utilized a blue light source in their study. Improvements

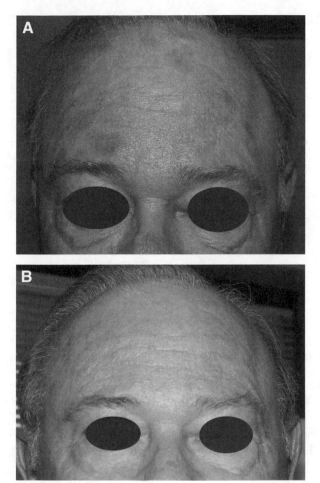

FIGURE 8.—Levulan PDT for AKs. Patient presented with AKs before treatment (A) and after treatment with Levulan PDT (B). (Reprinted by permission of Edizioni Minerva Medica from: Gold MH. Aminolevulinic acid photodynamic therapy for cosmetic uses on the skin. *G Ital Dermatol Venereol.* 2007;142:311-326.)

were noted in the sallowness of the skin, fine wrinkling, and mottled hyper-pigmentation of the skin with a 1-hour drug incubation.

The second very important study to be noted was from Ruiz-Rodriguez et al,[26] who studied a shorter drug incubation time (3 hours) with their ALA and utilized an IPL for their light source. The authors coined the therapy "photodynamic photorejuvenation" as a result of their findings. Seventeen patients were treated with ALA and an IPL device, and after 2 IPL treatments the cosmetic appearance was noted as excellent. All the AKs cleared with the IPL-PDT therapy and they reported an 87 percent improvement in skin texture, wrinkling, pigmentary changes, and telangiectasias.

A variety of other significant investigator-initiated clinical trials with a variety of lasers and light sources soon appeared in the literature (Table 3).[27-30]

TABLE 3.—Open-Label Clinical Trials with ALA-PDT

Trial	Light Source	Drug Incubation (No. of Patients)	Significant Results	Other Significant Notes
Gold[27]	Blue Light	30-60 minutes (10)	83% AKs responded; crow's feet, 90%; skin roughness, 100%; hyperpigmentation, 90%; facial erythema, 70%	
Goldman et al[28]	Blue Light	1 hour (32)	90% AKs responded; improvement in skin texture, 72%; pigment change, 59%	62.5% preferred ALA-PDT over cryotherapy
Avram et al[29]	IPL	1 hour (17)	69% AK response; telangiectasia, 55%; pigment change, 48%; skin texture, 25%	1 treatment with ALA-PDT/IPL compatible to 5 IPL-alone treatments
Alexiades-Armenakas et al[30]	PDL	2-3 hours (19)	Actinic chelitis, 68% clearance at 12 months	

The results of these clinical trials clearly demonstrated that through the use of full-face ALA application and exposure to a variety of lasers and light sources, a photorejuvenation response can be commonly seen and AKs will respond as well. The studies also pointed out that by using ALA-PDT, "typical" photorejuvenation treatment protocols could be modified; that is, for the most part, 1 or 2 ALA-PDT therapies were equivalent to, if not superior to, the routine 5 to 6 IPL photorejuvenation treatments typically performed by most physicians performing photorejuvenation.

LEVULAN PDT CLINICAL TRIALS: SPLIT FACE FOR AKS

To verify the open-label clinical trials, 5 split-face clinical trials have been published (Table 4). The first, by Alster et al,[31] compared ALA and an IPL on one side of the face to IPL alone on the other side of the face in 10 individuals. They found that those receiving the ALA-IPL therapy improved more so in the parameters of photorejuvenation compared with the IPL-treated side. Key[32] examined subjects utilizing a PDL with ALA on one half of the face; the ALA-PDL side improved in parameters of photorejuvenation more than the PDL side alone. Marmur et al[33] looked at a split-face ALA-IPL versus IPL alone and through skin biopsies and ultrastructural analyses examined the production of type I and type III collagen production. They found a greater increase in type I and type III collagen production in those patients receiving ALA-IPL over IPL alone, helping explain the texture changes commonly seen in patients receiving ALA-PDT treatments.

Dover et al[34] reported on their ALA-IPL split-face protocol in which patients received 3 split-face ALA-IPL treatments at 3-week intervals followed by 2 additional IPL full-face treatments. The patients were then evaluated at

4 weeks following the last IPL treatment. They found an improvement in the global score for photoaging (80 percent vs 50 percent), mottled hyperpigmentation (95 percent vs 65 percent), and improvement in fine lines (55 percent vs 20 percent). Interestingly, in their group of 29 individuals there was no statistical change in tactile skin roughness or sallowness over baseline.

Gold et al[35] reported their split-face analysis utilizing ALA-IPL on half of the face with only an IPL on the other half. The protocol included 3 split-face treatments at 4-week intervals, with follow-up at 1 and 3 months following the last treatment. Of the 13 individuals studied, this group found changes in the ALA-IPL side versus the IPL side of improvement in AKs (78 percent vs 53.6 percent), crow's feet (55 percent vs 28.5 percent), tactile skin roughness (55 percent vs 29.5 percent), mottled hyperpigmentation (60.3 percent vs

TABLE 4.—Split-Face ALA-PDT Clinical Trials

Trial	Light Source	Drug Incubation (No Patients)	Significant Results	Other Significant Notes
Alster et al[31]	IPL	1 hour (10)	ALA-IPL side higher clinical scores for photorejuvenation	
Key[32]	PDL	1 hour (14)	ALA-PDL more significant than PDL alone for photorejuvenation	
Marmur et al[33]	IPL	1 hour (7)	Ultrastructural analysis: increase in type I collagen, more so when pretreated with ALA	
Dover et al[34]	IPL	1 hour (20)	Improvement in global protoaging scale for ALA-IPL side (80% vs 50%), hyperpigmentation (95% vs 65%), fine lines (55% vs 20%)	3 split-face treatments, then 2 full-face IPLs
Gold et al[35]	IPL	1 hour (13)	Improvements on ALA-IPL side versus IPL alone: AKs (78% vs 54%), crow's feet (55% vs 20%), skin roughness (55% vs 30%), hyperpigmentation (60% vs 37%), facial erythema (85% vs 54%)	

37.2 percent), and improvement in erythema (84.6 percent vs 53.8 percent). No adverse effects were noted and no PDT effect was seen in the treated individuals—once again significant with the newer paradigm of short-contact, full-face treatments with a variety of lasers and light sources.

NEWER STUDIES OF ALA-PDT OF SIGNIFICANCE

Over the past year or so, there have been several important contributions to the literature that warrant mention at this time.

The first, by Redbord and Hanke,[36] reported on a series of patients treated with short-contact, full-face therapy utilizing ALA and a blue light source. Of significance was that the PDT effects, so commonly seen in the early clinical trials, were virtually absent in this group of patients. Gold[37] looked at the pharmacoeconomics associated with this kind of therapy for the treatment of AKs versus the traditional choices for AKs, including cryotherapy, 5-fluorouracil, and imiquimod. The findings, based on models, showed the cost effectiveness of ALA-PDT in today's health care environment.

Examples of ALA-PDT photorejuvenation are seen in Figs 9 and 10.

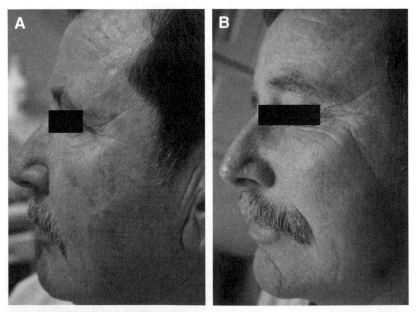

FIGURE 9.—Levulan PDT for photorejuvenation. Before treatment (A) and after Levulan PDT treatment (B). (Reprinted by permission of Edizioni Minerva Medica from: Gold MH. Aminolevulinic acid photodynamic therapy for cosmetic uses on the skin. *G Ital Dermatol Venereol.* 2007;142:311-326.)

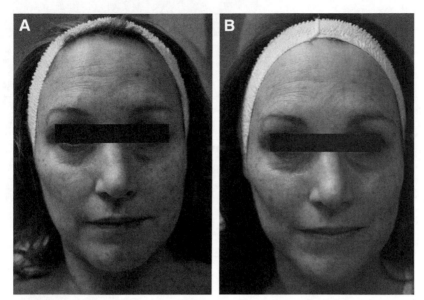

FIGURE 10.—Levulan PDT for photorejuvenation. Before treatment (A) and after Levulan PDT treatment (B). (Courtesy of Gold MH. Photodynamic therapy update 2007. *J Drugs Dermatol.* 2007;6:1131-1137. Reprinted with permission from the *Journal of Drugs in Dermatology.*)

METVIX/METVIXIA FOR AKS AND SUPERFICIAL SKIN CANCERS

The second photosensitizer, Metvix/Metvixia (MAL), is available in Europe and Australia as well as in several other countries around the world. It has European Union clearance for the treatment of nonhyperkeratotic AKs of the face and scalp and basal cell carcinomas that are not suitable for conventional surgery. In the United States, FDA approval, at the time of this writing, is for the treatment of nonhyperkeratotic AKs of the face and scalp. MAL is still not available for use in the United States. MAL is best utilized with a red light source at 630 nm. Clinical trials supporting its effectiveness in the treatment of AKs are numerous and well designed, with convincing results (Table 5).[38-45] Most of the current recommendations for MAL-PDT recommend that the treatment areas be prepared by gentle curetting before application of the MAL. Once applied, a 3-hour drug incubation under occlusion is recommended. Again, a red light source is recommended and, through the European consensus study,[46] treatments are usually recommended to be performed twice, 1 week apart.

Clinical trials for photorejuvenation with MAL are just beginning. The first of these trials has now been published. Zane et al[47] reported on the use of MAL red light in 20 patients with 137 AKs who had severe photodamage. Using the 3-hour drug incubation under occlusion, red light, and 2 therapies 1 week apart, they were able to show an 88.3 percent clearance of the AKs. In

TABLE 5.—Metvix for AKs

Study	No. Patients	No. Lesions Treated with MAL PDT (PP*)	Dosage Regimen	Results (Lesion CR**) at 3 Months
Phase II study: Braathen[39]	110	384 MAL PDT	Dose and regime finding study	Metvix 160 mg/g for 3 hours optimal (compared: 1 and 3 hours, 80 and 160 mg/g) Second Metvix PDT increased CR from 67% to 89% (lesions were prepared) Efficacy is better with lesion preparation than without
1x Metvix PDT vs double freeze-thaw cryotherapy: Szeimies[40]	202 (102)	367 MAL PDT	1 MAL PDT session vs double cycle cryotherapy For lesions on face and scalp, 93% of lesions	Complete lesion response at 3 months: 1 Metvix session (69%) as effective as double freeze-thaw cryotherapy (75%) 96% patients had excellent or good cosmetic outcome vs 81% with cryotherapy 74% patients preferred Metvix PDT to previous other therapies
European double-blind, placebo-controlled trial[41]	39		1 MAL PDT session vs placebo	Complete lesion response at 3 months: 1 Metvix session (76%) > placebo (18%)
2 Metvix PDT vs single cryotherapy, placebo controlled: Freeman[42]	200 (88)	295 MAL PDT	2 MAL PDT sessions 7 days apart vs single-cycle cryotherapy	Complete lesion response at 3 months: 2 Metvix sessions (91%) > cryotherapy (68%) placebo (30%) 84% of patients had an excellent cosmetic outcome with Metvix PDT vs cryotherapy (51%) 98% had excellent or good cosmesis with Metvix 85% of patients rated Metvix better (61%) or equal 14%) to previous treatments
US double-blind, 2 Matvix PDT vs placebo-controlled trial: Pariser[43]	80 (42)	260 MAL PDT	2 MAL PDT sessions 7 days apart vs placebo	Complete lesion response at 3 months: 2 Metvix sessions (89%) > placebo (38%) 97% of patients had excellent or good cosmetic outcome with Metvix PDT 73% of patients preferred Metvix PDT to other previous therapies

(*Continued*)

addition, there was improvement in photoaging, mottled hyperpigmentation, fine lines, roughness, and sallowness of the skin. They found no change in deep wrinkles, telangiectasia and facial erythema, or sebaceous hyperplasia.

TABLE 5 (cont.)

Study	No. Patients	No. Lesions Treated with MAL PDT (PP*)	Dosage Regimen	Results (Lesion CR**) at 3 Months
Single Metvix PDT vs dual Metvix PDT: Tarstedt[44]	211 (105)	400 MAL PDT	1 MAL PDT session, retreat only noncomplete responding lesions at 3 months (19%) (regimen I) vs 2 MAL PDT 7 days apart (regimen II)	At 3 months: For thin lesions, complete lesion response similar with 1 Metvix (93%) and 2 Metvix (89%) For thicker lsesions, CR better with 2 Metvix (84%) than 1 Metvix (70%), which improved after repeat treatment at 3 months (88%) regimen I is not inferior to regimen II Overall: regimen I: 92% (81% after first session); regimen II: 87% For thin lesions: regimen I: 97%; regimen II: 89% For thicker lesions: regimen I: 88%; regimen II: 84%
Intraindividual (right-left) comparison 1 Metvix PDT vs double cryotherapy[15] Aktion Study, Morton[45]	119	758	1 MAL PDT session vs double freeze-thaw cryotherapy Noncomplete responding lesions retreated at 3 months MAL PDT 14, 9% Cryotherapy 26, 8%	Complete lesion response at 3 months: 83% 1 Metvix session 72% double freeze-thaw cryotherapy Half as many lesions (10% vs 20%) required retreatment at 3 months with Melvix to achieve similar CR rates at 6 months (86% Metvix PDT vs 83% cryotherapy) "Excellent" cosmetic outcome 71% Metvix PDT, 57% cryotherapy Overall patient preference was significantly higher with Metvix (45% vs 10%; $P < .001$)

*Per protocol.
**Complete Response.

A recent study by Ruiz-Rodriguez et al[48] is very significant and needs to be further evaluated. In this study, they looked at the use of a nonablative fractional device before drug incubation in the hopes of enhancing drug penetration and improving clinical outcomes. In a split-face analysis, one side of the face received the nonablative fractional device therapy before the application of MAL. After the usual drug incubation and red light therapy, they were able to show that with the use of the fractional device there was more of a photorejuvenation effect seen on the fractionated PDT side than on the side not treated with the fractional device.

COMPARISON OF ALA AND MAL

Over the past several years there have been several reports trying to compare the 2 photosensitizers, especially in regard to pain as well as efficacy.

Although these reports appear in the literature,[49,50] it is important to keep in mind that there has never been a study utilizing the branded products of both drugs, and that the comparisons do not routinely use the "standard" protocols currently being used.[51] One day, hopefully, we will have a true comparative study of the photosensitizers; until then, keep standards in mind, keep brand drug versus compounded drug in mind, and be careful in drawing conclusions.

ACNE VULGARIS AND RELATED DISORDERS

Acne vulgaris remains one of the most common reasons patients seek care by dermatologists; up to 30 percent of all dermatologist visits are related to acne vulgaris and its sequelae.[52] Acne vulgaris is a multifactorial disease with genetics, hormonal factors and, at times, environmental concerns playing a role. Acne vulgaris is a disorder of the sebaceous glands in which hormonal activity causes dilation and then obstruction of the sebaceous glands, which lead to the production and proliferation of bacteria within the glands, predominantly *Propionibacterium acnes (P acnes)*. Further proliferation of the bacteria results in an inflammatory response and the production of inflammatory papules, pustules, and cystic acne vulgaris lesions.[53]

Medical therapy for acne vulgaris remains the gold standard. Both topical and systemic therapies exist that have shown their place in treating acne lesions. These therapies will not be reviewed here. However, several recent developments may change how clinicians approach patients with inflammatory acne vulgaris. This includes resistance to our currently used systemic antibiotics (up to 60 percent being reported), a recent report linking breast cancer to long-term antibiotic use, and the continued restrictions being placed on isotretinoin.[54]

P acnes have a photodynamic response naturally in the skin. During the growth cycle, *P acnes* naturally produce porphyrins, predominately PpIX and coproporphyrin III. These have absorption spectra peaks in the blue light range, and so exposure of inflammatory acne vulgaris to a blue light source should be and has been shown effective in the treatment of mild to moderate inflammatory acne vulgaris.

A group of investigators has looked at adding ALA to the treatment of moderate to severe inflammatory acne vulgaris to further understand its role in treatment. Once again, the concept of short-contact, full-face therapy has played a principal role in the investigations to be presented. Further, a variety of lasers and light sources have been used in the treatment of inflammatory acne vulgaris with ALA-PDT.

The first report describing the use of ALA-PDT in the treatment of inflammatory acne vulgaris was by Hongcharu et al[55] in 2000. The group used a broadband light source (500-700 nm) and 3-hour ALA drug incubation in 22 patients with inflammatory acne vulgaris. They showed significant clearance after 4 weeks that persisted up to 20 weeks in those who had multiple treatments or 10 weeks in those who had a single treatment. A PDT effect was described that consisted in this patient population of an acneiform folliculitis, postinflammatory hyperpigmentation, superficial peeling, and crusting.

Itoh et al[56] have also reported findings with ALA and inflammatory acne vulgaris. In 2000, they reported on the use of ALA and a 635-nm PDL in an intractable case of inflammatory acne vulgaris. The treated area remained disease free for 8 months; a classic PDT effect was noted. The group's second report in 2001 looked at a single ALA treatment in 13 patients using a polychromatic visible light (600 to 700 nm).[57] The inflammatory acne vulgaris lesions improved, and new-lesion acne vulgaris was reduced through the 6-month follow-up period. A classic PDT effect, however, was once again described.

Goldman and Boyce[58] reported on the use of short-contact (1-hour drug incubation) 5-ALA and treatment with both the IPL and blue light source in the treatment of acne vulgaris and SGH. PDT effects were not seen, and "relative" clearing of the inflammatory acne vulgaris occurred within 2 to 4 weeks. Gold[59] evaluated 10 patients with moderate to severe inflammatory acne vulgaris utilizing short-contact (30-minute drug incubation) and a high-intensity blue light source. Four treatments at 1-week intervals yielded a 60 percent response rate (compared with 43 percent with blue light alone). No PDT effects were reported. Goldman and Boyce[60] described their experiences with blue light in a group of 22 patients with and without ALA. A greater response to therapy was seen in the ALA blue light group than in the blue light group alone. Again, no PDT effects were observed. Gold[61] reported moderate to severe inflammatory acne vulgaris responding to an IPL device, with 72 percent clearance in 12 patients. Again, the short-contact, full-face therapies were well tolerated with no PDT effects seen. Taub[62] also reported success in treating inflammatory acne vulgaris with either a blue light source or an IPL with no PDT effect.

Further studies have also shown the success of ALA-PDT in the treatment of inflammatory acne vulgaris with other light sources. Alexiades-Armenakas[63] presented data with the PDL and ALA in inflammatory acne vulgaris. A drug incubation average time of 45 minutes and an average 3 PDL sessions cleared all the 14 patients involved in this clinical trial. Miller and Van Camp[64] reported on the successful use of ALA and the KTP laser in patients with inflammatory acne vulgaris.

In 2 recent split-face ALA-IPL analyses, Santos et al,[65] utilizing 13 patients, and Rojanamatin et al,[66] with 14 patients, demonstrated that by utilizing ALA with the IPL device, statistical improvements in inflammatory acne vulgaris can be seen with ALA-IPL over IPL alone.

At the time of this writing, the use of ALA-PDT in the treatment of moderate to severe inflammatory acne vulgaris is under Phase II investigations with 20 percent 5-ALA and blue light, utilizing multiple-drug incubation and blue light time periods. Guidance derived from these multicenter clinical trials will yield further insight for the use of ALA-PDT in acne vulgaris. From this author's personal perspective, ALA-PDT is useful for moderate to severe inflammatory acne vulgaris using a variety of lasers and light sources. Clinical examples of utilizing ALA-PDT in inflammatory acne vulgaris are shown in Figs 11 and 12.

The use of MAL in acne vulgaris has begun to be evaluated. A report by Wiegell et al[67] showed that inflammatory acne vulgaris and the red light source yielded significant clinical improvement, but noticeable discomfort was described in most of the patients (13 of 21 with severe pain, 6 of 21 with moderate pain). A PDT effect was also described that included pustular reactions in almost all the patients lasting 2 to 3 days. Exfoliation occurred in most of the patients at day 4. Horfelt et al[68] and Mavilia et al[69] have also reported the use of MAL in inflammatory acne vulgaris with good clinical re-

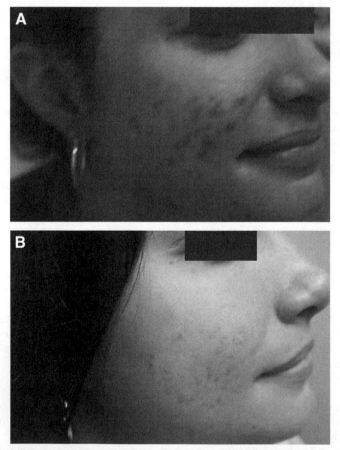

FIGURE 11.—Levulan PDT for acne. Before treatment (A) and after Levulan PDT treatment (B). (Photos courtesy Michael H. Gold, MD, The Laser and Rejuvenation Center, Nashville, TN.)

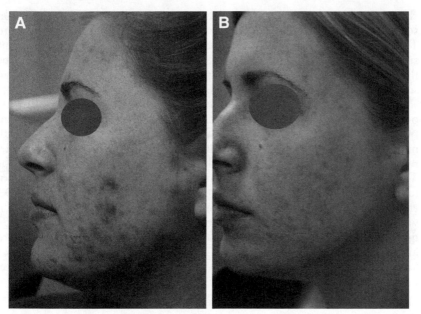

FIGURE 12.—Levulan PDT for acne. Before treatment (**A**) and after Levulan PDT treatment (**B**). (Reprinted by permission of Edizioni Minerva Medica from: Gold MH. Aminolevulinic acid photodynamic therapy for cosmetic uses on the skin. *G Ital Dermatol Venereol.* 2007;142:311-326.)

sults but still with a PDT effect. Further work will need to be performed with regard to MAL and its potential role in inflammatory acne vulgaris.

Clinical investigations have also looked at SGH and HS as possible entities that can be routinely treated with ALA-PDT.

Several investigations have looked at SGH with ALA-PDT. Horio et al[70] were the first to report on SGH and ALA-PDT using a slide projector as a light source. They treated SGH lesions in a patient 3 times at 1-week intervals. The lesions became smaller but never resolved. Alster and Tanzi[71] reported on the use of the PDL on lesions of SGH with ALA. One-hour drug incubation was used, and 7 patients cleared with 1 treatment; 3 others required 2 treatments with the PDL. The ALA-PDL–treated lesions were also found to be more successful than PDL alone–treated lesions. Richey and Hopson,[72] using a blue light source and 1-hour drug incubation, treated 10 patients with SGH. These patients received 3 to 6 treatments once per week and were followed for 6 months after the last treatment. A 70 percent clearance rate was reported, with 20 percent recurrence at 3 to 4 months. Gold et al[73] reported their findings with ALA, SGH, and either an IPL or blue light source. Patients received short-contact (30- to 60-minute drug incubation) and were treated with an IPL (n = 5) or a blue light (n = 6). Results showed SGH clearances of 55 percent with either therapy at the follow-up 3-month time period.

Recalcitrant HS has also been reported to respond to ALA-PDT. Gold et al[74] has reported the successful use of ALA-PDT and blue light. Strauss et al[75] failed, however, to verify these results. Strauss reported on their experiences with 4 patients with HS. These individuals received MAL under occlusion for 4 hours before local anesthesia and exposure to either a red light source (n = 3) or a broadband light source (570 to 670 nm) in 1 patient. Their group of patients showed mixed results. Only 1 patient found some success with the treatment; 1 dropped out of the trial before finishing the therapy and the others were either unable to tolerate the treatment or had some worsening of the disease process.

Gold et al[74] had completely the opposite results with blue light in the group of individuals they treated with recalcitrant HS. Four individuals were identified with recalcitrant HS and were treated with short-contact (15- to 30-minute drug incubation) and exposure to a blue light source. The patients received either weekly or biweekly therapy for up to 4 treatments. At the 3-month follow-up period there was noted a 75 percent to 100 percent resolution in disease activity. The treatments were well tolerated with no PDT effects observed. From personal experience of this author, 3 of the 4 individuals have remained disease free for upwards of 2 years, with 1 patient requiring intermittent therapy for disease control. A further study by Rivard and Ozog[76] confirmed the work of Gold et al in recalcitrant HS. Further, larger clinical trials are warranted to further explain the role of PDT in recalcitrant HS.

How I Use Levulan PDT in my Clinical Practice

There are no set standards that state empirically one way or another is the best or only way clinicians should approach the utilization of ALA-PDT in the United States for their patients who are preparing for ALA-PDT. Each clinician will develop guidelines and procedures that will optimize the use of PDT in their offices. The US Consensus Paper[77] and other reports[78,79] outline steps to follow when beginning PDT in the clinical setting. The following description shows how my clinic utilizes ALA-PDT.

The first thing we do in our office is to explain all the risks and benefits of the procedure you are going to be performing on the patient on that given day. You must explain every detail and document this thoroughly. A signed, written informed consent will verify that you have reviewed the necessary information and potential sequelae with the patient. Remember that ALA-PDT utilized for photorejuvenation, acne vulgaris, SGH, and HS is an off-label use of ALA according to the FDA, and this, too, must be explained. The use of ALA for AKs is an approved use for ALA, although with shorter drug incubation times and varying light sources this, too, is considered off-label.

Because the majority of PDT treatments are performed on the face, the face will be used as the example for the procedure. The face must be thoroughly cleansed with a mild cleanser. A degreasing procedure is performed next to enhance the skin's absorption of ALA. There are 2 major ways to degrease the skin: microdermabrasion or an acetone scrub. Our clinic uses an acetone scrub as it is a less expensive procedure than microdermabrasion, but there is growing evidence that the use of microdermabrasion enhances the penetration of ALA.[80] If a microdermabrasion is to be done, there are options here as well, including standard microdermabrasion with crystals, crystal-less microdermabrasion, paddle-enhanced microdermabrasion, and microdermabrasion with iontophoresis to enhance ALA's penetration into the skin. We utilize crystal-less microdermabrasion systems, the paddle method, or the iontophoresis system when we choose to use microdermabrasion in our patient population.

Next, the Levulan Kerastick is mixed (Fig 3). The Levulan Kerastick is a 20 percent weight/volume 5-ALA solution with 48 percent alcohol. It has a special roll-on dermatologic applicator at one end to allow easy and accurate application of the medicine to the area(s) being treated. This applicator tip is applied to a flexible glass tubing that contains two glass vials. One of the vials contains the ALA in a powder form; the other contains the ethanol. Light manual pressure on the glass vials in the Kerastick will break the vials, allowing mixture of the 2 by gentle rotation in a back-and-forth direction. Three minutes of mixing is recommended before the application of the 20 percent 5-ALA.

Once the Kerastick is prepared, it will be painted onto the skin in a uniform manner, covering the forehead, cheeks, chin, and nose area. If there are AKs or inflammatory acne lesions present, a second coat of medicine is routinely applied to those lesions. The drug is then allowed to incubate on the skin. For all practical indications, drug incubation is 1 hour for photorejuvenation and AKs, 30 to 45 minutes for inflammatory acne vulgaris, and 1 hour for SGH. For each successive treatment, drug incubation may be increased by approximately 15 to 30 minutes.

The patient is now ready for light or laser administration. If an IPL light source is going to be used, it is recommended that the skin be once again cleansed before the use of the light source. One will find that the coupling medium, or gel, will not remain on the skin surface after the application of the ALA. If a blue light source or PDL is to be used, most would still recommend the skin be cleansed once again, although it is not mandatory. All our treatments are carried out with the aid of cold air cooling, which the patient holds and uses as needed. The treatment settings for a variety of devices are shown in Table 6.

After the therapy is completed, there are several very important steps to be performed before discharging the patient from your clinic. First, any remaining ALA needs to be thoroughly removed from the skin. Many clinicians are finding that if they perform an IPL or PDL treatment they next perform a short, 5-minute blue light "quenching" that will, for all practical purposes, remove any excess ALA. It may also serve to give an additional benefit to the patient, although clinical trials with regard to this concept have not been performed. Next, we use ice on the treated areas, which helps with any patient discomfort or skin burning. During this time we begin our discussions of proper skin care and sun protection, which are crucial for the patient to follow to avoid the only real adverse effect of the procedure, phototoxicity. Phototoxicity can be minimized or totally taken care of by following several very simple rules. The patient must remain out of the sun for the first 24 to 48 hours following the procedure. Sunscreen use, with a minimum SPF of 30, is required and is applied in our office before the patient leaves. There are many new creams and lotions that are being evaluated to help reduce any erythema that may be associated with lasers and light

TABLE 6.—Parameters for Lasers/Light Sources Useful for PDT

Device (Company)	Treatment Parameters
IPL Quantum SR (Lumenis Ltd., Yokneam, Israel)	1. 560-nm filter 2. Double pulse (2.4/4.0 msec with 10-msec delay) 3. Single pass with no overlap 4. 25-35 J/cm^2
Lumenis One* (Lumenis Ltd.)	1. 560-nm filter 2. Double pulse (4.0/4/0 msec with 20-msec delay) 3. Single pass with no overlap 4. 15-25 J/cm^2
VascuLight SR* (Lumenis Ltd.)	1. 560-nm filter 2. Double pulse (3.0/6.0 msec with 10-msec delay) 3. Single pass with no overlap 4. 30-35 J/cm^2
EsteLux Pulsed Light System* (Palomar Medical Technologies, Burlington, Mass.)	1. 20 msec 2. 19-30 J/cm^2 3. Single pass with no overlap
Photogenica V Star* (Cynosure Inc., Chelmsford, Mass.)	1. 585-nm or 595-nm wavelength PDL 2. 10-mm spot size 3. 40-msec pulse width 4. 7.5 J/cm^2 5. 2 passes with 50% overlap
V Beam (Candela Corp., Wayland, Mass.)	1. 595-nm PDL 2. 10-mm spot size 3. 6-msec pulse width 4. 7.5 J/cm^2 5. 2 passes with 50% overlap
ClearLight* (Lumenis Ltd.)	1. 405-420 nm blue light 2. 8-10 minutes under light
BluU* (DUSA Pharmaceuticals, Wilmington, Mass.)	1. 417 nm ±5-nm blue light 2. 8-15 minutes under light
SkinStation* (Radiancy, Orangeburg, NY)	1. 500-1200 nm pulsed light 2. 2 passes 3. 45 J/cm^2
Aurora (Syneron Medical Ltd., Yokneam, Isreal)	1. 580-980 nm 2. Optical energy of 16-22 J/cm^2; RF energy of 16-22 J/cm^2 3. Single pass
PhotoLight* (Cynosure Inc.)	1. 550-nm filter 2. 8 J/cm^2 3. 15-20 msec 4. Single pass
Sciton BBL* (Sciton Inc., Palo Alto, Calif.)	1. 560-nm BBL filter 2. 14 J/cm^2 3. 12 msec 4. Single pass

*Devices used by author; other settings from recognized experts in the laser field.

sources without the use of ALA; these are also being investigated for their potentials with ALA as well. These have included Neocutis Bio-restorative Skin Cream,[81] Biafine,[82] and Avene Gel Deau.[83]

As noted, phototoxicity is the only major concern that may be seen following an ALA-PDT procedure. By following the simple rules outlined above, this is routinely minimized in our clinical setting. Patients may note some desquamation of the skin after several days, but proper use of moisturizers or "spray" waters will minimize this effect. A phototoxic effect from ALA-PDT is shown in Fig 13.

Patients also must have a thorough understanding of how many treatments with ALA-PDT they will require for a given effect. This remains an elusive answer at this time, and further clinical studies will help give guidelines as to what has been found in clinical trial work. However, clinical trials do not always correlate into real-world experiences, so it is not possible to give a precise answer when asked how many treatments one will require to achieve a certain result. Each patient must be treated as an individual, and clinical trial results should be used as guidelines for a given patient's need. Also, skin care is a must with patients who undergo an ALA-PDT procedure; maintenance therapy will be required, although no clinical trials have demonstrated when or how many sessions.

ALA-PDT is a procedure that has created a new buzz in dermatology—both in the medical and cosmetic dermatology world. AKs, as well as mod-

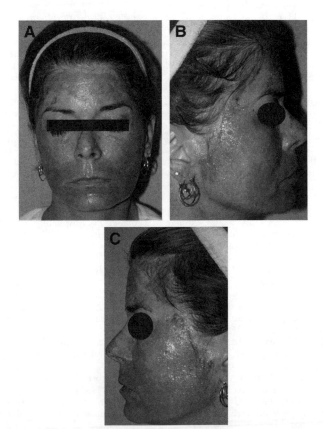

FIGURE 13. Phototoxicity effect after ALA-PDT treatment. (Photos courtesy of Michael H. Gold, MD, The Laser and Rejuvenation Center, Nashville, TN.)

erate to severe inflammatory acne vulgaris, SGH, and HS can be successfully treated with Levulan PDT and a variety of lasers and light sources. Future research endeavors will further define clinical protocols and entities for which Levulan PDT is useful and continue to allow us to offer new therapies for our patients.

References

1. Raab O. Ueber die wirkung fluoreszierenden stoffe auf infusorien. *Z Biol.* 1900; 39:524-526.
2. Von Tappeiner H, Jodblauer A. Uber die wirkung der photodynamischen (fluorescierenden) staffe auf protozoan und enzyme. *Dtsch Arch Klin Med.* 1904;80:427-487.
3. Jesionek A, Von Tappeiner H. Behandlung der hautcarcinome nut fluorescierenden stoffen. *Dtsch Arch Klin Med.* 1905;85:223-227.
4. Hausman W. Die sensibilisierende wirkung des hamatoporphyrins. *Biochem Zeit.* 1911:276-316.
5. Meyer-Betz F. Untersuchungen uber die bioloische (photodynamische) wirkung des hamatoporphyrins und anderer derivative des blut-und gallenfarbstoffs. *Dtsch Arch Klin Med.* 1913;112:476-503.
6. Auler H, Banzer G. Untersuchungen ueber die rolle der porphyrine bei geschwulstkranken menschen und tieren. *Z Krebsforsch.* 1942;53:65-68.
7. Figge FHJ, Weiland GS, Manganiello LDJ. Cancer detection and therapy. Affinity of neoplastic embryonic and traumatized tissue for porphyrins and metalloporphyrins. *Proc Soc Exp Biol Med.* 1948;68:640.
8. Dougherty TJ, Kaufman JE, Goldfarb A, et al. Photoradiation therapy for the treatment of malignant tumors. *Cancer Res.* 1978;38:2628-2635.
9. Kennedy JC, Pottier RH, Pross DC et al. Photodynamic therapy with endogenous protoporphyrin IX: basic principles and present clinical experiences. *J Photochem Photobiol B.* 1990;6:143-148.
10. Gold MH, Goldman MP. 5-Aminolevulinic acid photodynamic therapy: where we have been and where we are going. *Dermatol Surg.* 2004;30:1077-1084.
11. Jeffes EW, McCullough JL, Weinstein GD, et al. Photodynamic therapy of actinic keratoses with topical aminolevulinic acid hydrochloride and fluorescent blue light. *J Am Acad Dermatol.* 2001;45:96-104.
12. Jeffes EW. Levulan: the first approved topical photosensitizer for the treatment of actinic keratosis. *J Dermatolog Treat.* 2002;13:S19-S23.
13. Nestor MS, Goldberg DJ, Goldman MP, et al. Photorejuvenation: non-ablative skin rejuvenation using intense pulsed light. *Skin Aging.* 2003;3:8.
14. Goldman M, Eckhouse S. Photothermal sclerosis of leg veins. *Dermatol Surg.* 1996;22:323-30.
15. Anderson RR, Parish JA. Selective photothermolysis: precise microsurgery by selective absorption of pulsed radiation. *Science.* 1983;220:524-527.
16. Biter PH. Noninvasive rejuvenation of photodamaged skin using serial, full-face intense pulsed light treatments. *Dermatol Surg.* 2000;26:835-842.
17. Goldberg DJ, Cutler KB. Non-ablative treatment of rhytids with intense pulsed light. *Lasers Surg Med.* 2000;26:196-200.
18. Weiss RA, Weiss MA, Beasley KL. Rejuvenation of photoaged skin: 5 years results with intense pulsed light of the face, neck and chest. *Dermatol Surg.* 2002;28: 115-119.
19. Negishi K, Tezuka Y, Kushikata N, et al. Photorejuvenation for Asian skin by intense pulsed light. *Dermatol Surg.* 2001;27:627-631.
20. Hernandez-Perez E. Gross and microscopic findings in patients submitted to nonablative full-face resurfacing using intense pulsed light: a preliminary study. *Dermatol Surg.* 2002;28:651-655.

21. Town G, Ash C, Eadie E, et al. Measuring key parameters of intense pulsed light (IPL) devices. *J Cosmet Laser Ther.* 2007;9:148-160.
22. Nestor MS, Gold MH, Kauvar AN. The use of photodynamic therapy in dermatology: results of a consensus conference. *J Drugs Dermatol.* 2006;5:140-154.
23. Alexiades-Armenakas MR, Geronemus RG. Laser-mediated photodynamic therapy of actinic keratoses. *Arch Dermatol.* 2003;139:1313-1320.
24. Gold MH. The evolving role of aminolevulinic acid hydrochloride with photodynamic therapy in photoaging. *Cutis.* 2002;69:8-13.
25. Touma D, Yaar M, Whitehead S, et al. A trial of short incubation, broad-area photodynamic therapy for facial actinic keratoses and diffuse photodamage. *Arch Dermatol.* 2004;140:33-40.
26. Ruiz-Rodriguez R, Sanz-Sanchez T, Cordoba S. Photodynamic photorejuvenation. *Dermatol Surg.* 2002;28:742-774.
27. Gold MH, Bradshaw VL, Boring MM, et al. Treatment of sebaceous gland hyperplasia by photodynamic therapy with 5-aminolevulinic acid and a blue light source or intense pulsed light source. *J Drugs Dermatol.* 2004;3:S6-S9.
28. Goldman MP, Atkin D, Kincad S. PDT/ALA in the treatment of actinic damage: real world experience. *J Lasers Surg Med.* 2002;14:24.
29. Avram DK, Goldman MP. Effectiveness and safety of ALA-IPL in treating actinic keratoses and photodamage. *J Drugs Dermatol.* 2004;3:S36-S39.
30. Alexiades-Armenakas MR, Geronemus RG. Laser-mediated photodynamic therapy of actinic chelitis. *J Drugs Dermatol.* 2004;3:548-551.
31. Alster TS, Tanzi EL, Welch EC. Photorejuvenation of facial skin with topical 20% 5-aminolevulinic acid and intense pulsed light treatment: a split-face comparison study. *J Drugs Dermatol.* 2005;4:35-38.
32. Key DJ. Aminolevulinic acid-pulsed dye laser photodynamic therapy for the treatment of photoaging. *Cosmetic Derm.* 2005;18:31-36.
33. Marmur ES, Phelps R, Goldberg DJ. Ultrastructural changes seen after ALA-IPL photorejuvenation: a pilot study. *J Cosmet Laser Ther.* 2005;7:21-24.
34. Dover JS, Bhatia AC, Stewart B, et al. Topical 5-aminolevulinic acid combined with intense pulsed light in the treatment of photoaging. *Arch Dermatol.* 2005;141:1247-1252.
35. Gold MH, Bradshaw VL, Boring MM, et al. Split-face comparison of photodynamic therapy with 5-aminolevulinic acid and intense pulsed light versus intense pulsed light alone for photodamage. *Dermatol Surg.* 2006;32:795-801.
36. Redbord KP, Hanke CW. Topical photodynamic therapy for dermatologic disorders: results and complications. *J Drugs Dermatol.* 2007;6:1197-1202.
37. Gold MH. 5-Aminolevulinic acid photodynamic therapy versus methyl aminolevulinate photodynamic therapy for inflammatory acne vulgaris. *J Am Acad Dermatol.* 2008;58:S60-S62.
38. Gold MH. Aminolevulinic acid photodynamic therapy for actinic keratoses and photorejuvenation. *Exp Rev Dermatol.* 2007;2:391-402.
39. Data on file. Galderma. http://www.galderma.com/. Accessed June 3, 2008.
40. Szeimies RM, Karrer S, Radakovic-Fijan S, et al. Photodynamic therapy using topical methyl 5-aminolevulinate compared with cryotherapy for actinic keratosis: a prospective, randomized study. *J Am Acad Dermatol.* 2002;47:258-262.
41. Bjerring P, Funk J, Poed-Petersen J, et al. Randomized double blind study comparing photodynamic therapy (PDT) with Metvix to PDT with placebo cream in actinic keratosis [abstract]. 29th Nordic Congress of Dermatology and Venereology, Gothenborg, 2001.
42. Freeman M, Vinciullo C, Francis D, et al. A comparison of photodynamic therapy using topical methyl aminolevulinate (Metvix) with single cycle cryotherapy in patients with actinic keratosis: a prospective, randomized study. *J Dermatolog Treat.* 2003;14:99-106.
43. Pariser DM, Lowe NJ, Stewart DM, et al. Photodynamic therapy with topical methyl aminolevulinate (Metvix) is effective and safe in the treatment of actinic keratosis: results of a prospective randomized trial. *J Am Acad Dermatol.* 2003;48:227-232.

44. Tarstedt M, Rosdahl I, Berne B, et al. A randomized multicenter study to compare two treatment regimens of topical methyl aminolevulinate (Metvix)-PDT in actinic keratosis of the face and scalp. *Acta Derm Venereol.* 2005;85:424-428.
45. Morton C, Campbell S, Gupta G, et al. Intraindividual, right-left comparison of topical methyl aminolevulinate-photodynamic therapy and cryotherapy in subjects with actinic keratoses: a multicentre, randomized controlled study. *Br J Dermatol.* 2006;155:1029-1036.
46. Braathen LR, Szeimies RM, Basset-Seguin N, et al. Guidelines on the use of photodynamic therapy for nonmelanoma skin cancer: an international consensus. *J Am Acad Dermatol.* 2007;56:125-143.
47. Zane C, Capezzera R, Sala R, et al. Clinical and echographic analysis of photodynamic therapy using methylaminolevulinate as sensitizer in the treatment of photodamaged facial skin. *Lasers Surg Med.* 2007;39:203-209.
48. Ruiz-Rodriguez R, López L, Candelas D, et al. Enhanced efficacy of photodynamic therapy after fractional resurfacing: fractional photodynamic rejuvenation. *J Drugs Dermatol.* 2007;6:818-820.
49. Wiegell SR, Wulf HC. Photodynamic therapy of acne vulgaris using 5-aminolevulinic acid versus methyl aminolaevulinate. *J Am Acad Dermatol.* 2006;54:647-651.
50. Kashe A, Luderschmidt S, Ring J et al. Photodynamic therapy induces less pain in patients treated with methyl aminolaevulinate compared to aminolaevulinic acid. *J Drugs Dermatol.* 2006;5:353-356.
51. Gold MH. Pharmacoeconomic analysis of the treatment of multiple actinic keratoses. *J Drugs Dermatol.* 2008;7:23-25.
52. Del Rosso J. Acne in the adolescent patient: interrelationship of psychological impact and therapeutic options. *Today Ther Trends.* 2001;19:473-484.
53. Leyden JJ. Therapy for acne vulgaris. *N Engl J Med.* 1997;336:1156-1162.
54. Coates P, Vyakrnam S, Eady EA, et al. Prevalence of antibiotic-resistant propionibacteria on the skin of acne patients: 10-year surveillance data and snapshot distribution study. *Br J Dermatol.* 2002;146:840-848.
55. Hongcharu W, Taylor CR, Chang Y, et al. Topical ALA-photodynamic therapy for the treatment of acne vulgaris. *J Invest Dermatol.* 2000;115:183-192.
56. Itoh Y, Ninomiya Y, Tajima S, et al. Photodynamic therapy for acne vulgaris with topical 5-aminolevulinic acid. *Arch Dermatol.* 2000;136:1093-1095.
57. Itoh Y, Ninomiya Y, Tajima S, et al. Photodynamic therapy of acne vulgaris with topical delta aminolevulinic acid and incoherent light in Japanese patients. *Br J Dermatol.* 2001;144:575-579.
58. Goldman MP, Boyce SM. A single-center study of aminolevulinic acid and 417 NM photodynamic therapy in the treatment of moderate to severe acne vulgaris. *J Drugs Dermatol.* 2003;2:393-396.
59. Gold MH. The utilization of ALA-PDT and a new photoclearing device for the treatment of severe inflammatory acne vulgaris—results of an initial clinical trial. *J Lasers Surg Med.* 2003;15:46.
60. Goldman MP, Boyce S. A single-center study of aminolevulinic acid and 417 nm photodynamic therapy in the treatment of moderate to severe acne vulgaris. *J Drugs Dermatol.* 2003;2:393-396.
61. Gold MH. The use of a novel intense pulsed light and heat source and ALA-PDT in the treatment of moderate to severe inflammatory acne vulgaris. *J Drugs Dermatol.* 2004:3:S14-S18.
62. Taub AF. PDT for the treatment of acne: a pilot study. *J Drugs Dermatol.* 2004; 3:S10-S14.
63. Alexiades-Armenakas MR. Long pulsed dye laser-mediated photodynamic therapy combined with topical therapy for mild-to-severe comedonal, inflammatory and cystic acne. *J Drugs Dermatol* 2006;5:45-55.
64. Miller A, Van Camp A. Treatment of acne vulgaris with photodynamic therapy: the use of aminolevulinic acid and green light. *Cosmet Derm.* 2006;19:624-627.

65. Santos AV, Belo VG, Santos G. Effectiveness of photodynamic therapy with topical 5-aminolevulinic acid and intense pulsed light versus intense pulsed light along in the treatment of acne vulgaris: comparative study. *Dermatol Surg.* 2005;31: 910-915.

66. Rojanamatin J, Choawawanich P. Treatment of inflammatory facial acne vulgaris with intense pulsed light (IPL) and short contact of topical 5-aminolevulinc acid (ALA): a pilot study. *Dermatol Surg.* 2006;32:991-997.

67. Wiegell SR, Wulf HC. Photodynamic therapy of acne vulgaris using methyl aminolaevulinate: a blinded, randomized controlled trial. *Br J Dermatol.* 2006;154: 969-976.

68. Horfelt C, Funk J, Frohm-Nilsson M, et al. Topical methyl aminolaevuninate photodynamic therapy for treatment of facial acne vulgaris: results of a randomized, controlled study. *Br J Dermatol.* 2006;155:608-613.

69. Mavilia L, Malara G, Moretti G, et al. Photodynamic therapy of acne using methyl aminolaevulinate diluted to 4% together with low doses of red light. *Br J Dermatol.* 2007;157:799-846.

70. Horio T, Horio O, Miyauchi-Hashimoto H, et al. Photodynamic therapy of sebaceous hyperplasia with topical 5-aminolevulinic acid and slide projector. *Br J Dermatol.* 2003;148:1274-1276.

71. Alster T, Tanzi E. Photodynamic therapy with topical aminolevulinic acid and pulsed dye laser irradiation for sebaceous hyperplasia. *J Drugs Dermatol.* 2003; 2:501-504.

72. Richey DF, Hopson B. Treatment of sebaceous hyperplasia by photodynamic therapy. *Cosmetic Derm.* 2004;17:525-529.

73. Gold MH, Boring MM, Bridges TM, et al. Treatment of sebaceous hyperplasia by photodynamic therapy with 5-aminolevulinic acid and a blue light source or intense pulsed light source. *J Drugs Dermatol.* 2004;3:S5-S8.

74. Gold MH, Bridges TM, Bradshaw VL, et al. ALA-PDT and blue light therapy for hidradenitis suppurativa. *J Drugs Dermatol.* 2004;3:32-35.

75. Strauss RM, Pollock B, Stables GI, et al. Photodynamic therapy using aminolevulinic acid does not lead to clinical improvement in hidradenitis suppurativa. *Br J Dermatol.* 2005;152:803-804.

76. Rivard J, Ozog D. Henry Ford Hospital dermatology experience with Levulan Kerastick and blue light photodynamic therapy. *J Drugs Dermatol.* 2006;5: 556-561.

77. Nestor M, Gold MH, Kauvar A, et al. The use of photodynamic therapy in dermatology: results of a consensus conference. *J Drugs Dermatol.* 2006;5: 140-154.

78. Gold MH, Nestor MS. Current treatments of actinic keratosis. *J Drugs Dermatol.* 2006;5:17-25.

79. Gold MH, Biron JA, Boring M, et al. Treatment of moderate to severe inflammatory acne vulgaris: photodynamic therapy with 5-aminolevulinic acid and a novel advanced fluorescence technology pulsed light source. *J Drugs Dermatol.* 2007;6: 319-322.

80. Fang JY, Lee WR, Shen SC, et al. Enhancement of topical 5-aminolaevulinic acid delivery by erbium:YAG laser and microdermabrasion: a comparison with iontophoresis and electroporation. *Br J Dermatol.* 2004;151:132-140.

81. Gold MH, Biron JA. A novel skin cream containing a mixture of human growth factors and cytokines for the treatment of adverse events associated with photodynamic therapy. *J Drugs Dermatol.* 2006;5:796-798.

82. Gold MH. Single-center, split-face, double-blind, randomized clinical trial of the efficacy of a trolamine-containing topical emulsion and a topical petrolatum-based product in reducing redness and peeling after treatment with a microlaser peel [poster]. Presented at the American of Academy Dermatology Annual Meeting 2006, San Francisco, CA.

83. Gold MH, Ribet V, Gral N, et al. Calming efficacy and tolerance of Avene spring water gel after epilatory laser treatment combined to healing cream in adults [poster]. Presented at the American of Academy Dermatology Annual Meeting 2006, San Francisco, CA.

---

*Dr Gold is a consultant for DUSA Pharmaceuticals, Alma Lasers, Aesthera, Cynosure, Sciton, Lumenis, and Neocutis. He also owns in DUSA and Lumenis as well as Neocutis.

Statistics of Interest to the Dermatologist

MARTIN A. WEINSTOCK, MD, PHD, AND MARGARET M. BOYLE, BS
Brown University Dermatoepidemiology Unit, Providence, Rhode Island

Morbidity and Mortality

Health Care Delivery in the United States

Miscellaneous

TABLE 1.—New Cases of Selected Reportable Infectious Diseases in the United States

	1940	1950	1960	1970	1980	1990	2000	2005	2007*
AIDS	***	***	***	***	***	41,595	40,758	30,568**	***
Anthrax	76	49	23	2	1	0	1	***	0
Congenital Rubella	***	***	***	77	50	11	9	1	0
Congenital Syphilis	***	***	***	***	***	3865	529	273	492
Diphtheria	15,536	5796	918	435	3	4	1	0	0
Gonorrhea	175,841	286,746	258,933	600,072	1,004,029	690,169	358,995	314,370	332,511
Hansen's Disease	0	44	54	129	223	198	91	89	60
Lyme Disease	0	0	0	0	0	0	17,730	21,304	20,599
Measles	291,162	319,124	441,703	47,351	13,506	27,786	86	62+++	30
Plague	1	3	2	13	18	2	6	7	6
Rocky Mountain Spotted Fever	457	464	204	390	1163	651	495	1843	2106
Syphilis (primary and secondary)	***	23,939	16,145	21,982	27,204	50,223	5979	8020	10,417
Toxic Shock Syndrome	***	***	***	***	***	322	135	96	79
Tuberculosis+	102,984++	121,742++	55,494	37,137	27,749	25,701	16,377	11,547	***
U.S. Population (millions)	132	151	179	203	227	249	281	296	302

Key:
*For 52 weeks ending December 29, 2007. Incidence data for reporting year 2007 are provisional.
**Last update December 3, 2005.
***Data not available.
+Reporting criteria changed in 1975.
++Data include newly reported active and inactive cases.
+++Of 62 cases reported, 51 were indigenous, and 11 were imported from another country.

Sources:
Centers for Disease Control and Prevention: Summary of Notifiable Diseases, United States, 2007. *Morbidity and Mortality Weekly Report* 56[51&52]:1360-1369, 2008.
Centers for Disease Control and Prevention: Summary of Notifiable Diseases, United States, 2005. *Morbidity and Mortality Weekly Report* 54[51&52]:1320-1330, 2006.
Centers for Disease Control and Prevention: Summary of Notifiable Diseases, United States, 2000. *Morbidity and Mortality Weekly Report* 49[51&52]:1167-1174, 2001.
Centers for Disease Control and Prevention: Annual Summary 1994: Reported morbidity and mortality. *Morbidity and Mortality Weekly Report* 1994;43(53):[70-71].
Centers for Disease Control and Prevention: Annual Summary 1984: Reported morbidity and mortality. *Morbidity and Mortality Weekly Report* 33:124-129, 1986.

TABLE 2.—Estimates of HIV/AIDS, 2007

Region	Adults and Children Living With HIV	Adults and Children Newly Infected With HIV	Adult Prevalence (%)	Adult and Child Deaths Due to AIDS
Sub-Saharan Africa	20.9 million–24.3 million	1.4 million–2.4 million	4.6–5.5	1.5 million–2.0 million
Middle East and North Africa	270,000–500,000	16,000–65,000	0.2–0.4	20,000–34,000
South and South-East Asia	3.3 million–5.1 million	180,000–740,000	0.2–0.4	230,000–380,000
East Asia	620,000–960,000	21,000–220,000	<0.2	28,000–49,000
Oceania	53,000–120,000	11,000–26,000	0.3–0.7	<500–2,700
Latin America	1.4–1.9 million	47,000–220,000	0.4–0.6	49,000–91,000
Caribbean	210,000–270,000	15,000–23,000	0.9–1.2	9,800–18,000
Eastern Europe and Central Asia	1.2 million–2.1 million	70,000–290,000	0.7–1.2	42,000–88,000
Western and Central Europe	600,000–1.1 million	19,000–86,000	0.2–0.4	<15,000
North America	480,000–1.9 million	38,000–68,000	0.5–0.9	18,000–31,000
Total	33.2 million 30.6 million–36.1 million	2.5 million 1.8–4.1 million	0.80% 0.7–0.9%	2.1 million 1.9 million–2.4 million

Source: AIDS Epidemic Update, Joint United Nations Programme on HIV/AIDS (UNAIDS) World Health Organization (WHO), December 2007.

TABLE 3.—AIDS Cases by Age Group and Exposure Category, and
Cumulative Totals Through 2006, United States

	2006 No.	2006 (%)	Cumulative Total* No.	Cumulative Total* (%)
Adult/adolescent exposure category				
Male-to-male sexual contact	13,775	(35%)	429,897	(44%)
Injection drug use	5239	(13%)	230,763	(23%)
Male-to-male sexual contact and injection drug use	1603	(4%)	65,524	(7%)
Hemophilia/coagulation disorder	54	(0%)	5524	(1%)
Heterosexual contact	7836	(20%)	134,796	(14%)
Receipt of blood transfusion, blood components, or tissue**	131	(0%)	9389	(1%)
Other/risk factor not reported or identified***	10,278	(26%)	107,450	(11%)
Adult/adolescent SUBTOTAL	38,916	(100%)	983,343	(100%)
Pediatric exposure category (<13 years at diagnosis)				
Hemophilia/coagulation disorder	0	(0%)	229	(2%)
Mother with/at risk for HIV infection	74	(86%)	8738	(92%)
Receipt of blood transfusion, blood components, or tissue+	1	(1%)	387	(4%)
Other/risk not reported or identified++	11	(13%)	168	(2%)
Pediatric SUBTOTAL	86	(100%)	9522	(100%)
TOTAL	39,002	(100%)	992,865	(100%)

*From the beginning of the epidemic through 2006. Includes 3 persons of unknown sex.

**AIDS developed in 47 adults/adolescents after they received blood that tested negative for HIV antibodies. AIDS developed in 14 additional adults after they received tissue, organs, or artificial insemination from HIV-infected donors. Four of the 14 received tissue or organs from a donor who was negative for HIV antibody at the time of donation.

***Includes 37 adults/adolescents who were exposed to HIV-infected blood, body fluids, or concentrated virus in health care, laboratory, or household settings, as supported by seroconversion, epidemiologic, and/or laboratory evidence. One person was infected after intentional inoculation with HIV-infected blood. Includes an additional 740 persons who acquired HIV infection perinatally but who were more than 12 years of age when AIDS was diagnosed. These 740 persons are not counted in the values for the pediatric transmission category.

+AIDS developed in 3 children after they received blood that had tested negative for HIV antibodies.

++Includes 5 children who were exposed to HIV-infected blood, as supported by seroconversion, epidemiologic, and/or laboratory evidence: 1 child was infected after intentional inoculation with HIV-infected blood, and 5 children were exposed to HIV-infected blood in a household setting. Of the 168 children, 26 had sexual contact with an adult with, or at high risk for, HIV infection.

Source:
Centers for Disease Control and Prevention: *HIV/AIDS Surveillance Report, 2006* Vol. 18. Atlanta: U.S. Department of Health and Human Services, Centers for Disease Control and Prevention; 2007:37. Also available at: http://www.cdc.gov/hiv/topics/surveillance/resources/reports/.

TABLE 4.—Selected Causes of Death, United States, 1995 and 2005

Cause of Death	Number of Deaths 1995	Number of Deaths 2005
Malignant melanoma	6907	8345
Infections of the skin	864	1702
Motor vehicle traffic accidents	43,363	45,343
Accident involving animal being ridden	86	120
Accidental drowning and submersion	3790	3582
Victim of lightning	76	48
Homicide and legal intervention	22,895	18,538
All cancer	538,455	559,312
All causes	2,312,132	2,448,017

Source:
National Center for Health Statistics, Division of Vital Statistics, personal communication, February 2008.

TABLE 5.—Annual Change in Cancer Incidence in the United States

Top 20 Highest Incidence Sites	Average Annual Percent Change	
	1992-2005	1975-1991
Thyroid	5.2	0.8
Liver and Intrahepatic Bile Duct	3.1	3.0
Melanoma of the Skin	2.7	3.7
Kidney and Renal Pelvis	1.9	2.4
Non-Hodgkin Lymphoma	0.5	3.6
Esophagus	0.4	0.7
Pancreas	0.3	−0.2
Urinary Bladder	0.1	0.6
Hodgkin Lymphoma	0.0	0.4
Brain and Other Nervous System	−0.2	1.2
Myeloma	−0.2	1.2
Leukemia	−0.4	0.1
Corpus Uteri	−0.4	−2.1
Breast	−0.5	2.2
Lung and Bronchus	−0.9	1.5
Ovary	−1.3	0.0
Colon and Rectum	−1.3	−0.1
Prostate	−1.3	4.9
Oral Cavity and Pharynx	−1.3	−0.6
Stomach	−1.6	−1.5
All sites	−0.5	1.3

Note:
SEER 9 registries and NCHS public use data file for the total U.S. Rates are per 100,000 and age-adjusted to the 2000 U.S. Standard Population (19 age groups-Census P25-1130) standard.
Rates are for invasive cancers only.

Source:
Surveillance Research Program, National Cancer Institute SEER*Stat Software (*www.seer.cancer.gov/seerstat*) version 6.40-beta.
Surveillance, Epidemiology, and End Results Program (*www.seer.cancer.gov*) SEER*Stat Database: Incidence - SEER 9 REgs. Limited–Use, Nov. 2007 (1973-2005) <Katrina/Rita Population Adjustment>Linked to County Attributes–Total U.S. 1969-2005 Counties, National Cancer Institute, DCCPS, Surveillance Research Program, Cancer Statistics Branch, released April 2008, based on the November 2007 submission.
Ries LAG, Melbert D, Krapcho M, Stinchcomb DG, Howlader N, Horner MJ, Mariotto A, Miller BA, Feuer EJ, Altekruse SF, Lewis DR, Clegg L, Eisner MP, Reichman M, Edwards BK (eds). *SEER Cancer Statistics Review: 1975-2005*, National Cancer Institute, Bethesda, MD, http://seer.cancer.gov/csr/1975-2004/, based on November 2007 SEER data submission, posted to the SEER website, 2008.

TABLE 6.—Melanoma Incidence and Mortality Rates, United States

Year	Incidence*	Mortality**
1975	7.9	2.1
1976	8.1	2.2
1977	8.9	2.3
1978	8.9	2.3
1979	9.5	2.4
1980	10.5	2.3
1981	11.1	2.4
1982	11.2	2.5
1983	11.1	2.5
1984	11.4	2.5
1985	12.8	2.6
1986	13.3	2.6
1987	13.7	2.7
1988	12.9	2.7
1989	13.7	2.7
1990	13.8	2.8
1991	14.6	2.7
1992	14.8	2.7
1993	14.6	2.7
1994	15.6	2.7
1995	16.4	2.7
1996	17.2	2.8
1997	17.7	2.7
1998	17.8	2.8
1999	18.2	2.6
2000	18.8	2.7
2001	19.5	2.7
2002	18.9	2.6
2003	19.2	2.7
2004	20.1	2.7
2005	21.5	2.7

+2008 estimate: 62,480 newly diagnosed cases and 8420 deaths

Note:
    *SEER 9 areas. Rates are per 100,000 and are age-adjusted to the 2000 US Standard population (19 age groups-Census P25-1130) standard.
    **National Center for Health Statistics public use data file for the total US. Rates per 100,000 and age-adjusted to the 2000 U.S. standard population. (19 age groups-Census P25-1130) standard.
    +Melanoma *in situ* accounts for about 54,020 new cases annually.
Source:
    American Cancer Society, Inc., Surveillance Research. *Cancer Facts & Figures 2008:4:2008.*
    Reis LAG, Melbert D, Krapcho M, Stinchcomb DG, Howlader N, Horner MJ, Mariotto A, Miller BA, Feuer EJ, Altekruse SF, Lewis DR, Clegg L, Eisner MP, Reichman M, Edwards BK (eds). *SEER Cancer Statistics Review: 1975-2005,* National Cancer Institute, Bethesda, MD, *http://seer.cancer.gov/csr/1975-2005/,* based on November 2007 SEER data submission posted to the SEER website, 2008.
    Surveillance Research Program, National Cancer Institute SEER*Stat (*www.seer.cancer.gov/seerstat*) version 6.4.0-beta.
    Surveillance, Epidemiology, and End-Results (SEER) Program, (www.seer.cancer.gov) SEER*Stat Database: Incidence-SEER 9 Regs Limited-Use November 2007 Sub. (1973-2005) <Katrina/Rita Population Adjustment>-Linked to County Attributes—Total U.S., 1969-2005 Counties, National Cancer Institute DCCPS, Branch, released April 2008, based on the November 2007 submission.
    Surveillance, Epidemiology, and End-Results (SEER) Program, SEER* Stat Database:Mortality-All COD, Total US (1969-2005) Linked to County Attributes—Total U. S., 1969-2005 Counties. National Cancer Institute DCCPS, Surveillance Research Program, Cancer Statistics Branch, released January 2008. Underlying mortality data provided by the National Center for Health Statistics (*www.cdc.gov/nchs*).

TABLE 7.—Melanoma Five-Year Relative Survival

Year	Whites	Blacks
	By Year at Diagnosis	
1960-1963*	60%	—
1970-1973*	68%	—
1975-1977+	82%	60%
1978-1980+	83%	60%
1981-1983+	83%	61%
1984-1986+	87%	70%
1987-1989+	88%	80%
1990-1992+	90%	61%
1993-1995+	90%	67%
1996-2004+	92%	78%
	By Stage at Diagnosis (1996-2004)	
Local	99%	95%
Regional	65%	47%
Distant	15%	24%

Key:
—Insufficient data.
*Rates are based on the End Results data from a series of hospital registries and one population-based registry.
+Rates are from the SEER 9 registries. Rates are based on follow-up of patients into 2005.
Notes:
Relative survival is the observed survival divided by the survival expected in a demographically similar subgroup of the general population.
Survival estimates among blacks are imprecise due to small numbers of cases observed.
Source:
Ries LAG, Melbert D, Krapcho M, Stinchcomb DG, Howlader N, Mariotto A, Miller BA, Feuer EJ, Altekruse SF, Lewis DR, Clegg L, Eisner MP, Reichman M, Edwards BK (eds). *SEER Cancer Statistics Review: 1975-2005,* National Cancer Institute, Bethesda, MD, *http://seer.cancer.gov/csr/1975-2005/,* based on November 2007 SEER data submission posted, to the SEER website, 2008.

TABLE 8.—Contact Dermatitis in Belgium: Proportion of Positive Patch Tests to Standard Chemicals in 295 Patients With at Least 1 Positive Reaction (Among 520 Patients Tested in 2007)

	Chemical	(%)
1.	Nickel sulphate	33.10
2.	Cobalt chloride	13.20
3.	Fragrance mix I	12.50
4.	Potassium dichromate	11.80
5.	Balsam of Peru	10.80
6.	Paraphenylenediamine	8.30
7.	Fragrance mix II	7.60
8.	Formaldehyde	6.90
9.	Colophonium	4.90
10.	Hydroxyisohexyl-3-cyclohexene carboxaldehyde	4.90
11.	Methyldibromo glutaronitrile	4.20
12.	Epoxy resin	3.85
13.	Thiuram mix	3.80
14.	Wood alcohols	3.80
15.	Methyl(chloro)isothiazolinone	3.50
16.	Benzocaine	3.10
17.	Budesonide	3.10
18.	Neomycin sulphate	3.10
19.	Quaternium-15	2.80
20.	Paratertiarybutylphenol-formaldehyde resin	2.40
21.	Mercaptobenzothiazole	2.10
22.	Sesquiterpene lactone mix	2.10
23.	Mercapto mix	1.70
24.	Isopropyl-phenylparaphenylenediamine	1.05
25.	Paraben mix	1.00
26.	Tixocortol pivalate	1.00
27.	Clioquinol	0.35
28.	Primin	0.35

(From Goossens A, University Hospital, Katholieke Universiteit Leuven, Belgium, personal communication, January 2008.)

TABLE 9.—Dermatology Trainees in the United States

Year Residency to Be Completed	Male Residents	Female Residents	Unknown	Total
MD Programs				
2008	127	242		369
2009	147	234		381
2010	137	235		372
2011	1	4		5
2012	0	1		1
DO Programs				
2008	18	9		27
2009	14	13		27
2010	15	19	1	35

Source:
American Academy of Dermatology, personal communication, January 2008.

TABLE 10.—Diplomates Certified by The American Board of Dermatology
From 1933 to 2007

Decade Totals (Inclusive Dates)	Average Number Certified per Year
1933-1940	69
1941-1950	74
1951-1960	76
1961-1970	112
1971-1980	247
1981-1990	271
1991-2000	295
2001-2007	323
TOTAL 1933 through 2007	13,570
Individual Year Totals	**Actual Number Certified**
1999	286
2000	283
2001	305
2002	309
2003	307
2004	329
2005	352
2006	319
2007	342

Source:
The American Board of Dermatology, Inc. personal communication, January 2008.

TABLE 11.—Physicians Certified in Dermatologic Subspecialties

A. Physicians Certified for Special Qualification in Dermatopathology, 1974-2007

Year	Average Number Certified per year		Total
	Dermatologists	Pathologists	
1974-1975	108	44	302
1976-1980	54	49	515
1981-1985	37	34	351
1986-1990	11	14	125
1991-1995	20	20	196
1996-2000	14	32	227
	Actual Number Certified		
2001	10	34	44
2002	14	55	69
2003	14	48	62
2004	16	45	61
2005	23	47	70
2006	32	37	69
2007	26	50	76
Total Number Certified 1974 through 2007	1028	1142	2170

B. Dermatologists Certified for Special Qualification in Clinical and Laboratory Dermatological Immunology, 1985-2007

Year	Number Certified
1985	52
1987	16
1989	22
1991	15
1993	5
1997	5
2001	6
Total 1985-2007	121

C. Dermatologists Certified for Special Qualification in Pediatric Dermatology, 2004 and 2006

2004	90
2006	41
Total 2004 through 2007	131

Notes:
—No special qualification examination for Dermatopathology was administered in 1992, 1994, and 1996.
—No special qualification examination in Clinical and Laboratory Dermatological Immunology was administered in 1986, 1988, 1990, 1992, 1994, 1995, 1996, 1998, 1999, 2000, 2002, 2003, 2004, 2005, 2006 or 2007.
—Special qualification in Pediatric Dermatology began in 2004. No special qualification examination in Pediatric Dermatology was administered in 2005 or 2007.
Source:
American Board of Dermatology and American Board of Pathology, personal communication, January, 2008.

TABLE 12.—Visits to Non-Federal Office-Based Physicians in the United States, 2005

Diagnosis	Dermatologist		Type of Physician Other		All Physicians	
	Number of Visits (1000's)	Percent	Number of Visits (1000's)	Percent	Number of Visits (1000's)	Percent
Acne vulgaris	3676	11.3	*	*	5017	0.5
Eczematous dermatitis	2001	6.2	7320	0.8	9321	1.0
Warts	1547	4.8	1987	0.2	3535	0.4
Skin cancer	3242	10.0	2927	0.3	6169	0.6
Psoriasis	1141	3.5	*	*	1439	0.2
Fungal infections	*	*	2287	0.3	3021	0.3
Hair disorders	862	2.7	*	*	1243	0.1
Actinic keratosis	3234	10.0	*	*	3838	0.4
Benign neoplasm of the skin	3236	10.0	*	*	4346	0.5
All disorders	32,442	100.0	931,175	100.0	963,617	100.0

*Figure suppressed due to small sample size.

Figures may not add to totals because of rounding.

Source:

Centers for Disease Control and Prevention, National Center for Health Statistics, 2005 National Ambulatory Medical Care Survey, personal communication, March, 2008.

TABLE 13.—Health Insurance Coverage of the United States Population, 2006

	Children 1-17 Years	Adults 18-64 Years	Adults 65 Years and Over
Individually Purchased Insurance	8%	7%	25%
Employment-based Coverage	57%	62%	37%
Public Insurance, All types	30%	18%	96%
Medicaid	27%	13%	10%
No Health Insurance	12%	18%	2%

Note: Some individuals have both public and private insurance, so the numbers will not add to 100%.
Source:
Employee Benefit Research Institute, *Issue Brief No. 310,* "Sources of Health Insurance and Characteristics of the Uninsured: Analysis of the March 2007 Current Population Survey," October, 2007, Washington, DC, personal communication, February, 2008.

TABLE 14.—Nonelderly Population With Selected Sources of Health Insurance, by Family Income, 2006

Yearly Family Income Level	Employment-Based Coverage %	Individually Purchased %	Public %	Uninsured %	Total %
under $10,000	11	10	47	36	100
$10,000-$19,999	21	9	40	34	100
$20,000-$29,999	39	8	27	31	100
$30,000-$39,999	52	7	22	24	100
$40,000-$49,999	64	7	15	19	100
$50,000-$74,000	75	6	11	13	100
$75,000 and over	85	5	6	7	100
TOTAL	62	7	18	18	100

Note: Details may not add to totals because individuals may receive coverage from more than one source.
Source:
Fronstin P, "Sources of Coverage and Characteristics of the Uninsured: Analysis of the March 2007 Current Population Survey." *EBRI Issue Brief*, No. 310 (Washington, DC. Employee Benefit Research Institute), October, 2007.

TABLE 15.—Health Maintenance Organization (HMO)
Market Penetration in the United States,
January 1, 2007

HMO Penetration in Region	
Pacific	41%
Northeast	30%
Mid-Atlantic	29%
Mountain	22%
East North Central	19%
South Atlantic	17%
West North Central	13%
East South Central	11%
West South Central	10%

HMO Penetration Top Ten Most Highly Penetrated Metropolitan Statistical Areas	
Tallahassee, FL	75%
Madison, WI	61%
Buffalo-Cheektowaga-Tonawanda, NY	60%
Rochester, NY	60%
Visalia-Porterville, CA	56%
Santa Ana-Anaheim-Irvine, CA	53%
Fresno, CA	52%
Sacramento—Arden-Arcade—Roseville, CA	49%
Santa Barbara-Santa Maria, CA	49%
Modesto, CA	48%

Source:
2007 HealthLeaders-Interstudy Publications, *Managed Care Census,* Nashville, TN. Personal communication, March, 2008.

TABLE 16.—National Health Expenditure Amounts: Selected Calendar Years

(Billions of Dollars)

Spending Category	1980	1990	2000	2010*	2011*
Total National Health Expenditures	246	696	1310	2776	2966
Health Services and Supplies	234	670	1262	2601	2778
Personal Health Care	215	609	1138	2313	2473
Hospital Care	102	254	417	861	922
Professional Services	67	217	425	862	919
Physician and Clinical Services	47	158	289	577	613
Other Professional Services	4	18	39	78	83
Dental Services	13	32	61	118	126
Other Personal Health Care	3	10	37	89	98
Nursing Home and Home Health	20	65	126	226	239
Home Health Care	2	13	32	73	78
Nursing Home Care	18	53	94	153	161
Retail Outlet Sale of Medical Products	26	73	171	364	392
Prescription Drugs	12	40	122	292	318
Other Medical Products	14	33	49	72	75
Durable Medical Equipment	4	11	18	29	31
Other Non-Durable Medical Products	10	23	31	43	44
Program Administration and Net Cost of Private Health Insurance	12	40	81	206	218
Government Public Health Activities	7	20	44	82	88
Investment	12	26	48	176	188
Research+	6	13	29	52	56
Structures and Equipment	7	14	19	124	133

Note: Numbers may not add to totals because of rounding.
*Projected values. The health spending projections were based on the 2005 version of the National Health Expenditures (NHE) released in January, 2007.
+Research and development expenditures of drug companies and other manufacturers and providers of medical equipment and supplies are excluded from research expenditures. These research expenditures are implicitly included in the expenditure class in which the product falls, in that they are covered by the payment received for that product.

Source:
Centers for Medicare and Medicaid Services, Office of the Actuary, January, 2008.

TABLE 17.—Spending on Consumer Advertising of
Prescription Products, United States

Year	(Annual Dollars in Millions)
2007	4905
2006	4745
2005	4132
2004	4084
2003	3082
2002	2514
2001	2479
2000	2150*
1999	1590
1998	1173
1997	844
1996	595
1995	313
1994	242
1993	165
1992	156
1991	56
1990	48
1989	12

*Estimated.
Source: TNS Media Intelligence Copyright 2008, Magazine Publishers of America,
Inc. Personal communication, March 2008.

TABLE 18.—Results of the American Academy of Dermatology Skin Cancer
Screening Program, 1985-2007

Year	Number Screened	Basal Cell Carcinoma	Squamous Cell Carcinoma	Malignant Melanoma
1985	32,000	1056	163	97
1986	41,486	3049	398	262
1987	41,649	2798	302	257
1988	67,124	4457	474	435
1989	78,486	6266	761	593
1990	98,060	7959	1069	872
1991	102,485	8110	1193	1062
1992	98,440	8403	1280	1054
1993	97,553	7067	1068	2465+
1994	86,895	6908	1235	1010
1995	88,934	7503	1317	1353
1996	94,363	8713	1656	1399
1997	99,554	8730	1685	1469
1998	89,536	6687	1308	1078
1999	89,916	5790	1136	635
2000	65,854	5074	1053	653
2001	70,562	5192	1102	642
2002	64,492	4733	1009	692
2003	70,692	4481	1032	489
2004	71,243	4891	1165	760
2005	82,532	5659	1411	794
2006	85,272	6354	1649	876
2007	90,484	6193	1852	883
TOTAL	1,807,612	136,073	25,318	19,830

Key:
+Number of cases included melanoma, "rule out melanoma," and lentigo maligna.
Source:
American Academy of Dermatology: *2007 Skin Cancer Screening Program Statistical Summary Report*, February 2008.

TABLE 19.—Leading Dermatology Journals

Journal	Total Citations in 2006	Number of Articles Published in 2006
Journal of Investigative Dermatology	17,757	285
Journal of the American Academy of Dermatology	14,545	343
British Journal of Dermatology	14,099	353
Archives of Dermatology	11,004	188
Dermatology	4174	156
Contact Dermatitis	4072	95
Dermatologic Surgery	3495	162
International Journal of Dermatology	3485	262
Acta Dermato-Venereologica	2801	71
Clinical and Experimental Dermatology	2647	145
Burns	2590	185
Archives of Dermatological Research	2040	77
Journal of Cutaneous Pathology	2023	146
American Journal of Dermatopathology	1888	57
Pigment Cell Research	1668	52
Cutis	1639	102
Experimental Dermatology	1593	99
Journal of the European Academy of Dermatology	1512	209
Pediatric Dermatology	1475	112
Melanoma Research	1471	70
Journal of Dermatological Science	1409	76
Mycoses	1397	105
Journal of Dermatology	1389	152
Wound Repair and Regeneration	1339	90
European Journal of Dermatology	1303	94

Source:
  Journal Citation Reports Web Version 2006: JCR, Science Edition. Philadelphia: The Thomson Corporation, January, 2008.

CLINICAL DERMATOLOGY

1 Urticarial and Eczematous Disorders

Null Mutations in the Filaggrin Gene (*FLG*) Determine Major Susceptibility to Early-Onset Atopic Dermatitis that Persists into Adulthood
Barker JNWN, Palmer CNA, Zhao Y, et al (King's College London; Univ of Dundee, Scotland; Univ of Newcastle upon Tyne, England)
J Invest Dermatol 127:564-567, 2007

Atopic dermatitis (AD) is a common disease with a complex etiology in childhood and adult life. A significant proportion of childhood AD is transient, but in many cases it persists into adulthood. We have recently shown that null mutations in the filaggrin gene (*FLG*) are an important predisposing factor for childhood eczema and eczema-associated asthma, but persistence to adulthood has not been analyzed. Here we studied a cohort of adult patients with persistent AD, which had been present since early childhood. In this cohort, the combined allele frequency of the two common *FLG* null variants was 0.270 (cf. population frequency 0.046). This represents an odds ratio of 7.7 with 95% confidence interval of 5.3–10.9 and a χ^2 P-value of 1.7×10^{-53}. Our data conclusively demonstrate that identification of *FLG* null alleles is an indicator of a poor prognosis in AD, predisposing to a form of eczema that starts in early infancy and persists into adulthood. This study helps to further define the nature of the AD phenotype associated with *FLG* null alleles.

▶ The filaggrin gene (*FLG*) is located in the epidermal differentiation complex 1q21. Profilaggrin is the main protein component of keratohyalin granules. On terminal differentiation of keratinocytes, profilaggrin is dephosphorylated and cleaved into 10 to 12 essentially identical 37 kd filaggrin peptides that subsequently aggregate into the keratin filament cytoskeleton, causing the collapse of the granular layer into flattened squames. The collapsed cytoskeleton is then cross-linked to form a barrier to the outside world. It has also been suggested that degradation products of filaggrin contribute to moisture retention in the cornified layers of the epidermis.[1]

In 2006, Smith et al[2] identified 2 null mutations, R501X and 2282del4, in the *FLG* in Scottish, Irish, and European American patients with ichthyosis vulgaris. Smith et al[2] estimated that approximately 10% of persons of European origin carry 1 of the 2 loss-of-function mutations in the *FLG*. Both of the above mutations lead to premature termination codons resulting in complete absence of processed filaggrin in the epidermis. Less-common mutations located centrally in the filaggrin domain have been identified by Sandilands et al.[3] These mutations cause mild disease in heterozygotes and more severe disease in homozygotes. It is postulated that the compromised epidermal barrier that results from mutations in the *FLG* leads to increased passage of antigens, allergens, and chemicals into the skin, which, in turn, can provoke an immune response. Barker et al noted that 42% of the patients studied with childhood onset, adult persistent atopic dermatitis had 1 or more filaggrin null alleles, and in a report by Nomura et al,[4] the investigators described 2 novel mutations, 3321delA and S2554X, in the *FLG* in Japanese patients. Additional mutations in the *FLG* will almost certainly be discovered in the future.

These studies document a genetic link to the formation of an ineffective epidermal barrier. Clinically, it has been noted that liberally applied moisturizers, which improve barrier function, are often of benefit. Topical agents designed to specifically improve barrier function will likely continue to be developed in the future. We now have scientific evidence to share with patients and parents of patients with atopic dermatitis indicating that the skin barrier function abnormality is the primary problem of many if not most patients with atopic dermatitis. This differs from the belief (and hope) of many patients that some specific antigen can be found and eliminated to cure their disease. Emphasizing this might encourage patients to be more compliant with their use of topical medication and moisturizers.

S. Raimer, MD

References

1. Rawlings AV, Harding CR. Moisturization and skin barrier function. *Dermatol Ther.* 2004;17:43-48.
2. Smith FJD, Irvine AD, Terron-Kwiatkowski A, et al. Common loss-of-function mutations in the gene encoding filaggrin cause ichthyosis vulgaris. *Nat Genet.* 2006;38:337-342.
3. Sandilands A, O'Regan GM, Liao H, et al. Prevalent and rare mutations in the gene encoding filaggrin cause ichthyosis vulgaris and predispose individuals to atopic dermatitis. *J Invest Dermatol.* 2006;126:1770-1775.
4. Nomura T, Sandilands A, Akiyama M, et al. Unique mutations in the filaggrin gene in Japanese patients with ichthyosis vulgaris and atopic dermatitis. *J Allergy Clin Immunol.* 2007;119:434-440.

Unique mutations in the filaggrin gene in Japanese patients with ichthyosis vulgaris and atopic dermatitis

Nomura T, Sandilands A, Akiyama M, et al (Hokkaido Univ, Sapporo, Japan; Univ of Dundee, Scotland; Tayside Univ Hospitals Natl Health Service Trust, Dundee, Scotland; et al)

J Allergy Clin Immunol 119:434-440, 2007

Background.—Filaggrin is a key protein involved in skin barrier function. Recently, mutations in the filaggrin gene, *FLG*, were identified in European families with ichthyosis vulgaris (IV) and shown to be an important predisposing factor for atopic dermatitis (AD).

Objective.—To study the role of *FLG* mutations in IV/AD in Japan.

Methods.—The known filaggrin mutations were studied by genotyping and new mutations identified by DNA sequencing.

Results.—The European-specific mutations R501X and 2282del4 were absent from 253 Japanese individuals. We therefore sequenced the *FLG* gene in 4 Japanese families with IV and identified 2 novel mutations, 3321delA and S2554X. Immunohistologic and ultrastructural observations indicated that both truncation mutations lead to a striking reduction of keratohyalin granules in the epidermis. We screened 143 Japanese patients with AD for these *FLG* null mutations and identified them in 8 patients with AD (5.6%), including S2554X in 6 patients (4.2%) and 3321delA in 2 patients (1.4%). Both null variants were absent from 156 unrelated Japanese nonatopic and nonichthyotic controls, giving a significant statistical association between the *FLG* mutations and AD ($\chi^2 P$ value, .0015). This is the first report of *FLG* mutations in a non-European population.

Conclusion.—Our data indicate that *FLG* mutations in Japan are unique from those found in European-origin populations.

Clinical Implications.—Filaggrin null variants are also significant predisposing factors for AD in Japan and, on the basis of the recent European studies, may predict a more severe and persistent form of atopy.

▶ The filaggrin gene (*FLG*) is located in the epidermal differentiation complex 1q21. Profilaggrin is the main protein component of keratohyalin granules. On terminal differentiation of keratinocytes, profilaggrin is dephosphorylated and cleaved into 10 to 12 essentially identical 37 kd filaggrin peptides that subsequently aggregate the keratin filament cytoskeleton, causing the collapse of the granular layer into flattened squames. The collapsed cytoskeleton is then cross-linked to form a barrier to the outside world. It has also been suggested that degradation products of filaggrin contribute to moisture retention in the cornified layers of the epidermis.[1]

In 2006, Smith et al[2] identified 2 null mutations, R501X and 2282del4, in the *FLG* in Scottish, Irish, and European American patients with ichthyosis vulgaris. Smith et al[2] estimated that approximately 10% of persons of European origin carry 1 of the 2 loss-of-function mutations in the *FLG*. Both of the above mutations lead to premature termination codons resulting in complete absence of processed filaggrin in the epidermis. Less common mutations located centrally in the filaggrin domain have been identified by Sandilands et al.[3] These mutations cause mild disease in heterozygotes and more severe disease in homozygotes. It is postulated that the compromised epidermal barrier that results from mutations in the *FLG* leads to increased passage of antigens, allergens, and chemicals into the skin, which, in turn, can provoke an immune response. In a report by Barker et al,[4] the investigators noted that 42% of the patients studied with childhood onset, adult persistent atopic dermatitis had 1 or more filaggrin null alleles, and Nomura et al described 2 novel mutations, 3321delA and S2554X, in the *FLG* in Japanese patients. Additional mutations in the *FLG* will almost certainly be discovered in the future.

These studies document a genetic link to the formation of an ineffective epidermal barrier. Clinically, it has been noted that liberally applied moisturizers, which improve barrier function, are often of benefit. Topical agents designed to specifically improve barrier function will likely continue to be developed in the future. We now have scientific evidence to share with patients and parents of patients with atopic dermatitis indicating that the skin barrier function abnormality is the primary problem of many if not most patients with atopic dermatitis. This differs from the belief (and hope) of many patients that some specific antigen can be found and eliminated to cure their disease. Emphasizing this might encourage patients to be more compliant with their use of topical medication and moisturizers.

S. Raimer, MD

References

1. Rawlings AV, Harding CR. Moisturization and skin barrier function. *Dermatol Ther*. 2004;17:43-48.
2. Smith FJD, Irvine AD, Terron-Kwiatkowski A, et al. Common loss-of-function mutations in the gene encoding filaggrin cause ichthyosis vulgaris. *Nat Genet*. 2006;38:337-342.
3. Sandilands A, O'Regan GM, Liao H, et al. Prevalent and rare mutations in the gene encoding filaggrin cause ichthyosis vulgaris and predispose individuals to atopic dermatitis. *J Invest Dermatol*. 2006;126:1770-1775.
4. Barker JNWN, Palmer CNA, Zhao Y, et al. Null mutations in the filaggrin gene (*FLG*) determine major susceptibility to early-onset atopic dermatitis that persists into adulthood. *J Invest Dermatol*. 2007;127:564-567.

Lifetime prevalence of self-reported atopic diseases in a population-based sample of elderly subjects: results of the ESTHER study
Wolkewitz M, Rothenbacher D, Löw M, et al (Ruprecht-Karls-Univ Heidelberg, Germany; Saarland Ministry for Public Health, Saarbrücken, Germany)
Br J Dermatol 156:693-697, 2007

Background.—Prevalence studies of atopic diseases such as atopic dermatitis (AD), hay fever and allergic asthma have mostly been performed in children. Studies in the adult population are still rare.

Objectives.—We estimated the lifetime prevalence of different atopic diseases in an elderly population in Saarland, Germany. Additionally we investigated the association between atopic diseases and sociodemographic factors including age, gender, duration of school education (as a proxy measure of socioeconomic status), family history, and size of place of residence.

Methods.—This study was conducted between June 2000 and December 2002 in the State of Saarland, Germany. Participants aged 50–75 years (n = 9961) were recruited by their general practitioner in the context of a general health screening examination. All filled out a standardized questionnaire and reported whether a physician had ever diagnosed an atopic disease (hay fever, AD or asthma).

Results.—Overall, 9949 subjects (mean age 62 years, 45% men) were included in this analysis. The lifetime prevalence of reported AD, hay fever and asthma was 4.3%, 8.3% and 5.5%, respectively. Lifetime prevalence of AD and asthma among women, and lifetime prevalence of hay fever among both genders, strongly decreased with age. Duration of school education (≤ 9 years, 10–11 years, > 11 years) was strongly associated with AD (3.7%, 5.7%, 6.8%; P trend < 0.0001) and hay fever (7.2%, 11.2%, 12.8%; P trend < 0.0001), but only tentatively with asthma.

Conclusions.—The lifetime prevalence of AD is considerably lower in the elderly compared with the prevalence reported among younger adults in recent studies. Adults with a longer duration of school education appeared to have a higher risk for atopic diseases.

▶ Although the prevalence of atopic diseases in children and adolescents has steadily increased, only a few studies have examined their prevalence in adults. Previous investigations seem to indicate a strong and consistent association of socioeconomic status and atopy. Wolkewitz et al sought to estimate the lifetime prevalence of atopic diseases in adults aged 50 to 74 years and to investigate the relationship between atopic diseases and sociodemographic factors in these individuals. They found that the incidence of such diseases was considerably lower in older compared with younger subjects and that the prevalence of atopic disease and hay fever decreased with increasing age. They also concluded that the duration of school education was a useful marker for various lifestyle and environmental factors that affect the risk for various atopic diseases, especially AD and hay fever.

B. H. Thiers, MD

Early allergen exposure and atopic eczema
Harris JM, Williams HC, White C, et al (Imperial College School of Medicine, London; Univ of Nottingham, England)
Br J Dermatol 156:698-704, 2007

Background.—The relationship between exposure to indoor aeroallergens in early life and subsequent eczema is unclear. We have previously failed to show any significant associations between early life exposure to house dust mite and cat fur allergens and either sensitization to these allergens or wheeze. We have also previously reported a *lower* prevalence of parent reported, doctor-diagnosed eczema by age 2 years for children exposed to higher concentrations of house dust mite, but no other associations with other definitions of eczema or for exposure to cat allergen.

Objectives.—To extend the exposure–response analysis of allergen exposure and eczema outcomes measured up to age 8 years, and to investigate the role of other genetic and environmental determinants.

Methods.—A total of 593 children (92.4% of those eligible) born to all newly pregnant women attending one of three general practitioner surgeries in Ashford, Kent, were followed from birth to age 8 years. Concentrations of house dust mite and cat allergen were measured in dust samples collected from the home at 8 weeks after birth. The risk of subsequent eczema as defined by the U.K. diagnostic criteria was determined according to different levels (quintiles) of allergen exposure at birth.

Results.—By age 8 years, 150 (25.3%) children had met the diagnostic criteria for eczema at least once. Visible flexural dermatitis was recorded at least once for 129 (28.0%). As in other studies, parental allergic history was positively associated with most eczema outcomes, as were higher maternal education and less crowded homes. No clear linear associations between early exposure to house dust mite or cat allergen were found, regardless of the definition of eczema used. The risk of eczema appeared to increase for the three lowest quintiles of house dust mite allergen exposure (odds ratio, OR 1.37 for third quintile compared with first), and then to fall for the two highest quintiles (OR 0.66 and 0.71) even after controlling for confounding factors.

Conclusions.—The lack of any clear exposure–disease relationship between allergens in early life and subsequent eczema argues against allergen exposure being a major factor causing eczema. If the lower levels of eczema at higher levels of house dust mite are confirmed, then interventions aimed at reducing house dust mite in early infancy could paradoxically increase the risk of subsequent eczema.

▶ This is a carefully conducted study with a good retention rate. Harris et al found no clear-cut evidence of a relationship between exposure to antigens early in life and subsequent development of eczema. Interestingly, there was a tendency for children exposed to the highest level of dust mites to have the least chance of developing eczema. The results of this study would argue against trying to use mattress covers and other methods to prevent exposure of young children to dust mites in an effort to prevent atopic dermatitis.

S. Raimer, MD

Stealth monitoring of adherence to topical medication: Adherence is very poor in children with atopic dermatitis

Krejci-Manwaring J, Tusa MG, Carroll C, et al (Wake Forest Univ School of Medicine, Winston-Salem, NC; Ohio State Univ School of Medicine and Public Health, Columbus)

J Am Acad Dermatol 56:211-216, 2007

Background.—Atopic dermatitis is a common problem for which topical agents are the primary treatment. When topical medications fail, further therapy may include systemic agents with the potential for greater toxicity. Adherence to topical treatment of atopic dermatitis has not been well characterized. Poor adherence to topical medication could account for failure of topical therapy.

Purpose.—To determine adherence to topical treatment in patients with atopic dermatitis.

Methods.—Thirty-seven children were given 0.1% triamcinolone ointment and were counseled to use it twice daily. They were told to return in 4 weeks, at which time they were told to continue treatment for another 4 weeks. Electronic monitors were used to measure adherence over the entire 8 week study. Patients were not informed of the compliance monitoring until the end of the study.

Results.—Twenty-six patients completed 8 weeks of treatment. Mean adherence from the baseline to the end of the study was 32%. Adherence was higher on or near office visit days and subsequently decreased rapidly.

Limitations.—This study was limited by the large number of subjects who failed to return for follow-up appointments or withdrew from the study.

Conclusions.—Adherence to topical medications is very poor in a clinic population of children with atopic dermatitis. Office visits are one means to increase adherence. If adherence to topical treatment can be improved, exposure to more costly and potentially toxic systemic agents may be avoidable.

▶ This study is important in that it documented by the use of electronic monitors that adherence to prescribed topical treatments is poor in children with atopic dermatitis. Poor adherence is therefore a more likely explanation for treatment failure than lack of effectiveness of any specific preparation. Because compliance improves near the time of an office visit, asking patients to return for an initial follow-up visit approximately 1 week after initiation of treatment is recommended. Most patients (or parents) will be reasonably compliant with treatment for 1 week. If definite improvement can be seen in a child's condition, then patients may be more likely to use topical medication appropriately when treatment for atopic dermatitis is needed.

S. Raimer, MD

Low basal serum cortisol in patients with severe atopic dermatitis: potent topical corticosteroids wrongfully accused

Haeck IM, Timmer-de Mik L, Lentjes EGWM, et al (Univ Med Centre Utrecht, The Netherlands)
Br J Dermatol 156:979-985, 2007

Background.—Topical corticosteroids are used extensively to treat inflammatory skin disorders including atopic dermatitis (AD). Several studies have described temporary reversible suppression of hypothalamic–pituitary–adrenal function. However, sound evidence of permanent disturbance of adrenal gland function is lacking.

Objectives.—To relate basal cortisol levels to prior use of topical corticosteroids and disease activity in patients with moderate to severe AD and to investigate the effect on basal serum cortisol levels of topical corticosteroid treatment during hospitalization.

Methods.—Two groups of patients with AD were evaluated: 25 inpatients with severe AD who required hospitalization (group 1) and 28 outpatients with moderate to severe AD (group 2). In group 1, morning basal serum cortisol levels were measured twice, at admission and at discharge; in group 2, morning basal serum cortisol levels were measured once. Use of topical corticosteroids in the 3 months prior to the cortisol measurement was recorded and disease activity was monitored using the Six Area, Six Sign Atopic Dermatitis (SASSAD) score and serum thymus and activation-regulated chemokine (TARC) levels.

Results.—On admission, basal cortisol levels in group 1 were significantly ($P < 0.001$) decreased in 80% of the patients. In group 2, the basal cortisol levels were normal in all but three patients. Comparing the two groups, group 1 on admission had a significantly lower cortisol level than that of group 2 ($P < 0.001$). Disease activity in group 1 on admission was significantly higher than that of group 2 ($P < 0.001$). There was no difference in use of topical corticosteroids in the 3 months before cortisol measurement. At discharge in group 1 there was a significant increase ($P < 0.0001$) of basal cortisol levels and a significant ($P < 0.001$) decrease in disease activity reflected by the decrease in serum TARC levels and SASSAD score.

Conclusions.—Disease activity, rather than the use of topical corticosteroids, is responsible for the low basal cortisol values in patients with severe AD.

▶ Dermatologists have significant concern about percutaneous absorption when topical steroids are applied to large body surface areas. The problem is potentially greatest in children, especially when the topical preparations are applied to inflamed skin where absorption may be increased because of the compromised epidermal barrier. Haeck et al investigated basal serum cortisol levels in adult patients with moderate-to-severe AD and attempted to correlate their findings with the total amount of topical corticosteroid used and to disease activity during the previous 3 months. They also investigated the effect of intensive topical corticosteroid treatment on basal serum cortisol levels and disease activity in hospitalized patients with severe AD. The investigators demonstrated that low basal serum cortisol levels were not caused by prior use of potent topical corticosteroids in patients with moderate-to-severe skin disease. No significant correlation was found between the amount of corticosteroids applied and basal serum cortisol values. Although inpatients with active disease had significantly lower basal serum cortisol levels than did outpatients with controlled disease, there was no significant difference in topical corticosteroid use in the 2 groups. Interestingly, the basal serum cortisol levels in inpatients increased dramatically during intensive treatment with large amounts of potent topical corticosteroid preparations. The authors concluded that treatment with potent topical corticosteroids does not suppress function of the HPA access.

B. H. Thiers, MD

Targeting calcineurin activation as a therapeutic strategy for T-cell acute lymphoblastic leukemia
Medyouf H, Alcalde H, Berthier C, et al (Institut Curie, Orsay, France; Université Paris VII)
Nature Med 13:736-741, 2007

Calcineurin is a calcium-activated serine/threonine phosphatase critical to a number of developmental processes in the cardiovascular, nervous and immune systems. In the T-cell lineage, calcineurin activation is important for pre–T-cell receptor (TCR) signaling, TCR-mediated positive selection of thymocytes into mature T cells, and many aspects of the immune response. The critical role of calcineurin in the immune response is underscored by the fact that calcineurin inhibitors, such as cyclosporin A (CsA) and FK506, are powerful immunosuppressants in wide clinical use. We observed sustained calcineurin activation in human B- and T-cell lymphomas and in all mouse models of lymphoid malignancies analyzed. In intracellular NOTCH1 (ICN1)- and TEL-JAK2–induced T-cell lymphoblastic leukemia, two mouse models relevant to human malignancies, *in vivo* inhibition of calcineurin activity by CsA or FK506 induced apoptosis of leukemic cells and rapid tumor clearance, and substantially prolonged mouse survival. In contrast, ectopic expression of a constitutively activated mutant of calcineurin favored leukemia progression. Moreover, CsA treatment induced apoptosis in human lymphoma and leukemia cell lines. Thus, calcineurin activation is critical for the maintenance of the leukemic phenotype *in vivo*, identifying this pathway as a relevant therapeutic target in lymphoid malignancies.

▶ What a surprise! Much of the negative publicity surrounding the topical calcineurin inhibitors involves their alleged association with lymphoma. Medyouf and colleagues present data that suggest a role for calcineurin inhibition for the treatment of lymphoid malignancy; this would seem to imply that calcineurin inhibition provides a protective rather than a permissive effect with regard to the development of lymphoproliferative disorders. Medyouf et al even sug gest clinical trials that combine calcineurin inhibitors with currently available chemotherapy regimens for patients with those leukemia and lymphoma subtypes that demonstrate calcineurin activation. The feasibility of manipulating the calcineurin signaling pathway was discussed in an accompanying article.[1] The data presented in an article by Arellano and colleagues[2] show no increased risk of lymphoma in patients with atopic dermatitis who are treated with topical calcineurin inhibitors; this seems to indicate that the severity of the skin disease may be the main factor associated with the perceived risk of lymphoma. Arellano et al suggest studies to evaluate the relative influence of the severity of atopic dermatitis, the use of high-potency topical steroids, and the use of corticosteroids in general on the development of lymphoma in patients with atopic dermatitis.

B. H. Thiers, MD

References

1. Müeller MR, Rao A. Linking calcineurin activity to leukemogenesis. *Nat Med.* 2007;13:669-671.
2. Arellano FM, Wentworth CE, Arana A, Fernández C, Paul CF. Risk of lymphoma following exposure to calcineurin inhibitors and topical steroids in patients with atopic dermatitis. *J Invest Dermatol.* 2007;127:808-816.

Risk of Lymphoma Following Exposure to Calcineurin Inhibitors and Topical Steroids in Patients with Atopic Dermatitis
Arellano FM, Wentworth CE, Arana A, et al (Risk Management Resources, Bridgewater, NJ; UNSW, Sydney, Australia; Risk Management Resources–EU, Zaragoza, Spain; et al)
J Invest Dermatol 127:808-816, 2007

Systemic use of immunosuppressant agents increases the risk of lymphoma in transplantation. We performed a nested case-control study in the PharMetrics database to evaluate the association between topical immunosuppressants and lymphoma in a cohort of patients with atopic dermatitis. We identified cases of lymphoma and randomly selected four controls for each case, matched by length of follow-up. We used conditional logistic regression to calculate odds ratio (OR) and 95% confidence intervals (CIs) of the association between topical immunosuppressants and lymphoma. Two hundred and ninety-four cases of lymphoma occurred in 293,253 patients, 81 in patients younger than 20 years. The adjusted analysis yielded the following OR (95% CI) for: severity (OR 2.4; 95% CI 1.5–3.8), oral steroids 1.5 (1.0–2.4), "super potent" topical steroids 1.2 (0.8–1.8) , "low potency" topical steroids OR 1.1 (0.7–1.6); pimecrolimus 0.8 (0.4–1.6), tacrolimus OR 0.8 (0.4–1.7), and concomitant topical steroids, pimecrolimus, and tacrolimus 1.0 (0.3–4.1). We did not find an increased risk of lymphoma in patients treated with topical calcineurin inhibitors. It is difficult to disentangle the effects of severity of disease on outcome *versus* the true effects of drugs.

However, in the adjusted analysis, severity of AD was the main factor associated with an increased risk of lymphoma.

▶ What a surprise! Much of the negative publicity surrounding the topical calcineurin inhibitors involves their alleged association with lymphoma. In an article by Medyouf and colleagues,[1] data are presented that suggest a role for calcineurin inhibition for the treatment of lymphoid malignancy; this would seem to imply that calcineurin inhibition provides a protective rather than a permissive effect with regard to the development of lymphoproliferative disorders. Meydouf et al even suggest clinical trials that combine calcineurin inhibitors with currently available chemotherapy regimens for patients with those leukemia and lymphoma subtypes that demonstrate calcineurin activation. The feasibility of manipulating the calcineurin signaling pathway was discussed in an accompanying article.[2] The data presented by Arellano and colleagues show no increased risk of lymphoma in patients with atopic dermatitis who are treated with topical calcineurin inhibitors; this seems to indicate that the severity of the skin disease may be the main factor associated with the perceived risk of lymphoma. Arellano et al suggest studies to evaluate the relative influence of the severity of atopic dermatitis, the use of high-potency topical steroids, and the use of corticosteroids in general on the development of lymphoma in patients with atopic dermatitis.

B. H. Thiers, MD

References

1. Medyouf H, Alcalde H, Berthier C, et al. Targeting calcineurin activation as a therapeutic strategy for T-cell acute lymphoblastic leukaemia. *Nature Med.* 2007;13:736-741.
2. Müeller MR, Rao A. Linking calcineurin activity to leukemogenesis. *Nat Med.* 2007;13:669-671.

Topical Application with a New NF-κB Inhibitor Improves Atopic Dermatitis in NC/NgaTnd Mice

Tanaka A, Muto S, Jung K, et al (Tokyo Univ of Agriculture and Technology; Inst of Medicinal Molecular Design Inc, Tokyo)
J Invest Dermatol 127:855-863, 2007

Growing evidence has demonstrated the crucial role of NF-κB activation on disease severity in allergic disorders. In this study, we examined the clinical relevance of a novel NF-κB inhibitor, IMD-0354, for atopic dermatitis (AD) by its topical application. To investigate the *in vivo* efficacy, 1% IMD-0354 ointment was applied daily to NC/NgaTnd mice with severe dermatitis, which served as a model for human AD. During 2 weeks of treatment, scratching behavior decreased and severity of dermatitis reduced in mice treated with IMD-0354 as well as FK506 without diverse effects. Based on histological examinations, the hyperplasia of keratinocytes and infiltration of inflammatory cells were significantly reduced in the skin of IMD-0354-

treated mice. The expressions of T-helper 2 cytokines and tumor necrosis factor-α at the affected skin sites were downregulated in IMD-0354-treated mice. Furthermore, IMD-0354 suppressed the proliferation of various immunocompetent cells, neurite outgrowth of nerve growth factor-stimulated pheochromocytoma cells, IgE production from splenic B cells, and IgE-mediated activation of mast cells *in vitro*. IMD-0354 effectively reduced the allergic inflammation in NC/NgaTnd mice *in vivo*. Thus, a drug that interferes with NF-κB activity may provide an alternative therapeutic strategy for the treatment of AD.

▶ The activation of NF-κB enhances the production of inflammatory cytokines and chemokines, thereby suggesting that this transcription factor may represent a viable therapeutic target for inflammatory skin diseases. No direct evidence relates NF-κB to the pathogenesis of atopic dermatitis, although some reports have suggested that it may play a role in the underlying immunologic disturbance. Tanaka and colleagues demonstrate the activation of NF-κB in the skin of patients who are affected with atopic dermatitis, and they show that the topical application of an NF-κB inhibitor is effective for suppressing this transcription factor and for reducing the clinical symptoms of the disease. NF-κB may be an important molecular target for controlling atopic dermatitis, although human studies will obviously be required to confirm the therapeutic usefulness of any compound that interferes with its activity.

B. H. Thiers, MD

Systemic Treatment of Severe Atopic Eczema: A Systematic Review
Schmitt J, Schäkel K, Schmitt N, et al (Univ Hosp Carl Gustav Carus, Dresden, Germany; Technical Univ, Dresden, Germany)
Acta Derm Venereol 87:100-111, 2007

Systemic immunosuppressive agents are recommended for patients with atopic eczema in whom disease activity cannot be controlled adequately with topical treatments. Guidelines do not give clear advice on which agents to prefer. We systematically reviewed clinical trials on systemic treatment for severe atopic eczema to provide evidence-based treatment recommendations. Standardized literature search, independent standardized assessment of eligibility and data abstraction was performed by 2 reviewers. Twenty-seven studies totalling 979 patients were included. Eleven studies consistently showed effectiveness of cyclosporine. Cyclosporine is recommended as first option for patients with atopic eczema refractory to conventional treatment. Evidence from randomized controlled trials also exists for interferon-γ and azathioprine. Although frequently used in clinical practice, systemic glucocorticosteroids have not been assessed adequately in studies. Mycophenolate mofetile showed effectiveness in 2 small uncontrolled studies. Intravenous immunoglobulins and infliximab are not recommended based on published data.

▶ Schmitt et al found that current guidelines for the treatment of patients with atopic dermatitis do not always reflect published evidence, which endorses the use of systemic steroids, cyclosporine, methotrexate, or azathioprine for patients whose disease is resistant to topical therapy.[1] They also found that evidence for these treatments varies greatly in terms of quality, quantity, and results and that no algorithm exists for the preference of systemic treatments for the disease. They conclude by recommending that treatment guidelines for atopic dermatitis be updated.

B. H. Thiers, MD

Reference

1. Ellis C, Luger T, Abeck D, et al. International Consensus Conference on Atopic Dermatitis II (ICCAD II): clinical update and current treatment strategies. *Br J Dermatol.* 2003;148:3-10.

An open-label, dose-ranging study of methotrexate for moderate-to-severe adult atopic eczema

Weatherhead SC, Wahie S, Reynolds NJ, et al (Royal Victoria Infirmary, Newcastle upon Tyne, England)
Br J Dermatol 156:346-351, 2007

Background.—Treatment options for moderate-to-severe atopic eczema are limited. Although methotrexate (MTX) is a widely used and effective treatment for psoriasis, there have been no previous prospective trials of its use in refractory atopic eczema, despite a few small, retrospective reports suggesting that it is a well-tolerated and effective treatment.

Objectives.—We have assessed the safety and efficacy of oral MTX in 12 adults with moderate-to-severe atopic eczema in an open-label, dose-ranging, prospective trial using objective outcome measures.

Methods.—All patients had previously received other second-line therapies and had disease only partially responsive to potent topical steroids and emollients. During the 24-week MTX treatment period, unrestricted use of standard topical therapy was permitted. We used an incremental MTX dose regime, starting at 10 mg per week (following a 5-mg test dose) and increasing by 2.5 mg weekly until response was achieved or treatment was limited by toxicity. Disease activity [six area six sign atopic dermatitis (SASSAD) score] was assessed every 4 weeks during treatment and 12 weeks after stopping MTX. The primary endpoint was 24-week change in disease activity.

Results.—On average, disease activity improved by 52% from baseline (95% confidence interval 45–60%). There were significant improvements in quality of life, body surface area affected and loss of sleep and itch scores. Global response was rated as 'marked improvement' in five of 12 and six of 12 patients, by investigators and patients, respectively. In all patients, the majority of improvement in disease activity was seen by week 12, and, interestingly, patients who had not responded well over this period despite reaching a dose of 15 mg weekly failed to improve with further dose escalation.

Only one patient withdrew due to minor adverse effects. MTX was well tolerated by the remaining 11 patients, all of whom completed treatment, achieving a median dose of 15 mg weekly. Importantly, eight of nine patients had a persistent improvement 12 weeks after stopping MTX, with mean disease activity remaining 34% below baseline.

Conclusions.—We have shown that MTX is an effective, well-tolerated treatment for moderate-to-severe atopic eczema, and response appears to compare favourably with other second-line therapies. A randomized, controlled trial is now warranted.

▶ Topical corticosteroids are the mainstay of treatment for patients with atopic dermatitis. Other topical preparations such as the calcineurin inhibitors are more suited for maintenance therapy and have made an uncertain impact on the control of more severe or acute disease. But what is the most prudent course of action for the patient with severe or extensive disease who did not respond to conservative measures? This is a question faced regularly by many of us who work in tertiary care facilities and indeed by many of our brethren in private practice. UV light therapy is often recommended, with narrow-band UVB treatment being much less cumbersome, apparently safer, and just as effective as photochemotherapy. However, to many of our patients, the inconvenience of visiting a physician's office or hospital facility for treatment is a significant compliance barrier. The next step in the therapeutic ladder is often system immunosuppressive therapy. A variety of agents have been proposed, including azathioprine, methotrexate, mycophenolate mofetil, and cyclosporine. Which of these is the "best" in terms of safety and efficacy will be impossible to determine barring the unlikely commissioning of a large-scale randomized, double-blind trial featuring a head-to-head comparison of these drugs. Physicians using these drugs should clearly be well-schooled in their potential side effects and the need for appropriate monitoring.

B. H. Thiers, MD

Mycophenolate mofetil for severe childhood atopic dermatitis: experience in 14 patients

Heller M, Shin HT, Orlow SJ, et al (New York Univ; Hackensack Univ, NJ)
Br J Dermatol 157:127-132, 2007

Background.—Reports of successful treatment of atopic dermatitis (AD) with mycophenolate mofetil (MMF) have thus far been limited to adults. Considering that the condition typically develops during childhood and is most active during this period, MMF would represent a valuable addition to the therapeutic armamentarium for paediatric AD.

Objectives.—To evaluate the safety and efficacy of MMF in the treatment of severe childhood AD.

Methods.—A retrospective analysis was performed of all children treated with MMF as systemic monotherapy for severe, recalcitrant AD between

August 2003 and August 2006 at New York University Medical Center. Fourteen patients meeting these criteria were identified.

Results.—Four patients (29%) achieved complete clearance, four (29%) had > 90% improvement (almost complete), five (35%) had 60–90% improvement and one (7%) failed to respond. Initial responses occurred within 8 weeks (mean 4 weeks), and maximal effects were attained after 8–12 weeks (mean 9 weeks) at MMF doses of 40–50 mg kg^{-1} daily in younger children and 30–40 mg kg^{-1} daily in adolescents. The medication was well tolerated in all patients, with no infectious complications or development of leucopenia, anaemia, thrombocytopenia or elevated aminotransferases.

Conclusions.—This retrospective case series demonstrates that MMF can be a safe and effective treatment for severe, refractory AD in children. MMF represents a promising therapeutic alternative to traditional systemic immunosuppressive agents with less favourable side-effect profiles, and prospective controlled studies are warranted, further to assess its benefits in paediatric AD.

▶ This retrospective analysis of 14 children with severe recalcitrant atopic dermatitis treated with MMF at New York University Medical Center between 2003 and 2006 showed very good results. The dosage recommended by the authors is 1200 mg/m^2 or 40-50 mg/kg for younger children (who have a faster hepatic metabolism of the drug) and 30-40 mg/kg for older children and adolescents. The immunomodulary effects of MMF result from the inhibition of the inosine monophosphate dehydrogenase enzyme. This blocks the de nova pathway of purine synthesis, preferentially inhibiting the proliferation of B and T lymphocytes, which lack a purine salvage pathway and therefore depend on de novo synthesis. Because lymphocytes are the primary target of MMF, unwanted effects on other cell types are minimized. Therefore, MMF appears to be a safer drug than many other immunosuppressive agents and might be considered for treatment of severe atopic dermatitis unresponsive to topical therapy. The cost of the drug may be prohibitive for some patients.

S. Raimer, MD

Clinical and immunopathologic findings during treatment of recalcitrant atopic eczema with efalizumab
Hassan AS, Kaelin U, Braathen LR, et al (Univ of Bern, Switzerland)
J Am Acad Dermatol 56:217-221, 2007

Background.—Atopic eczema is seen most commonly in infants and children but can persist or develop in adulthood. In addition to the most typical eczematous flexural lesions, patients may have a nonflexural distribution and other morphologic variants such as the nummular or prurigo-like patterns. Systemic therapy may be needed to treat widespread moderate-to-severe atopic eczema, but such therapy can be associated with serious side effects. Efalizumab is a recombinant humanized monoclonal IgG$_1$antibody that blocks multiple T cell–dependent functions. The clinical response of re

C

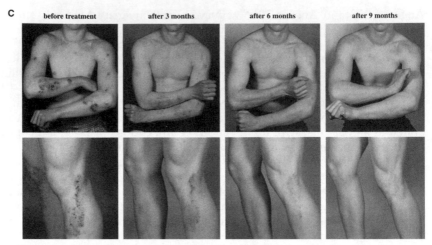

FIGURE 1C.—Eczematous skin lesions including discoid pattern over trunk and extremities before treatment and after 3, 6, and 9 months of efalizumab monotherapy. (Courtesy of Hassan AS, Kaelin U, Braathen LR, et al. Clinical and immunopathologic findings during treatment of recalcitrant atopic eczema with efalizumab. *J Am Acad Dermatol.* 2007;56:217-221. Copyright Elsevier, 2007.)

calcitrant atopic eczema (AE) with efalizumab was assessed, and the inflammatory infiltrate during treatment was characterized.

Case Report.—Man, 19, with a flare up of his AE was admitted to hospital for additional evaluation. The patient had experienced AE since childhood and when seen had numerous itchy, erythematous and partly oozing, impetiginized, eczematous lesions on the head, neck, trunk, and flexural and extensor surfaces of the upper and lower extremities. He had previously been treated with topical corticosteroids, calcineurin inhibitors, and phototherapy, with poor improvement of his condition. Two 5-mm punch biopsy specimens were obtained from eczematous skin lesions on the thigh before treatment was initiated with efalizumab. Another biopsy specimen was obtained after 6 months of treatment from slightly erythematous infiltrated skin adjacent to the previous biopsy site. Routine histopathologic examination and immunohistochemical analyses were performed.

Results.—A significant clinical improvement was observed after 3, 6, and 9 months of efalizumab therapy (Fig 1C). At last report, the patient was in the 11th month of therapy and had not received any other treatment modality, other than an emollient, for 10 months. The patient was highly satisfied with the efalizumab therapy, particularly, because no flare-ups occurred, even during the winter months.

Conclusions.—Efalizumab monotherapy may result in a significant reduction of the inflammatory cellular infiltrate in skin lesions of AE.

Efalizumab could be a valuable therapeutic option in the management of severe recalcitrant forms of AE.

▶ Although Hassan et al reported impressive results in a single case (Fig 1C), a small series reported by Takiguchi et al[1] showed mixed results. Clearly, this treatment shows promise but, as conceded by Takiguchi et al, a larger scale, randomized, double-blind, placebo-controlled trial will be needed to accurately assess the place of efalizumab therapy in the care of patients with severe AD. As is the case with psoriasis, the larger societal question to be addressed is what degree of clinical response and what safety profile should be required to justify the use of this costly drug versus older, admittedly imperfect and occasionally hazardous therapies.

B. H. Thiers, MD

Reference

1. Takiguchi R, Tofte S, Simpson B, et al. Efalizumab for severe atopic dermatitis: a pilot study in adults. *J Am Acad Dermatol.* 2007;56:222-227.

Efalizumab for severe atopic dermatitis: A pilot study in adults
Takiguchi R, Tofte S, Simpson B, et al (Oregon Health & Science Univ, Portland)
J Am Acad Dermatol 56:222-227, 2007

Background.—Severe atopic dermatitis (AD) often cannot be adequately controlled with topical agents. The continuous use of current systemic therapies for AD is limited by end-organ toxicities. A safe and effective systemic therapy for patients with recalcitrant AD is greatly needed.

Objective.—To evaluate the potential safety and efficacy of efalizumab, an inhibitor of T cell activation and migration, in adults with severe AD.

Methods.—An investigator-initiated, prospective, open-label, pilot study was conducted involving ten subjects with severe AD. Subjects received an initial conditioning subcutaneous dose of efalizumab of 0.7 mg/kg followed by 1.0 mg/kg weekly for another 11 weeks for a total of 12 doses. The primary efficacy outcome was the change in the mean Eczema Area and Severity Index (EASI) score from baseline as measured at week 12. Monitoring of adverse events continued for 8 weeks after discontinuation of therapy.

Results.—EASI scores improved from a mean baseline score of 37.1 ± 13.5 to 17.6 ± 14.5 at week 12 (52.3% improvement; $P < .0001$). Six out of ten subjects reached at least a 50% improvement in EASI score by week 12. Pruritus levels decreased from 6.9 cm ± 1.8 cm to 4.9 cm ± 2.5 cm utilizing a visual analogue score ($P < .015$). Overall, efalizumab was well tolerated. There were three significant adverse events during the course of this study, including thrombocytopenia, viral gastroenteritis, and a subject with worsening of disease beyond baseline levels after drug discontinuation.

Limitations.—It is difficult to apply these findings to larger populations of patients with AD because this study lacked a control group and involved a small number of subjects with very severe disease. Long-term efficacy and safety of efalizumab in this population is not known.

Conclusions.—Efalizumab therapy resulted in significant clinical improvements in six of ten subjects with severe AD. Efalizumab may serve as a good alternative to current systemic immunosuppressants used for AD; however, double-blind placebo-controlled studies are needed to test its efficacy and safety.

▶ Although Hassan et al[1] reported impressive results in a single case, the small series reported by Takiguchi et al showed mixed results. Clearly, this treatment shows promise but, as conceded by Takiguchi et al, a larger scale, randomized, double-blind, placebo-controlled trial will be needed to accurately assess the place of efalizumab therapy in the care of patients with severe AD. As is the case with psoriasis, the larger societal question to be addressed is what degree of clinical response and what safety profile should be required to justify the use of this costly drug versus older, admittedly imperfect and occasionally hazardous therapies.

B. H. Thiers, MD

Reference

1. Hassan AS, Kaelin U, Braathen LR, Yawalkar N. Clinical and immunopathologic findings during treatment of recalcitrant atopic eczema with efalizumab. *J Am Acad Dermatol.* 2007;56:217-221.

Dominant-negative mutations in the DNA-binding domain of STAT3 cause hyper-IgE syndrome
Minegishi Y, Saito M, Tsuchiya S, et al (Tokyo Med and Dental Univ; Tokyo Univ, Sendai, Japan; Fujita Health Univ, Aichi, Japan; et al)
Nature 448:1058-1062, 2007

Hyper-immunoglobulin E syndrome (HIES) is a compound primary immunodeficiency characterized by a highly elevated serum IgE, recurrent staphylococcal skin abscesses and cyst-forming pneumonia, with disproportionately milder inflammatory responses, referred to as cold abscesses, and skeletal abnormalities. Although some cases of familial HIES with autosomal dominant or recessive inheritance have been reported, most cases of HIES are sporadic, and their pathogenesis has remained mysterious for a long time. Here we show that dominant-negative mutations in the human signal transducer and activator of transcription 3 (*STAT3*) gene result in the classical multisystem HIES. We found that eight out of fifteen unrelated nonfamilial HIES patients had heterozygous *STAT3* mutations, but their parents and siblings did not have the mutant *STAT3* alleles, suggesting that these were *de novo* mutations. Five different mutations were found, all of which were located in the STAT3 DNA-binding domain. The patients' peripheral blood cells showed defective responses to cytokines, including interleukin (IL)-6 and IL-10, and the DNA-binding ability of STAT3 in these cells was greatly diminished. All five mutants were non-functional by themselves and showed dominant-negative effects when co-expressed with wild-type *STAT3*. These results highlight the multiple roles played by STAT3 in humans, and underline the critical involvement of multiple cytokine pathways in the pathogenesis of HIES.

▶ The JAK-STAT pathways mediate intracellular signaling by a wide variety of external stimuli. The specificity of the response is determined in large part by the binding of the individual activated STAT proteins to selective DNA sequences in the target gene promoter regions. Of the 7 human STAT proteins, STAT3 is particularly interesting in that it mediates the signaling of numerous cytokines and growth factors, including those of the IL-6 and interferon families; furthermore, in mice, *STAT3* gene deletion is incompatible with life.

In this study by Minegishi et al and in a study by Holland et al,[1] both groups of investigators elected to explore the role of *STAT3* in the hyper-IgE syndrome, a multisystem disorder in which they detected impaired responses to IL-6. This syndrome, which occurs in both inherited and sporadic forms, is characterized by increased IgE levels, eczema, superficial and pulmonary bacterial infections, and skeletal abnormalities.

In this study by Minegishi et al, the investigators examined STAT3 DNA sequences of 15 unrelated patients with sporadic hyper-IgE syndrome, and found 5 different heterozygous mutations within the DNA-binding domain in 8 of these subjects. These mutations were not found in the other 7 patients, any of the family members tested, or in 1000 unrelated control subjects. Further investigation revealed that the protein product of the mutant gene was nonfunctional alone, but that residual STAT3 DNA binding did occur in the patients' cells upon activation with interferon-γ, albeit at a much reduced level.

In the study by Holland et al,[1] the authors investigated STAT3 DNA sequences in a larger group of patients including those of sporadic and familial origin, and their family members where possible. These investigators identified 18 *STAT3* mutations in 50 patients and demonstrated autosomal dominant transmission of the mutation in 17 of these. Interestingly, in this study, mutations in both the DNA-binding and SH2 domains were found, but were dispersed between the familial and sporadic forms of disease.

The results presented in these studies are particularly compelling because they offer a rational explanation for many of the clinical features of the hyper-IgE syndrome. For example, impaired function of *STAT3* in bone physiology could account for the skeletal abnormalities found in this disease, and impairment of IL-10 function (within the IFN family) would be expected to lead to immune dysregulation. These data certainly further our understanding of the role of the JAK-STAT pathways in health and disease.

G. M. P. Galbraith, MD

Reference

1. Holland SM, DeLeo FR, Elloumi HZ, et al. *STAT3* mutations in the hyper-IgE syndrome. *N Engl J Med*. 2007;357:1-5.

STAT3 Mutations in the Hyper-IgE Syndrome

Holland SM, DeLeo FR, Elloumi HZ, et al (Natl Inst Allergy and Infectious Diseases, Bethesda, Md and Hamilton, Mont; Natl Human Genome Research Inst, Bethesda, Md; Natl Cancer Inst, Bethesda, Md; et al)
N Engl J Med 357:1-5, 2007

Background.—The hyper-IgE syndrome (or Job's syndrome) is a rare disorder of immunity and connective tissue characterized by dermatitis, boils, cyst-forming pneumonias, elevated serum IgE levels, retained primary dentition, and bone abnormalities. Inheritance is autosomal dominant; sporadic cases are also found.

Methods.—We collected longitudinal clinical data on patients with the hyper-IgE syndrome and their families and assayed the levels of cytokines secreted by stimulated leukocytes and the gene expression in resting and stimulated cells. These data implicated the signal transducer and activator of transcription 3 gene (*STAT3*) as a candidate gene, which we then sequenced.

Results.—We found increased levels of proinflammatory gene transcripts in unstimulated peripheral-blood neutrophils and mononuclear cells from patients with the hyper-IgE syndrome, as compared with levels in control cells. In vitro cultures of mononuclear cells from patients that were stimulated with lipopolysaccharide, with or without interferon-γ, had higher tumor necrosis factor α levels than did identically treated cells from unaffected persons (P=0.003). In contrast, the cells from patients with the hyper-IgE syndrome generated lower levels of monocyte chemoattractant protein 1 in response to the presence of interleukin-6 (P=0.03), suggesting a defect in interleukin-6 signaling through its downstream mediators, one of which is STAT3. We identified missense mutations and single-codon in-frame deletions in *STAT3* in 50 familial and sporadic cases of the hyper-IgE syndrome. Eighteen discrete mutations, five of which were hot spots, were predicted to directly affect the DNA-binding and SRC homology 2 (SH2) domains.

Conclusions.—Mutations in *STAT3* underlie sporadic and dominant forms of the hyper-IgE syndrome, an immunodeficiency syndrome involving increased innate immune response, recurrent infections, and complex somatic features.

▶ The JAK-STAT pathways mediate intracellular signaling by a wide variety of external stimuli. The specificity of the response is determined in large part by the binding of the individual activated STAT proteins to selective DNA sequences in the target gene promoter regions. Of the 7 human STAT proteins, STAT3 is particularly interesting in that it mediates the signaling of numerous cytokines and growth factors, including those of the IL-6 and interferon families; furthermore, in mice, *STAT3* gene deletion is incompatible with life.

In this study by Holland et al and in a study by Minegishi et al,[1] both groups of investigators elected to explore the role of STAT3 in the hyper-IgE syndrome, a multisystem disorder in which they detected impaired responses to IL-6. This syndrome, which occurs in both inherited and sporadic forms, is characterized by increased IgE levels, eczema, superficial and pulmonary bacterial infections, and skeletal abnormalities.

In the study by Minegishi et al,[1] the investigators examined STAT3 DNA sequences of 15 unrelated patients with sporadic hyper-IgE syndrome, and 5 different heterozygous mutations within the DNA-binding domain in 8 of these subjects. These mutations were not found in the other 7 patients, any of the family members tested, or in 1000 unrelated control subjects. Further investigation revealed that the protein product of the mutant gene was nonfunctional alone, but that residual STAT3 DNA binding did occur in the patients' cells upon activation with interferon-γ, albeit at a much reduced level.

In this study, Holland et al investigated STAT3 DNA sequences in a larger group of patients including those of sporadic and familial origin, and their family members where possible. These investigators identified 18 *STAT3* mutations in 50 patients, and demonstrated autosomal dominant transmission of the mutation in 17 of these. Interestingly, in this study, mutations in both the DNA-binding and SH2 domains were found, but were dispersed between the familial and sporadic forms of disease.

The results presented in these studies are particularly compelling because they offer a rational explanation for many of the clinical features of the hyper-IgE syndrome. For example, impaired function of *STAT3* in bone physiology could account for the skeletal abnormalities found in this disease, and impairment of IL-10 function (within the IFN family) would be expected to lead to immune dysregulation. These data certainly further our understanding of the role of the JAK-STAT pathways in health and disease.

G. M. P. Galbraith, MD

Reference

1. Minegishi Y, Saito M, Tsuchiya S, et al. Dominant-negative mutations in the DNA-binding domain of STAT3 cause hyper-IgE syndrome. *Nature.* 2007;448: 1058-1062.

Causes of death in hyper-IgE syndrome
Freeman AF, Kleiner DE, Nadiminti H, et al (NIH, Bethesda, Md; Univ of California, San Francisco)
J Allergy Clin Immunol 119:1234-1240, 2007

Background.—Hyper-IgE syndrome (HIES) is characterized by recurrent pyogenic infections, eczema, increased serum IgE levels, and a variety of connective tissue and skeletal system abnormalities. Little has been published regarding the causes of death in these patients or pathologic findings.

Objective.—To identify the cause of death in patients with HIES and to describe pathologic findings in fatal HIES.

Methods.—We reviewed the medical records and autopsy slides of 6 patients with HIES with autopsies performed at our institution.

Results.—All 6 patients with HIES were women and ranged in age from 24 to 40 years. All patients had a history of cystic lung disease and had pneumonia at the time of death, with *Pseudomonas aeruginosa* and fungal organisms predominating. Pulmonary fungal vascular invasion with fatal hemorrhage was observed in 3 patients, and metastatic fungal disease to the brain was observed in 2 patients caused by *Aspergillus fumigatus* and *Scedosporium prolificans*. Four patients had evidence of renal tubular injury, which was likely from amphotericin B toxicity; 3 patients had glomerulosclerosis; and 1 patient had 2 kidney angiomyolipomas.

Conclusions.—Our series highlights the important role *Pseudomonas* and *Aspergillus* species play in patients with HIES with cystic lung disease. Intensified antifungal and gram-negative bacterial prophylaxis need evaluation as possible strategies to prevent these infectious complications in patients with cystic lung disease.

Clinical Implications.—Fungal and *Pseudomonas* infection of cystic lung disease in HIES may be life threatening, and the proper management and prevention of these infections need continued investigation.

▶ In patients with hyper-IgE syndrome, pulmonary insufficiency often develops after many years of recurrent bouts of pneumonia. In this autopsy series presented by Freeman and colleagues, all patients died directly or indirectly of lung infection. The authors stress the importance of antistaphylococcal prophylaxis for preventing boils and pneumonia early during the course of hyper-IgE syndrome, and they raise the possibility of aggressive antifungal and gram-negative prophylaxis in adults with the condition.

B. H. Thiers, MD

Incidence of hand eczema in a population-based twin cohort: genetic and environmental risk factors
Lerbaek A, Kyvik KO, Ravn H, et al (Univ of Copenhagen; Univ of Southern Denmark, Odense; Statens Serum Institut, Copenhagen)
Br J Dermatol 157:552-557, 2007

Background.—Population-based studies on the incidence of hand eczema are sparse.

Objectives.—The aim of this prospective follow-up study was to determine the incidence rate of hand eczema in a population-based twin cohort. Secondly, the role of genetic factors and other potential risk factors for hand eczema was investigated.

Methods.—A questionnaire on self-reported hand eczema was answered by 5610 and 4128 twin individuals in 1996 and 2005, respectively. Data were analysed in a Poisson regression analysis.

Results.—The crude incidence rate was 8.8 cases per 1000 person-years (95% confidence interval, [CI] 7.7–9.9). Incidence rate ratios (IRRs) dependent on the co-twin's hand eczema status revealed a significant, doubled risk for monozygotic twin individuals with a co-twin affected by hand eczema, compared with dizygotic twin individuals with a co-twin affected by hand eczema (IRR 2.4, 95% CI 1.4–4.1). Also, significantly increased IRRs were found for positive patch test, atopic dermatitis, and wet work.

Conclusions.—Hand eczema is still a frequent disease and genetic factors are confirmed important risk factors. Positive patch test, atopic dermatitis and wet work were associated with an increased risk, whereas no association with age, sex, smoking or alcohol was found.

▶ The data presented by Lerbaek et al show that genetic factors are important risk factors for hand eczema, whereas sex or age do not influence the risk. They also found an association between an increased risk of hand eczema and positive patch test results, atopic dermatitis, and wet work. Smoking and alcohol were not significant risk factors. The authors warn that their results should be interpreted with caution, as their data were collected after the development of hand eczema and may be biased.

B. H. Thiers, MD

High frequency of contact allergy to gold in patients with endovascular coronary stents
Ekqvist S, Svedman C, Möller H, et al (Lund Univ, Malmö, Sweden; Blekinge Hosp, Karlskrona, Sweden; Lund Univ Hosp, Sweden)
Br J Dermatol 157:730-738, 2007

Background.—Stent implantation is an effective method for treatment of atherosclerotic disease. Factors predisposing to in-stent restenosis are still largely unknown. Contact allergy to metal ions eluted from the stent has been suggested to be a risk factor.

Objectives.—To explore whether there is a possible induction of contact allergy to metals used in stents among patients with a stainless steel stent containing nickel (Ni stent) and patients with a gold-plated stent (Au stent).

Methods.—Adults ($n = 484$) treated with coronary stent implantation participated in the study with patch testing. The study design was retrospective and cross-sectional with no assessment of contact allergy before stenting. Age- and sex-matched patch-tested patients with dermatitis ($n = 447$) served as controls.

Results.—Of Au-stented patients, 54 of 146 (37%) were allergic to gold compared with 85 of 447 (19%) controls ($P < 0.001$). Within the stented population there were no statistically significant differences in contact allergy to gold or nickel between Ni-stented and Au-stented patients. In multivariate models where other risk factors for contact allergy to gold were considered, the Au stent showed a trend towards statistical significance (odds ratio 1.43, 95% confidence interval 0.95–2.16; P = 0.09).

Conclusions.—As the frequency of contact allergy to gold is higher in stented patients independent of stent type it suggests a previous sensitization. However, several pieces of circumstantial evidence as well as statistical analysis indicate the possibility of sensitization in the coronary vessel by the

Au stent. Ni stents and Au stents should not be ruled out as risk factors for induction of contact allergy to these metals.

▶ Ekqvist et al noted that the frequency of contact allergy to gold is increased in patients with endovascular coronary stents, regardless of whether a gold- or nickel-containing stent is used. The explanation for this is unclear, although the authors suggest the possibility of previous sensitization. They do, however, point to circumstantial evidence and statistical findings that implicate induction of gold allergy after placement of a gold-plated stent in the coronary artery. A prospective longitudinal study would be necessary to prove that gold-plated stents are truly a risk factor for gold allergy.

B. H. Thiers, MD

Results of patch testing to a corticosteroid series: A retrospective review of 1188 patients during 6 years at Mayo Clinic

Davis MDP, el-Azhary RA, Farmer SA (Mayo Clinic, Rochester, Minn)
J Am Acad Dermatol 56:921-927, 2007

Background.—Allergy to topical corticosteroids is more common than previously realized. To detect this allergy, a corticosteroid series is used for patch testing in addition to corticosteroid screens on a standard series.

Objective.—We sought to review our experience with patch testing to corticosteroid series.

Methods.—We conducted a retrospective study of patch testing to our corticosteroid series over 6 years (January 1, 2000-December 31, 2005).

Results.—Of 1188 patients patch tested to corticosteroid series, 127 (10.69%) had allergic reaction to at least one corticosteroid; 56 reacted to multiple corticosteroids. Rates of allergic patch test reaction to 19,611 individual corticosteroids were 0.41% to 5.03%. Rates of reaction to corticosteroid groups were 1.10% to 5.72%; concomitant reactions between groups were noted. Present screens on our standard series identified 74% of those detected on the corticosteroid series; tixocortol pivalate alone detected less than 50%.

Limitations.—Limitations include that this study was retrospective and the possible interobserver variation in interpretation of patch tests.

Conclusion.—In patients suggested to have corticosteroid allergy, patch testing confirms allergy in 10.69%; allergy is often to multiple corticosteroids and across groups. Screens on a standard series may detect 74% of those detected on a corticosteroid series.

▶ The authors used a corticosteroid series comprised of 17 allergens to assess the possibility of topical corticosteroid allergy. They found that three or four screening allergens could detect approximately 70% of corticosteroid allergies. An extended series may be appropriate to help identify which corticosteroids a given patient could safely use. The use of corticosteroid groups is imprecise and would not be helpful for providing specific treatment recommendations.

B. H. Thiers, MD

Attenuation of Allergic Contact Dermatitis Through the Endocannabinoid System
Karsak M, Gaffal E, Date R, et al (Univ of Bonn, Germany; Life & Brain GmbH, Bonn, Germany; Consiglio Nazionale delle Ricerche, Napoli, Italy; et al)
Science 316:1494-1497, 2007

Allergic contact dermatitis affects about 5% of men and 11% of women in industrialized countries and is one of the leading causes for occupational diseases. In an animal model for cutaneous contact hypersensitivity, we show that mice lacking both known cannabinoid receptors display exacerbated allergic inflammation. In contrast, fatty acid amide hydrolase–deficient mice, which have increased levels of the endocannabinoid anandamide, displayed reduced allergic responses in the skin. Cannabinoid receptor antagonists exacerbated allergic inflammation, whereas receptor agonists attenuated inflammation. These results demonstrate a protective role of the endocannabinoid system in contact allergy in the skin and suggest a target for therapeutic intervention.

▶ Although no one is about to suggest the use of marijuana as a treatment for allergic contact dermatitis, the observation that the endocannabinoid system is activated in a murine model of contact hypersensitivity suggests that the endocannabinoid system may attenuate the inflammatory response in animals with topically induced allergic inflammation. This hypothesis is supported by the observation that genetic depletion or pharmacologic blockade of cannabinoid receptors enhances allergic inflammation, whereas stimulation of cannabinoid receptors has the opposite effect. The article by Karsak et al points to the possibility of future pharmacologic treatments for cutaneous inflammatory diseases using selective cannabinoid receptor agonists or inhibitors of the enzyme fatty acid amide hydrolase.

B. H. Thiers, MD

Allergy to tea tree oil: Retrospective review of 41 cases with positive patch tests over 4.5 years
Rutherford T, Nixon R, Tam M, et al (Skin and Cancer Found, Melbourne, Australia)
Australas J Dermatol 48:83-87, 2007

Tea tree oil use is increasing, with considerable interest in it being a 'natural' antimicrobial. It is found in many commercially available skin and hair care products in Australia. We retrospectively reviewed our patch test data at the Skin and Cancer Foundation Victoria over a 4.5-year period and identified 41 cases of positive reactions to oxidized tea tree oil of 2320 people patch-tested, giving a prevalence of 1.8%. The tea tree oil reaction was deemed relevant to the presenting dermatitis in 17 of 41 (41%) patients. Of those with positive reactions, 27 of 41 (66%) recalled prior use of tea tree oil and eight of 41 (20%) specified prior application of neat (100%) tea tree oil. Tea tree oil allergic contact dermatitis is under-reported in the literature but is sufficiently common in Australia to warrant inclusion of tea tree oil, at a concentration of 10% in petrolatum, in standard patch-test series. Given tea tree oil from freshly opened tea tree oil products elicits no or weak reactions, oxidized tea tree oil should be used for patch testing.

▶ Prepubertal gynecomastia is extremely uncommon, in contrast to pubertal gynecomastia, which occurs in more than 60% of males. Because prepubertal gynecomastia has no obvious physiologic explanation, pathologic causes should always be entertained. Nevertheless, prepubertal gynecomastia is found to be idiopathic in 90% of patients. Such cases may result from an environmental chemical that disrupts the endocrine system and leads to disproportionate estrogen and androgen pathway signaling. As demonstrated by Henley et al,[1] lavender and tea tree oils may possess such activity. Rutherford et al reminds us that allergy to tea tree oil is relatively common and is often relevant to the presenting dermatitis.

B. H. Thiers, MD

Reference

1. Henley DV, Lipson N, Korach KS, Block CA. Prepubertal gynecomastia linked to lavender and tea tree oils. *N Engl J Med.* 2007;356:479-485.

Prepubertal Gynecomastia Linked to Lavender and Tea Tree Oils
Henley DV, Lipson N, Korach KS, et al (Natl Inst of Environmental Health Sciences, Research Triangle Park, NC; Univ of Colorado School of Medicine, Denver; Pediatric Endocrine Associates, Greenwood Village, Colo)
N Engl J Med 356:479-485, 2007

Most cases of male prepubertal gynecomastia are classified as idiopathic. We investigated possible causes of gynecomastia in three prepubertal boys who were otherwise healthy and had normal serum concentrations of endogenous steroids. In all three boys, gynecomastia coincided with the topical application of products that contained lavender and tea tree oils. Gynecomastia resolved in each patient shortly after the use of products containing these oils was discontinued. Furthermore, studies in human cell lines indicated that the two oils had estrogenic and antiandrogenic activities. We conclude that repeated topical exposure to lavender and tea tree oils probably caused prepubertal gynecomastia in these boys.

▶ Prepubertal gynecomastia is extremely uncommon, in contrast to pubertal gynecomastia, which occurs in more than 60% of males. Because prepubertal gynecomastia has no obvious physiologic explanation, pathologic causes should always be entertained. Nevertheless, prepubertal gynecomastia is found to be idiopathic in 90% of patients. Such cases may result from an environmental chemical that disrupts the endocrine system and leads to disproportionate estrogen and androgen pathway signaling. As demonstrated by Henley et al, lavender and tea tree oils may possess such activity. Rutherford et al[1] remind us that allergy to tea tree oil is relatively common and is often relevant to the presenting dermatitis.

B. H. Thiers, MD

Reference

1. Rutherford T, Nixon R, Tam M, Tate B. Allergy to tea tree oil: retrospective review of 41 cases with positive patch tests over 4.5 years. *Australas J Dermatol.* 2007; 48:83-87.

Early Thimerosal Exposure and Neuropsychological Outcomes at 7 to 10 Years
Thompson WW, for the Vaccine Safety Datalink Team (Ctrs for Disease Control and Prevention, Atlanta, Ga; Abt Associates, Cambridge, Mass; Group Health Ctr for Health Studies, Seattle; et al)
N Engl J Med 357:1281-1292, 2007

Background.—It has been hypothesized that early exposure to thimerosal, a mercury-containing preservative used in vaccines and immune globulin preparations, is associated with neuropsychological deficits in children.

Methods.—We enrolled 1047 children between the ages of 7 and 10 years and administered standardized tests assessing 42 neuropsychological outcomes. (We did not assess autism-spectrum disorders.) Exposure to mercury from thimerosal was determined from computerized immunization records, medical records, personal immunization records, and parent interviews. Information on potential confounding factors was obtained from the interviews and medical charts. We assessed the association between current neuropsychological performance and exposure to mercury during the prenatal period, the neonatal period (birth to 28 days), and the first 7 months of life.

Results.—Among the 42 neuropsychological outcomes, we detected only a few significant associations with exposure to mercury from thimerosal. The detected associations were small and almost equally divided between positive and negative effects. Higher prenatal mercury exposure was associated with better performance on one measure of language and poorer performance on one measure of attention and executive functioning. Increasing levels of mercury exposure from birth to 7 months were associated with better performance on one measure of fine motor coordination and on one measure of attention and executive functioning. Increasing mercury exposure from birth to 28 days was associated with poorer performance on one measure of speech articulation and better performance on one measure of fine motor coordination.

Conclusions.—Our study does not support a causal association between early exposure to mercury from thimerosal-containing vaccines and immune globulins and deficits in neuropsychological functioning at the age of 7 to 10 years.

▶ The data presented by Thompson et al are consistent with that reported in a series of articles[1-3] reviewed in the 2005 YEAR BOOK OF DERMATOLOGY AND DERMATOLOGIC SURGERY. As noted then, thimerosal is more familiar to dermatologists as a cause of contact dermatitis, but it has also been used as a preservative in children's vaccines and has been implicated as a possible cause of autistic and neurodevelopmental disorders. Thimerosal contains ethyl mercury, an organic compound that is metabolized into mercury, whereas a related organic mercury-containing compound, methyl mercury, has been shown to have adverse effects on childhood development, especially with early exposure. Although some investigators believe that ethyl mercury might have a similar effect, little evidence supports that assertion. Moreover, ethyl mercury is more quickly metabolized and eliminated from the body than is methyl mercury. Nevertheless, the controversy over the toxicity of thimerosal-containing vaccines has continued despite the lack of evidence to support claims of adverse effects on children.[4,5]

B. H. Thiers, MD

References

1. Heron J, Golding J. Thimerosal exposure in infants and developmental disorders: a perspective cohort study in the United Kingdom does not support a cause or association. *Pediatrics.* 2004;114:577-583.
2. Andrews N, Miller E, Grant A, Stowe J, Osborne V, Taylor B. Thimerosal exposure in infants and developmental disorders: a retrospective cohort study in the United Kingdom does not support a cause or association. *Pediatrics.* 2004;114:584-591.
3. Parker SK, Schwartz B, Todd J, Pickering LK. Thimerosal-containing vaccines and autistic spectrum disorder: a critical review of published original data. *Pediatrics.* 2004;114:793-804.
4. Sugarman SD. Cases in vaccine court—legal battles over vaccines and autism. *N Engl J Med.* 2007;357:1275-1277.
5. Offit PA. Thimerosal and vaccines—a cautionary tale. *N Engl J Med.* 2007;357: 1278-1279.

The frequency of nasal carriage in chronic urticaria patients
Ertam I, Yuksel Biyikli SE, Yazkan FA, et al (Ege Univ Med Faculty, Izmir, Turkey)
J Eur Acad Dermatol Venereol 21:777-780, 2007

Objective.—Chronic urticaria is characterized by oedema of the skin and mucous membranes. Although many agents have been implicated, aetiology is unknown in 70 to 75% of patients. Infections and foci of chronic infections are most commonly held responsible for chronic urticaria. In this study, the frequency of nasal carriage as the occult focus of infection and sensitivity to antimicrobials are explored in patients with chronic urticaria.

Material and Method.—Ninety-four patients with chronic urticaria and 30 controls participated in the study, which was carried out at the Ege university medical faculty, department of dermatology between January 2004 and January 2005. Nasal swab specimens were taken from the patients and controls and incubated at 37 degrees C for 48 h, and inoculated on standard bacterial medium (blood agar). Antimicrobial susceptibility of a growth from isolates of the nasal swab specimens was conducted. Data were analysed statistically using chi-square and Mann–Whitney U-tests.

Results.—Ninety-four patients with chronic urticaria (72.3% female and 27.7% male) and 30 controls (63.3% female and 36.7% male) comprised the study group. Mean age of the patients and controls were 42.6 and 33.8 years, respectively. *Staphylococcus aureus* was detected in swab specimens from the nasal cavity in 50 of the 94 patients (53.2%) with chronic urticaria and four of the 30 controls (13.3%). Testing revealed that the most susceptible antibiotics were cefaclor, ceftriaxone, amoxycillin-clavulanic acid, amikacin, netilmicin, and fucidic acid.

Conclusion.—Growth on cultures prepared from nasal swab specimens of chronic urticaria patients was statistically higher than the control group. We detected resistance to growth against mupirocin, an antibiotic frequently used in nasal carriage. High nasal carriage of *Staphylococcus aureus* in patients with chronic urticaria compared to controls suggests that nasal carriage as a focus of infection should be kept in mind as aetiology.

▶ The authors found that nasal carriage of bacteria in patients with chronic urticaria was statistically higher than in controls. They suggest that nasal carriage might serve as a focus of infection and play a role in the etiology of that condition and its characteristic treatment resistance. One could argue that the nasal carriage and skin disease are unrelated. The obvious way to settle the issue would be to treat the colonizing organisms and assess the effect of such treatment on the underlying urticaria.

B. H. Thiers, MD

2 Psoriasis and Other Papulosquamous Disorders

Psoriasis: evolution of pathogenic concepts and new therapies through phases of translational research
Guttman-Yasskey E, Krueger JG (Rockefeller Univ, New York)
Br J Dermatol 157:1103-1115, 2007

Background.—Translational research is a process that uses scientific investigation to advance the understanding of human physiology or disease and then seeks to improve health by translating observations of experimental science to new therapies. A conventional view of translational research is that a disease is studied for cellular and molecular mechanisms in model systems and that the testing of new therapeutic approaches occurs in these models before proceeding to clinical trials in humans. Psoriasis may be unique in that it is a disease studied through translational science even though there is not an acceptable animal model. However, many rounds of bidirectional translation have taken place, and these have helped to define disease pathogenesis and to advance therapy for psoriasis. The purpose of this review was to describe the evolution of new pathogenic concepts and the testing of new therapeutic agents through translational research in humans.

Overview.—Psoriasis is a disease of many cell types, and recognition of abnormal growth/differentiation/structure formed by these cell types led to many pathogenic hypotheses. The first highly effective therapeutics for psoriasis such as ultraviolet (UV) B and psoralen plus UVA were developed through an empirical approach that was not based on specific hypotheses of disease pathogenesis or on mechanistic properties of the therapeutics. Development of a therapy for psoriasis based on a prior understanding of cellular pathogenesis could be considered to be the start of translational research. The therapeutic success achieved with methotrexate was the likely trigger for many clinical and laboratory investigations of altered keratinocyte growth and differentiation in psoriasis lesions. The production of monoclonal antibodies was first described in 1975 and led to the development of antibodies that could be used to mark specific populations of leukocytes in humans. The refinement of monoclonal antibody technologies and associated molecular biology led to development of key reagents for critical testing of hypotheses soon thereafter. Bidirectional translational research on psoriasis began in earnest when experiments on disease pathogenesis progressed to the point at which specific molecular or cellular alterations as disease causes could be proposed and experimental therapeutics to those pathways were available for testing in the clinic.

Conclusions.—The current view of disease pathogenesis presented in this report stems from research in patients and animal models, but with the perspectives that disease models can advance or hinder the overall translational enterprise and that the research process must be firmly grounded in the pathophysiology of the actual human condition.

▶ This is yet another of the many excellent review articles on the pathogenesis of psoriasis that have appeared in the past year. Guttman-Yassky and Krueger take a different approach, however, drawing parallels between the phases of translational research and the new concepts that have evolved to unlock the mysteries of this fascinating disease. As defined by the authors, translational research uses scientific investigation to translate basic science observations to clinically applicable therapies. Because the process can begin with either an interesting observation or with a basic laboratory finding, the authors' concept of translational research is that of a "bi-directional flow of information from the bedside or clinic to the laboratory and vice versa." In their article, Guttman-Yassky and Krueger trace the evolution of the immunological model of psoriasis from a focus on the epidermis and keratinocyte growth and differentiation to the new generation of disease-specific therapeutics. Many of these interfere with the activity of tumor necrosis factor-α, a key player in provoking the TH1 and TH17 immune response that characterizes the disease. As stated by the authors, "psoriasis is probably the best example of a common skin disease where rapid advances in pathogenic understanding and development of new therapies have occurred through the translational science approach."

B. H. Thiers, MD

Pathogenesis and therapy of psoriasis
Lowes MA, Bowcock AM, Krueger JG (Rockefeller Univ, New York; Washington Univ, St Louis)
Nature 445:866-873, 2007

Background.—Psoriasis is one of the most common human skin diseases. It is characterized by excessive growth and aberrant differentiation of keratinocytes, but it is fully reversible with appropriate therapy. Psoriasis is thought to have a key genetic base; the trigger of the keratinocyte response is thought to be activation of the cellular immune system, with T cells, dendritic cells, and a variety of immune–related cytokines and chemokines implicated in pathogenesis. The purpose of this report was to review the pathogenesis of psoriasis and the newest therapies, which target its immune components and may be predictive of potential treatments for other inflammatory human diseases.

Overview.—Psoriasis vulgaris is characterized by red, scaly, raised plaques. It can occur in children but it often begins in late adolescence or early adulthood and then usually persists for life. The disease has a tendency to develop in certain areas, such as the elbow, knee, and scalp. Histologically, there is a marked thickening of the epidermis, and epidermal rete become very elongated and form long, thin, downward projections into the dermis. Neutrophils are present within small foci in the stratum corneum, and there are significant mononuclear infiltrates in the epidermis, which are detectable with immunostaining. There are two fundamentally different cell types interacting in the formation of a psoriatic lesion–epidermal keratinocytes and mononuclear leukocytes. The development of effective therapies is dependent on understanding the molecular circuitry of inflammation in human autoimmune diseases. Previous conceptualizations of cytokine interactions in psoriasis have been based on a "type-1 pathway," which assumes a linear relationship between proximal inducers (IL-23 or IL-12), production of IFN-γ and TNF by type-1 cells, and downstream activation of numerous IFN-responsive genes through signal transducer and activation of transcription 1 (STAT1). This is a conceptually useful model, but it accounts for only a small proportion of the 1300-plus genes that become upregulated in psoriatic lesions. An alternative model is more of a network or interactive model. The choice of treatment is dependent on many factors, including extent of disease, the effects of psoriasis on a patient's life, and the patient's perception of their illness. In the past few years, biological therapies have been available for severe psoriasis. These agents are proteins or antibodies that target specific molecules thought to be essential in the pathogenesis of psoriasis.

Conclusions.—Unlike other autoimmune diseases in humans, it has been possible to study the cellular and genomic features of psoriasis in great detail. This review described how interactions between resident skin cells and elements of the immune system interact to produce a disease that can persist for decades in focal regions of the skin. The potential contributions of transmitted genes that increase susceptibility to psoriasis are also considered.

▶ Lowes et al offer a superb review of the state-of-the-art knowledge of the pathogenesis and treatment of psoriasis. The concepts are clearly presented and are accompanied by information-packed tables and illustrations (see Figs 2, 3, and Table 1 in the original article). Clearly this is a "must read" for anyone with a special research or clinical interest in the disorder. The authors conclude with a realistic assessment of unresolved issues and questions that must be answered to gain a greater understanding of this common disease and to improve its treatment.

B. H. Thiers, MD

Immunopathogenesis of psoriasis

Sabat R, Philipp S, Höflich C, et al (Univ Hosp Charité, Berlin; Schering AG, Berlin)
Exp Dermatol 16:779-798, 2007

Psoriasis is a chronic skin disease that affects about 1.5% of the Caucasian population and is characterized by typical macroscopic and microscopic skin alterations. Psoriatic lesions are sharply demarcated, red and slightly raised lesions with silver-whitish scales. The microscopic alterations of psoriatic plaques include an infiltration of immune cells in the dermis and epidermis, a dilatation and an increase in the number of blood vessels in the upper dermis, and a massively thickened epidermis with atypical keratinocyte differentiation. It is considered a fact that the immune system plays an important role in the pathogenesis of psoriasis. Since the early 1990s, it has been assumed that T1 cells play the dominant role in the initiation and maintenance of psoriasis. However, the profound success of anti-tumor necrosis factor-α therapy, when compared with T-cell depletion therapies, should provoke us to critically re-evaluate the current hypothesis for psoriasis pathogenesis. Recently made discoveries regarding other T-cell populations such as Th17 and regulatory T cells, dendritic cells, macrophages, the keratinocyte signal transduction and novel cytokines including interleukin (IL)-22, IL-23 and IL-20, let us postulate that the pathogenesis of psoriasis consists of distinct subsequent stages, in each of them different cell types playing a dominant role. Our model helps to explain the varied effectiveness of the currently tested immune modulating therapies and may enable the prediction of the success of future therapies.

▶ This is yet another of many excellent reviews of the immunopathogenesis of psoriasis that appeared during 2007. The authors postulate a "keratinocyte response stage" that is induced by the immune response and cutaneous inflammation. They suggest that therapies targeted at this stage would have the greatest chance of a rapid clinical response. They also comment that anti–TNF-α therapy is likely effective for 2 reasons: partial depletion of macrophages/dendritic cells and neutralization of TNF-α, the proinflammatory cytokine that powers the aberrant immune response in this disease.

B. H. Thiers, MD

Pathogenesis and clinical features of psoriasis

Griffiths CE, Barker JN (Univ of Manchester, England; King's College London)
Lancet 370:263-271, 2007

Psoriasis, a papulosquamous skin disease, was originally thought of as a disorder primarily of epidermal keratinocytes, but is now recognised as one of the commonest immune-mediated disorders. Tumour necrosis factor α, dendritic cells, and T-cells all contribute substantially to its pathogenesis. In early-onset psoriasis (beginning before age 40 years), carriage of HLA-Cw6 and environmental triggers, such as β-haemolytic streptococcal infections, are major determinants of disease expression. Moreover, at least nine chromosomal psoriasis susceptibility loci have been identified. Several clinical phenotypes of psoriasis are recognised, with chronic plaque (psoriasis vulgaris) accounting for 90% of cases. Comorbidities of psoriasis are attracting interest, and include impairment of quality of life and associated depressive illness, cardiovascular disease, and a seronegative arthritis known as psoriatic arthritis. A more complete understanding of underlying pathomechanisms is leading to new treatments, which will be discussed in the second part of this Series.

▶ This article by Griffiths and Barker and an article by Menter and Griffiths[1] appeared in the internal medicine journal, *Lancet*, and function as a compendium of current knowledge of the pathogenesis and treatment of psoriasis. Because they were published in a clinical journal that is read mostly by nondermatologists, concepts are presented in clearly understandable, straightforward terms without the confusing basic science that is found in some of our more esoteric publications. Nevertheless, the information presented here is relevant and important, and serves as a "must read" for all physicians interested in this disease, whether from the aspect of an academician or a practitioner. The authors are to be commended for their important contribution to the medical literature.

B. H. Thiers, MD

Reference

1. Menter A, Griffiths CE. Current and future management of psoriasis. *Lancet.* 2007;370:272-284.

Current and future management of psoriasis
Menter A, Griffiths CE (Southwestern Med School, Dallas; Univ of Manchester, England)
Lancet 370:272-284, 2007

Management of psoriasis begins with identification of the extent of cutaneous disease. However, a holistic, contractual approach to treatment is encouraged, with particular reference to psychosocial disability and quality-of-life issues. The presence of psoriasis on palms, soles, body folds, genitals, face, or nails, and concomitant joint disease, are also important when considering treatment options. An evidence-based approach is essential in delineating differences between the many available treatments. However, archaic approaches, especially combinational ones, are routinely used by some clinicians, with inadequate prospective or comparative evidence. Treatments currently available are: topical agents used predominantly for mild disease and for recalcitrant lesions in more severe disease; phototherapy for moderate disease; and systemic agents including photochemotherapy, oral agents, and newer injectable biological agents, which have revolutionised the management of severe psoriasis. Other innovative treatments are undergoing clinical studies, with the aim of maintaining safe, long-term control of the condition.

▶ This article by Menter and Griffiths and an article by Griffiths and Barker[1] appeared in the internal medicine journal, *Lancet*, and function as a compendium of current knowledge of the pathogenesis and treatment of psoriasis. Because they were published in a clinical journal that is read mostly by nondermatologists, concepts are presented in clearly understandable, straightforward terms without the confusing basic science that is found in some of our more esoteric publications. Nevertheless, the information presented here is relevant and important, and serves as a "must read" for all physicians interested in this disease, whether from the aspect of an academician or a practitioner. The authors are to be commended for their important contribution to the medical literature.

B. H. Thiers, MD

Reference

1. Griffiths CE, Barker JN. Pathogenesis and clinical features of psoriasis. *Lancet.* 2007;370:263-271.

$\alpha_1\beta_1$ integrin is crucial for accumulation of epidermal T cells and the development of psoriasis

Conrad C, Boyman O, Tonel G, et al (Univ Hosp of Zurich, Switzerland; King's College London School of Medicine; Biogen Idec Inc, Cambridge, Mass)
Nature Med 13:836-842, 2007

Psoriasis is a common T cell–mediated autoimmune inflammatory disease. We show that blocking the interaction of $\alpha_1\beta_1$ integrin (VLA-1) with collagen prevented accumulation of epidermal T cells and immunopathology of psoriasis. $\alpha_1\beta_1$ integrin, a major collagen-binding surface receptor, was exclusively expressed by epidermal but not dermal T cells. $\alpha_1\beta_1$-positive T cells showed characteristic surface markers of effector memory cells and contained high levels of interferon-γ but not interleukin-4. Blockade of $\alpha_1\beta_1$ inhibited migration of T cells into the epidermis in a clinically relevant xenotransplantation model. This was paralleled by a complete inhibition of psoriasis development, comparable to that caused by tumor necrosis factor-α blockers. These results define a crucial role for $\alpha_1\beta_1$ in controlling the accumulation of epidermal type 1 polarized effector memory T cells in a common human immunopathology and provide the basis for new strategies in psoriasis treatment focusing on T cell–extracellular matrix interactions.

▶ Conrad and colleagues present data that establish $\alpha_1\beta_1$-positive epidermal T cells as key players in the formation of the psoriatic lesion. They suggest new therapeutic approaches that target these cells in psoriasis and other autoimmune diseases. In addition to showing that these T cells are important effectors in the psoriatic disease process, these authors have also identified receptors on epidermal T cells that interact with connective tissue in the skin and that participate in T-cell–mediated inflammation. They suggest that further studies to characterize the molecular and functional characteristics of intraepithelial T cells in psoriasis, and their role in T-cell migration will provide new insight into the pathogenesis of the disease.[1]

B. H. Thiers, MD

Reference

1. Gudjonsson JE, Elder JT. The problem with upward mobility. *Nat Med.* 2007; 13:786-787.

A brief history of T_H17, the first major revision in the T_H1/T_H2 hypothesis of T cell–mediated tissue damage
Steinman L (Stanford Univ, Calif)
Nature Med 13:139-145, 2007

For over 35 years, immunologists have divided T-helper (T_H) cells into functional subsets. T-helper type 1 (T_H1) cells—long thought to mediate tissue damage—might be involved in the initiation of damage, but they do not sustain or play a decisive role in many commonly studied models of autoimmunity, allergy and microbial immunity. A major role for the cytokine interleukin-17 (IL-17) has now been described in various models of immune-mediated tissue injury, including organ-specific autoimmunity in the brain, heart, synovium and intestines, allergic disorders of the lung and skin, and microbial infections of the intestines and the nervous system. A pathway named T_H17 is now credited for causing and sustaining tissue damage in these diverse situations. The T_H1 pathway antagonizes the T_H17 pathway in an intricate fashion. The evolution of our understanding of the T_H17 pathway illuminates a shift in immunologists' perspectives regarding the basis of tissue damage, where for over 20 years the role of T_H1 cells was considered paramount.

▶ In recent years, a subset of CD4+ T cells designated T_H17 cells has been identified and so named because they produce interleukin-17 (IL-17), a pleiotropic inflammatory mediator; in addition, T_H17 cells produce IL-22. They are distinct from T_H1 and T_H2 cells and appear to be induced by IL-23. The list of human diseases in which IL-17 has been implicated includes multiple sclerosis, rheumatoid arthritis, Lyme disease, inflammatory bowel disease, and contact dermatitis. Steinman's review is a highly readable saga of this particular voyage of discovery to date, and includes a statement that for me is the quote of the year: "A historical perspective on the T_H1/T_H2 hypothesis is illuminating, both for its insights into important immunologic phenomena and for its revelations about how groups of highly trained intellectuals, in this case immunologists, can adhere to an idea for so many years, even in the face of its obvious flaws."

Psoriasis has for some time been considered to be a T_H1-associated disease. However, several previous studies have investigated the involvement of IL-17 and IL-23 in human psoriasis, and both cytokines have been shown to be abnormally expressed in psoriatic plaques.

In a study by Zheng et al,[1] the authors also examined the potential role of T_H17 cells in a murine model. These investigators showed that injection of IL-23 into the ears of mice resulted in epidermal hyperplasia similar to that found in psoriasis: this response was substantially reduced in IL-22 knockout mice, and by the administration of antibodies to IL-22, thus suggesting that the IL-23 effect was mediated by IL-22. They further showed that the expression of activated phospho-Stat3, a marker of keratinocyte proliferation, was also significantly reduced in IL-22 knockout mice treated with IL-23, suggesting the involvement of this transcription factor in the process. Thus, the evidence for a role of T_H17 cells in psoriasis is accumulating and will, no doubt, be the subject of further studies.

G. M. P. Galbraith, MD

Reference

1. Zheng Y, Danilenko DM, Valdez P, et al. Interleukin-22, a T_H17 cytokine, mediates IL-23-induced dermal inflammation and acanthosis. *Nature.* 2007;445:648-651.

Interleukin-22, a T_H17 cytokine, mediates IL-23-induced dermal inflammation and acanthosis
Zheng Y, Danilenko DM, Valdez P, et al (Genentech, Inc, South San Francisco)
Nature 445:648-651, 2007

Psoriasis is a chronic inflammatory skin disease characterized by hyperplasia of the epidermis (acanthosis), infiltration of leukocytes into both the dermis and epidermis, and dilation and growth of blood vessels. The underlying cause of the epidermal acanthosis in psoriasis is still largely unknown. Recently, interleukin (IL)-23, a cytokine involved in the development of IL-17-producing T helper cells (T_H17 cells), was found to have a potential function in the pathogenesis of psoriasis. Here we show that IL-22 is preferentially produced by T_H17 cells and mediates the acanthosis induced by IL-23. We found that IL-23 or IL-6 can directly induce the production of IL-22 from both murine and human naive T cells. However, the production of IL-22 and IL-17 from T_H17 cells is differentially regulated. Transforming growth factor-β, although crucial for IL-17 production, actually inhibits IL-22 production. Furthermore, IL-22 mediates IL-23-induced acanthosis and dermal inflammation through the activation of Stat3 (signal transduction and activators of transcription 3) *in vivo*. Our results suggest that T_H17 cells, through the production of both IL-22 and IL-17, might have essential functions in host defence and in the pathogenesis of autoimmune diseases such as psoriasis. IL-22, as an effector cytokine produced by T cells, mediates the crosstalk between the immune system and epithelial cells.

▶ In recent years, a subset of CD4+ T cells designated T_H17 cells has been identified and so named because they produce interleukin-17 (IL-17), a pleiotropic inflammatory mediator; in addition, T_H17 cells produce IL-22. They are distinct from T_H1 and T_H2 cells and appear to be induced by IL-23. The list of human diseases in which IL-17 has been implicated includes multiple sclerosis, rheumatoid arthritis, Lyme disease, inflammatory bowel disease and contact dermatitis. A review published in *Nature Medicine* by Steinman[1] is a highly readable saga of this particular voyage of discovery to date, and includes a statement that for me is the quote of the year: "A historical perspective on the T_H1/T_H2 hypothesis is illuminating, both for its insights into important immunologic phenomena and for its revelations about how groups of highly trained intellectuals, in this case immunologists, can adhere to an idea for so many years, even in the face of its obvious flaws." Psoriasis has for some time been considered to be a T_H1-associated disease. However, several previous studies have investigated the involvement of IL-17 and IL-23 in human psoriasis, and both cytokines have been shown to be abnormally expressed in psoriatic plaques. In this study, Zheng et al also examined the potential role of T_H17 cells in a murine model. These investigators showed that injection of IL-23 into the ears of mice resulted in epidermal hyperplasia similar to that found in psoriasis: this response was substantially reduced in IL-22 knockout mice, and by the administration of antibodies to IL-22, thus suggesting that the IL-23 effect was mediated by IL-22. They further showed that the expression of activated phospho-Stat3, a marker of keratinocyte proliferation, was also significantly reduced in IL-22 knockout mice treated with IL-23, suggesting the involvement of this transcription factor in the process. Thus, the evidence for a role of T_H17 cells in psoriasis is accumulating and will, no doubt, be the subject of further studies.

G. M. P. Galbraith, MD

Reference

1. Steinman L. A brief history of T_H17, the first major revision in the T_H1/T_H2 hypothesis of T cell–mediated tissue damage. *Nature Med.* 2007;13:139-145.

Polymorphisms in Interleukin-15 Gene on Chromosome 4q31.2 Are Associated with Psoriasis Vulgaris in Chinese Population
Zhang X-J, Yan K-L, Wang Z-M, et al (Anhui Med Univ, Hefei, China; Ministry of Education, Hefei, China; Chinese Natl Human Genome Ctr at Shanghai, China; et al)
J Invest Dermatol 127:2544-2551, 2007

Through a series of linkage analyses in a large Chinese family cohort of psoriasis, we previously identified and confirmed a non-HLA psoriasis linkage locus PSORS9 within a small region at 4q31.2-32.1. Within the critical region of the PSORS9 locus, IL-15 has been long recognized as a strong candidate gene for psoriasis. In this study, we investigated the association between IL-15 genetic polymorphisms and psoriasis in a large Chinese sample. Highly significant evidence for association was identified at a single-nucleotide polymorphism (SNP) (g.96516A →T) within the 3'-untranslated region (UTR) of the IL-15 gene ($P=0.00006$, after correction for multiple testing). Haplotype analysis using the SNPs within the 3'UTR region also provided strong supporting evidence for association ($P=0.00005$), where we identified a haplotype of the 3'UTR region of IL-15 associated with increased risk to psoriasis (odds ratio=1.65). This association was also supported by the results of our expression activity analyses, where we demonstrated that the identified risk haplotype is associated with an increased activity of IL-15. Therefore, we provided early evidence for the important role of IL-15 genetic variants in the pathogenesis of psoriasis, probably by increasing interleukin production and inflammation in the lesions of psoriasis.

▶ Considering the complexity of psoriasis, it is not surprising that virtually every known cytokine has been investigated for its potential pathogenic role. In this study, Zhang et al continued their studies of the genetic impact of interleukin 15 (IL-15) on this disease. IL-15 has been previously implicated because of its proinflammatory properties, the finding that it appears to be overexpressed in psoriatic lesions, and the inhibitory effect of antibodies to IL-15 on lesional severity in a mouse xenograft model. In the current study, the investigators examined the possible association between psoriasis and SNPs in the IL-15 gene, as they had predicted in a previous linkage analysis. The most significant association was found for the less common allele of a polymorphism located within the 3'UTR of the gene: possession of this allele was found to confer disease susceptibility with an odds ratio of 1.86. Functional studies provided evidence of increased IL-15 expression in cells with this allele. This study is also interesting because of the fact that IL-15 induces the production of IL-17 by human T-cell blast cells and, therefore, may be involved in the newly recognized role of T_H17 cells in psoriasis (see Zheng et al[1]).

G. M. P. Galbraith, MD

Reference

1. Zheng Y, Danilenko DM, Valdez P, et al. Interleukin-22, a T_H17 cytokine, mediates IL-23-induced dermal inflammation and acanthosis. *Nature.* 2007;445:648-651.

Antibodies to Complement Receptor 3 Treat Established Inflammation in Murine Models of Colitis and a Novel Model of Psoriasis Dermatitis
Leon F, Contractor N, Fuss I, et al (NIH, Bethesda, Md)
J Immunol 177:6974-6982, 2006

Prior studies indicated the ability of Abs to complement receptor 3 (CR3, CD11b/CD18) to suppress the production of IL-12 from immune cells. Therefore, we tested the ability of an anti-CR3 Ab (clone M1/70) to treat established IL-12-dependent Th1-mediated inflammation in murine models. Systemic administration of anti-CR3 significantly ameliorated established intestinal inflammation following the intrarectal administration of trinitrobenzene sulfonic acid (TNBS-colitis), as well as colitis and skin inflammation in C57BL/10 RAG-2$^{-/-}$ mice reconstituted with CD4$^+$CD45RB^{high} T cells. The hyperproliferative skin inflammation in this novel murine model demonstrated many characteristics of human psoriasis, and was prevented by the adoptive transfer of CD45RB^{low} T cells. In vitro and in vivo studies suggest that anti-CR3 treatment may act, at least in part, by directly inhibiting IL-12 production by APCs. Administration of anti-CR3 may be a useful therapeutic approach to consider for the treatment of inflammatory bowel disease and psoriasis in humans.

▶ This article and an article by Cargill et al[1] point toward inhibition of IL-12 production as a possible therapeutic target in treating psoriasis, a popular topic of debate in the recent literature.[2] The validity of this hypothesis is supported by a study published by Krueger et al,[3] demonstrating that an antibody against both IL-12 and IL-23 is quite effective in treating this condition. Although Cargill et al[1] emphasize the importance of genetic factors in psoriasis susceptibility, it must be remembered that other risk factors play a role as well.[4]

B. H. Thiers, MD

References

1. Cargill M, Schrodi SJ, Chang M, et al. A large-scale genetic association study confirms *IL12B* and leads to the identification of *IL23R* as psoriasis-risk genes. *Am J Hum Genet.* 2007;80:273-290.
2. Torti DC, Feldman SR. Interleukin12, interleukin-23, and psoriasis: current prospects. *J Am Acad Dermatol.* 2007;57:1059-1068.
3. Krueger GG, Langley RG, Leonardi C, et al. A human interleukin-12/23 monoclonal antibody for the treatment of psoriasis. *N Engl J Med.* 2007;356:580-592.
4. Huerta C, Rivero E, Rodríguez LA, et al. Incidence and risk factors for psoriasis in the general population. *Arch Dermatol.* 2007;143:1559-1565.

A Large-Scale Genetic Association Study Confirms *IL12B* and Leads to the Identification of *IL23R* as Psoriasis-Risk Genes
Cargill M, Schrodi SJ, Chang M, et al (Univ of Utah, Salt Lake City; LineaGen Research Corp, Salt Lake City; Genomics Collaborative Division of SeraCare Life Sciences, Cambridge, Mass)
Am J Hum Genet 80:273-290, 2007

We performed a multitiered, case-control association study of psoriasis in three independent sample sets of white North American individuals (1,446 cases and 1,432 controls) with 25,215 genecentric single-nucleotide polymorphisms (SNPs) and found a highly significant association with an *IL12B* 3'-untranslated-region SNP (*rs3212227*), confirming the results of a small Japanese study. This SNP was significant in all three sample sets (odds ratio [OR]$_{common}$ 0.64, combined P [P$_{comb}$] = 7.85 × 10^{-10}). A Monte Carlo simulation to address multiple testing suggests that this association is not a type I error. The coding regions of *IL12B* were resequenced in 96 individuals with psoriasis, and 30 additional *IL12B*-region SNPs were genotyped. Haplotypes were estimated, and genotype-conditioned analyses identified a second risk allele (*rs6887695*) located ~60 kb upstream of the *IL12B* coding region that exhibited association with psoriasis after adjustment for *rs3212227*. Together, these two SNPs mark a common *IL12B* risk haplotype (OR_{common} 1.40, $P_{comb} = 8.11 \times 10^{-9}$) and a less frequent protective haplotype (OR_{common} 0.58, $P_{comb} = 5.65 \times 10^{-12}$), which were statistically significant in all three studies. Since *IL12B* encodes the common IL-12p40 subunit of IL-12 and IL-23, we individually genotyped 17 SNPs in the genes encoding the other chains of these cytokines (*IL12A* and *IL23A*) and their receptors (*IL12RB1*, *IL12RB2*, and *IL23R*). Haplotype analyses identified two *IL23R* missense SNPs that together mark a common psoriasis-associated haplotype in all three studies (OR_{common} 1.44, $P_{comb} = 3.13 \times 10^{-6}$). Individuals homozygous for both the *IL12B* and the *IL23R* predisposing haplotypes have an increased risk of disease (OR_{common} 1.66, $P_{comb} = 1.33 \times 10^{-8}$). These data, and the previous observation that administration of an antibody specific for the IL-12p40 subunit to patients with psoriasis is highly efficacious, suggest that these genes play a fundamental role in psoriasis pathogenesis.

▶ This article and an article by Leon et al[1] point toward inhibition of IL-12 production as a possible therapeutic target in treating psoriasis, a popular topic of debate in the recent literature.[2] The validity of this hypothesis is supported by a study published by Krueger et al,[3] demonstrating that an antibody against both IL-12 and IL-23 is quite effective in treating this condition. Although Cargill et al emphasize the importance of genetic factors in psoriasis susceptibility, it must be remembered that other risk factors play a role as well.[4]

B. H. Thiers, MD

References

1. Leon F, Contractor N, Fuss I, et al. Antibodies to complement receptor 3 treat established inflammation in murine models of colitis and a novel model of psoriasis dermatitis. *J Immunol.* 2006;177:6974-6982.
2. Torti DC, Feldman SR. Interleukin12, interleukin-23, and psoriasis: current prospects. *J Am Acad Dermatol.* 2007;57:1059-1068.
3. Krueger GG, Langley RG, Leonardi C, et al. A human interleukin-12/23 monoclonal antibody for the treatment of psoriasis. *N Engl J Med.* 2007;356:580-592.
4. Huerta C, Rivero E, Rodríguez LA, et al. Incidence and risk factors for psoriasis in the general population. *Arch Dermatol.* 2007;143:1559-1565.

Endogenous IL-12 triggers an antiangiogenic program in melanoma cells
Airoldi I, Di Carlo E, Cocco C, et al (G Gaslini Inst, Genoa, Italy; "G d'Annunzio" Univ Found, Chieti, Italy; Istituto Nazionale per la Ricerca sul Cancro, Genoa, Italy; et al)
Proc Natl Acad Sci U S A 104:3996-4001, 2007

The IL12RB2 gene acts as a tumor suppressor in human B cell malignancies. Indeed, Il12rb2 knockout (KO) mice develop spontaneously B cell tumors, but also lung epithelial tumors. This latter phenotype may be related to (*i*) impairment of host IL-12-mediated immunosurveillance and/or (*ii*) IL-12 inability to inhibit directly the growth of IL-12 unresponsive malignant cells. To address this issue, we transplanted IL-12R$^+$ B16 melanoma cells into syngeneic Il12rb2 KO mice with the following rationale: (*i*) these mice have severe defects in IFN-γ production, as well as in cytotoxic T lymphocyte and natural killer cell cytotoxicity, and (*ii*) they produce but do not use IL-12 that can potentially bind to and target tumor cells only. Il12rb2 KO mice displayed higher endogenous serum levels of IL-12 and developed smaller B16 tumors than WT animals. These tumors showed reduced proliferation, increased apoptosis, and defective microvessel formation related to down-regulated expression of a set of proangiogenic genes previously unrelated to IL-12. Such effects depended on direct activity of endogenous IL-12 on tumor cells in KO mice, and hydrodynamic delivered IL-12 caused further reduced tumorigenicity of B16 cells in these mice. A previously undescribed mechanism of the IL-12 antitumor activity has been here identified and characterized.

▶ As noted by Krueger et al,[1] an aberrant type 1 helper cell immune response has been linked to the pathogenesis of psoriasis, and cytokines that can elicit such a response, such as interleukin-12 (IL-12) and interleukin-23 (IL-23), are being studied as potential therapeutic targets. In Krueger et al's report, the investigators report the results of a clinical trial by using a monoclonal antibody that recognizes both IL-12 and IL-23. This monoclonal antibody binds the p40 subunit shared by both interleukins. Psoriasis Area and Severity Index (PASI) 75 was achieved in approximately half the patients treated with the lowest doses and approximately 80% of those receiving the highest doses. The antibody is injected subcutaneously and serious adverse effects appear to be infrequent, although the trial was not designed to evaluate efficacy and safety of long-term use. And that, unfortunately, may be a significant issue. As shown by Airoldi et al, IL-12 appears to have antiangiogenic and antitumor activity. Is it possible that therapeutic interference with this cytokine activity may predispose to malignancy? Although it is extremely difficult to generalize findings in knock-out mice to humans, the lessons learned from cyclosporine may be worth remembering.

B. H. Thiers, MD

Reference

1. Krueger GG, Langley RG, Leonardi C, et al. A human interleukin-12/23 monoclonal antibody for the treatment of psoriasis. *N Engl J Med.* 2007;356:580-592.

A Human Interleukin-12/23 Monoclonal Antibody for the Treatment of Psoriasis

Krueger GG, for the CNTO 1275 Psoriasis Study Group (Univ of Utah, Salt Lake City; et al)

N Engl J Med 356:580-592, 2007

Background.—Skin-infiltrating lymphocytes expressing type 1 cytokines have been linked to the pathophysiology of psoriasis. We evaluated the safety and efficacy of a human interleukin-12/23 monoclonal antibody in treating psoriasis.

Methods.—In this double-blind, placebo-controlled trial, 320 patients with moderate-to-severe plaque psoriasis underwent randomization to treatment with the interleukin-12/23 monoclonal antibody (one 45-mg dose, one 90-mg dose, four weekly 45-mg doses, or four weekly 90-mg doses) or placebo; 64 patients were randomly assigned to each group. Patients assigned to the interleukin-12/23 monoclonal antibody received one additional dose at week 16 if needed. Patients assigned to placebo crossed over to receive one 90-mg dose of interleukin-12/23 monoclonal antibody at week 20.

Results.—There was at least 75% improvement in the psoriasis area-and-severity index at week 12 (the primary end point) in 52% of patients who received 45 mg of the interleukin-12/23 monoclonal antibody, in 59% of those who received 90 mg, in 67% of those who received four weekly 45-mg doses, and in 81% of those who received four weekly 90-mg doses, as compared with 2% of those who received placebo ($P<0.001$ for each comparison), and there was at least 90% improvement in 23%, 30%, 44%, and 52%, respectively, of patients who received the monoclonal antibody as compared with 2% of patients who received placebo ($P<0.001$ for each comparison). Adverse events occurred in 79% of patients treated with the interleukin-12/23 monoclonal antibody as compared with 72% of patients in the placebo group ($P=0.19$). Serious adverse events occurred in 4% of patients who received the monoclonal antibody and in 1% of those who received placebo ($P=0.69$).

Conclusions.—This study demonstrates the therapeutic efficacy of an interleukin-12/23 monoclonal antibody in psoriasis and provides further evidence of a role of the interleukin-12/23 p40 cytokines in the pathophysiology of psoriasis. Larger studies are needed to determine whether serious adverse events might limit the clinical usefulness of this new therapeutic target. (ClinicalTrials.gov number, NCT00320216.)

▶ As noted by Krueger et al, an aberrant type 1 helper cell immune response has been linked to the pathogenesis of psoriasis, and cytokines that can elicit such a response, such as interleukin-12 (IL-12) and interleukin-23 (IL-23), are being studied as potential therapeutic targets. Here, these investigators report the results of a clinical trial by using a monoclonal antibody that recognizes both IL-12 and IL-23. This monoclonal antibody binds the p40 subunit shared by both interleukins. Psoriasis Area and Severity Index (PASI) 75 was achieved in approximately half the patients treated with the lowest doses and approximately 80% of those receiving the highest doses. The antibody is injected subcutaneously and serious adverse effects appear to be infrequent, although the trial was not designed to evaluate efficacy and safety of long-term use. And that, unfortunately, may be a significant issue. As shown by Airoldi et al,[1] IL-12 appears to have antiangiogenic and antitumor activity. Is it possible that therapeutic interference with this cytokine activity may predispose to malignancy? Although it is extremely difficult to generalize findings in knock-out mice to humans, the lessons learned from cyclosporine may be worth remembering.

B. H. Thiers, MD

Reference

1. Airoldi I, Di Carlo E, Cocco C. Endogenous IL-12 triggers an antiangiogenic program in melanoma cells. *Proc Natl Acad Sci U S A.* 2007;104:3996-4001.

German evidence-based guidelines for the treatment of psoriasis vulgaris (short version)

Nast A, Kopp I, Augustin M, et al (Charité–Universitätsmedizin Berlin)
Arch Dermatol Res 299:111-138, 2007

Psoriasis vulgaris is a common and chronic inflammatory skin disease which has the potential to significantly reduce the quality of life in severely affected patients. The incidence of psoriasis in Western industrialized countries ranges from 1.5 to 2%. Despite the large variety of treatment options available, patient surveys have revealed insufficient satisfaction with the efficacy of available treatments and a high rate of medication noncompliance. To optimize the treatment of psoriasis in Germany, the Deutsche Dermatologische Gesellschaft and the Berufsverband Deutscher Dermatologen (BVDD) have initiated a project to develop evidence-based guidelines for the management of psoriasis. The guidelines focus on induction therapy in cases of mild, moderate, and severe plaque-type psoriasis in adults. The short version of the guidelines reported here consist of a series of therapeutic recommendations that are based on a systematic literature search and subsequent discussion with experts in the field; they have been approved by a team of dermatology experts. In addition to the therapeutic recommendations provided in this short version, the full version of the guidelines includes information on contraindications, adverse events, drug interactions, practicality, and costs as well as detailed information on how best to apply the treatments described.

▶ This is an incredibly well-done review of the available treatments for psoriasis coming from a somewhat different perspective than we use in the United States (see the Tables on p 114 in the original article). It has also been published in an expanded form in a German dermatology journal.[1] Clearly, treatment preferences vary from country to country, based on physician and patient preferences, costs, drug availability, and marketing practices of pharmaceutical companies. The authors of these evidence-based guidelines appear to believe that the new biological agents for psoriasis should be used as second-line systemic therapies after more traditional agents have proven ineffective. There are some in this country who would disagree.

B. H. Thiers, MD

Reference

1. Nast A, Kopp IB, Augustin M, et al. Evidence-based (S3) guidelines for the treatment of psoriasis vulgaris. *J Dtsch Dermatol Ges* 2007;5:1-119.

Polymorphisms in Folate, Pyrimidine, and Purine Metabolism Are Associated with Efficacy and Toxicity of Methotrexate in Psoriasis
Campalani E, Arenas M, Marinaki AM, et al (St John's Inst of Dermatology, London; Guy's and St Thomas' NHS Found Trust, London; King's College, London)
J Invest Dermatol 127:1860-1867, 2007

Methotrexate is the gold standard therapy for moderate to severe psoriasis, but there is marked interpersonal variation in its efficacy and toxicity. We hypothesized that in psoriasis patients, specific common polymorphisms in folate, pyrimidine, and purine metabolic enzymes are associated with methotrexate efficacy and/or toxicity. DNA from 203 retrospectively recruited psoriasis patients treated with methotrexate was collected and genotyped by restriction endonuclease digestion or length polymorphism assays. The reduced folate carrier (RFC) 80A allele and the thymidylate synthase (TS) 3'-untranslated region (3'-UTR) 6 bp deletion were associated with methotrexate-induced toxicity ($P=0.025$ and $P=0.025$, respectively). RFC 80A and 5-aminoimidazole-4-carboxamide ribonucleotide transformylase (ATIC) 347G were associated with methotrexate discontinuation ($P=0.048$ and $P=0.038$). The TS 5'-UTR 28 bp 3R polymorphism correlated with poor clinical outcome ($P=0.029$), however, this was not the case when patients with palmoplantar pustular psoriasis were not included in the analysis. Stronger associations between specific polymorphisms and methotrexate-induced toxicity and discontinuation were found in a subanalysis of patients on methotrexate not receiving folic acid supplementation. We have demonstrated preliminary evidence that specific polymorphisms of enzymes involved in folate, pyrimidine, and purine metabolism could be useful in predicting clinical response to methotrexate in patients with psoriasis.

▶ Previously, I've discussed the concept that gene testing can be used to predict patient response to certain drugs. Indeed, pharmacogenetics is the next frontier for dermatologic therapy and for medical therapy in general. Here, Campalani et al sought to investigate the role of common polymorphisms in folate, pyrimidine, and purine metabolic enzymes in predicting potential benefits and adverse events associated with methotrexate therapy for psoriasis.

They found several polymorphisms that have a significant impact on the clinical response to methotrexate and which therefore might act as predictive markers for methotrexate efficacy and toxicity. Pharmacogenetics will help clinicians make better and safer treatment choices in the future.

B. H. Thiers, MD

Psoriasis patients with diabetes type 2 are at high risk of developing liver fibrosis during methotrexate treatment
Rosenberg P, Urwitz H, Johannesson A, et al (Karolinska Univ, Stockholm; Lakarhuset Vallingby, Stockholm)
J Hepatol 46:1111-1118, 2007

Background/Aims.—We investigated the impact of diabetes mellitus type 2, overweight, alcohol over-consumption, and chronic hepatitis B or C as risk factors, for liver fibrosis in psoriasis patients treated with methotrexate.

Methods.—One hundred and sixty-nine liver biopsies from 71 patients who underwent liver biopsies as part of the monitoring of methotrexate treatment for psoriasis were reviewed. Fibrosis, steatosis and inflammation were staged according to the NAFLD activity score.

Results.—Twenty-six patients had one or more of the risk factors and 25 (96%) of these (median cumulative dose methotrexate 1500 mg) developed liver fibrosis. Of those without risk factor, 26 (58%) ($p = 0.012$) developed fibrosis (median cumulative dose methotrexate 2100 mg). Ten (38%) of the patients with risk factor(s) had severe fibrosis (stage 3–4) (mean cumulative dose methotrexate 1600 mg), while four (9%) ($p = 0.0012$) of those without risk factors had severe fibrosis (median cumulative dose methotrexate 1900 mg).

Conclusions.—Patients with methotrexate treated psoriasis and risk factors for liver disease, especially diabetes type 2 or overweight, are at higher risk of developing severe liver fibrosis compared to those without such risk factors, even when lower cumulative methotrexate doses are given.

▶ An increased risk of methotrexate-induced liver fibrosis in diabetic patients is really not surprising, given the hepatic changes that are known to occur in glucose-intolerant patients. Rosenberg et al found that this risk of severe fibrosis in methotrexate-treated patients was dependent on the presence of at least 1 of the following risk factors: obesity, high alcohol consumption, diabetes, or viral hepatitis. They showed a strong correlation between the presence of risk factors for steatohepatitis and the development of severe liver fibrosis in methotrexate-treated patients with psoriasis, but the development of advanced liver fibrosis during long-term treatment with methotrexate was less common in patients with rheumatoid arthritis. Studies such as those done by Sabat et al[1] and others[2,3] have shown an increased risk of diabetes, obesity, and cardiovascular disease in patients with psoriasis, and genetic factors may further increase the risk of liver fibrosis. The authors conclude that patients without risk factors could be monitored with noninvasive methods and could have their first liver biopsy after an accumulated dose of 3 to 4 g, but the guidelines issued by the American Academy of Dermatology seem more appropriate for monitoring patients with definable risk factors.[4] An interesting editorial accompanied this study.[5]

B. H. Thiers, MD

References

1. Sabat R, Philipp S, Höflich C, et al. Immunopathogenesis of psoriasis. *Exp Dermatol.* 2007;16:779-798.
2. Henseler T, Christophers E. Disease concomitance in psoriasis. *J Am Acad Dermatol.* 1995;32:982-986.
3. Mallbris L, Granath F, Hamsten A, Ståhle M. Psoriasis is associated with lipid abnormalities at the onset of skin disease. *J Am Acad Dermatol.* 2006;54:614-621.
4. Roenigk HH Jr, Auerbach R, Maibach H, Weinstein G, Lebwohl M. Methotrexate in psoriasis: consensus conference. *J Am Acad Dermatol.* 1998;38:478-485.
5. Aithal GP. Dangerous liaisons: drug, host and the environment. *J Hepatol.* 2007; 46:995-998.

Assessment of FIBRO*Spect* II to Detect Hepatic Fibrosis in Chronic Hepatitis C Patients

Zaman A, Rosen HR, Ingram K, et al (Oregon Health & Science Univ, Portland; Prometheus Labs, San Diego, Calif)
Am J Med 120:280.e9-14, 2007

Background.—The degree of liver fibrosis in patients with Hepatitis C (HCV) provides important prognostic information; however, the only current method available to obtain this information is by performing a liver biopsy. Liver biopsies are invasive, associated with complications, and costly. There has been recent interest in developing a panel of serum markers that can reliably predict the presence of fibrosis and, thus, obviate the need for a liver biopsy. Our objective was to prospectively validate a panel of serum fibrosis markers (FIBRO*Spect*[SM] II) that has been recently developed.

Methods.—Serum was obtained from 108 consecutive HCV (15% with HCV/ETOH) patients seen in a hepatology clinic at a single tertiary care center at the time of liver biopsy. The performance of FIBRO*Spect* II (consisting of 3 fibrosis markers: hyaluronic acid, tissue inhibitor of metalloproteinases 1, and alpha-2-macroglobulin) in differentiating mild (F0-F1) from significant (F2-F4) fibrosis was assessed by comparing the panel results with performed liver biopsy.

Results.—The prevalence of significant fibrosis in the study group was 36.1%. The diagnostic value of the serum marker panel to detect significant fibrosis as assessed by area under the receiver operating characteristic (ROC) curve was 0.826. Performance characteristics are as follows: sensitivity 71.8%, specificity 73.9%, positive predictive value 60.9%, negative predictive value 82.3%, and overall accuracy of 73.1%.

Conclusion.—This prospective study supports the clinical utility of serum markers in detecting fibrosis and validates the performance of FIBRO*Spect*

II in a prospective cohort of patients. The high negative predictive value of the test provides a reliable alternative to rule out severe fibrosis.

▶ Liver biopsy is the gold standard for determining the degree of hepatic fibrosis. However, it is an expensive and invasive procedure. The FIBRO*Spect* II panel measures the serum level of 3 fibrosis markers. Zaman et al show that in patients with chronic HCV, the test can effectively identify patients who do not have fibrosis, but it may not be useful in differentiating between intermediate stages of fibrosis.

Why should this be of interest to dermatologists? As a frequent prescriber of methotrexate for patients with severe psoriasis, I have often referred patients to our digestive disease service for a liver biopsy. Quite often, this test has been recommended as a preliminary screening device to assess whether liver biopsy is really needed. It must be emphasized, however, that the National Institutes of Health does not consider the FIBRO*Spect* II to be a substitute for a liver biopsy. Nevertheless, our digestive disease physicians agree with Zaman et al that a negative test does have good predictive value for ruling out the possibility of hepatic fibrosis. It also must be remembered that there are no data to evaluate the efficacy of the FIBRO*Spect* II in assessing the possibility of fibrosis in methotrexate-treated patients. Like this article, existing data are based on patients with documented HCV infection.

B. H. Thiers, MD

Adalimumab for severe psoriasis and psoriatic arthritis: An open-label study in 30 patients previously treated with other biologics
Papoutsaki M, Chimenti M-S, Costanzo A, et al (Univ of Rome "Tor Vergata"; Univ of Rome "La Sapienza")
J Am Acad Dermatol 57:269-275, 2007

Background.—Psoriasis is a chronic, genetically determined, immune-mediated, inflammatory skin disease affecting approximately 2% to 3% of the Caucasian population. Previously reported data demonstrated adalimumab to be an efficacious treatment of psoriatic arthritis and plaque-type psoriasis. Adalimumab is a fully human monoclonal antibody IgG1 against tumor necrosis factor alpha.

Objective.—To evaluate the efficacy and safety of adalimumab, in the treatment of psoriasis patients whose disease is refractory to treatment with other biologic agents.

Patients and Methods.—Thirty patients affected by plaque-type psoriasis with or without psoriatic arthritis, unresponsive to conventional and biologic systemic treatments were enrolled. Adalimumab was administered in monotherapy, at a dosage of 40 mg, subcutaneously, once a week.

Results.—At week 12, 26 of 30 patients (87%) achieved Psoriasis Area and Severity Index (PASI) 75; at week 24, 25 of 30 patients (83%) achieved PASI 75. Concerning psoriatic arthritis, at week 24, the mean Health Assessment Questionnaire score improved from 0.99 to 0.2, Ritchie articular in-

TABLE 1.—Type of Psoriasis, Previous Biological Treatments, Reason for Discontinuation, and Efficacy of Adalimumab Treatment at 24 Weeks*

Patient No.	Type of Psoriasis	Previous Biologic tx†	Duration of tx (wk)	Reason for Discontinuation	Efficacy of Adalimumab tx at wk 24
1	PsV	Ef-Et-*In*	22	AE (fever)	PASI 90
2	PsA	Et-*In*	38	LT lack of efficacy	PASI 90
3	PsV	In-Et-*Ef*	12	Lack of efficacy	PASI 90
4	PsA	Et-*In*	54	LT lack of efficacy	PASI 75
5	PsA	In-*Et*	12	Lack of efficacy	*Stopped at wk 12*
6	PA	In-*Et*	12	Lack of efficacy	PASI 90
7	PsA	In-*Et*	12	Lack of efficacy	PASI 90
8	PsV	Ef-Et-*In*	62	LT lack of efficacy	PASI 90
9	PsA	Et-*In*	70	LT lack of efficacy	PASI 90
10	PsA	Et-*In*	22	Lack of efficacy	PASI 90
11	PsA	In-*Et*	12	Lack of efficacy	<PASI 50
12	PsV	In-Et-*Ef*	9	AE (generalized inflammatory reaction)	PASI 90
13	PsV	Ef-Et-*In*	86	LT lack of efficacy	PASI 90
14	PsA	In-*Et*	24	LT lack of efficacy	PASI 75
15	PsV	In-Et-*Ef*	24	LT lack of efficacy	PASI 90
16	PsA	In-*Et*	4	Lack of efficacy	*Stopped at wk 20*
17	PsV	Ef-Et-*In*	70	LT lack of efficacy	PASI 90
18	PsA	In-*Et*	36	LT lack of efficacy	<PASI 90
19	PsV	Ef-Et-*In*	70	LT lack of efficacy	PASI 90
20	PsV	Ef-Et-*In*	62	LT lack of efficacy	PASI 90
21	PsA	In-*Et*	36	LT lack of efficacy	PASI 90
22	PsA	Et-*In*	38	LT lack of efficacy	PASI 90
23	PsA	Et-*In*	30	LT lack of efficacy	PASI 90
24	PsA	In-*Et*	12	Lack of efficacy	*Stopped at wk 16*
25	PsA	Et-*In*	2	AE (allergic reaction with asthma)	PASI 90
26	PsA	Et-*In*	22	Lack of efficacy	PASI 90
27	PsA	Et-*In*	22	Lack of efficacy	PASI 90
28	PsV	Ef-In-*Et*	12	Lack of efficacy	PASI 90
29	PsV	In-Et-*Ef*	12	Lack of efficacy	PASI 90
30	PsA	Et-*In*	22	Lack of efficacy	PASI 90

AE, Adverse event; *Ef*, efalizumab; *Et*, etanercept; *In*, infliximab; *LT*, long term; *PASI*, Psoriasis Area and Severity Index; *PsA*, psoriatic arthritis; *PsV*, plaque-type psoriasis; *tx*,therapy; *wk*,week(s).

*Infliximab and efalizumab were administered according to standard protocol for psoriasis (infliximab at 5 mg/kg at time 0 and at 2, 6, and every 8 weeks, efalizumab at a dosage of 1 mg/kg once a week); etanercept was administered at a dosage of 50 mg twice weekly.

†Italics shows last drug used prior to adalimumab.

(Courtesy of Papoutsaki M, Chimenti M-S, Costanzo A, et al. Adalimumab for severe psoriasis and psoriatic arthritis: an open-label study in 30 patients previously treated with other biologics. *J Am Acad Dermatol.* 2007;57:269-275. Copyright Elsevier, 2007.)

dex from 10.15 to 2, and Pain Visual Assessment Score from 6.32 to 1.2. Furthermore, therapy with adalimumab considerably enhanced patients' quality of life as assessed by two measures (Dermatology Life Quality Index, Psoriasis Disability Index). Adalimumab was generally safe and well tolerated.

Limitations.—This is not a randomized placebo-controlled study and is restricted to a small number of patients.

Conclusions.—In our experience, although preliminary, monotherapy with adalimumab 40 mg weekly proved to be an effective and safe treatment for the management of plaque-type psoriasis and psoriatic arthritis, with a rapid onset of action in patients whose disease had been refractory to both conventional and biologic agents (Table 1).

▶ Adalimumab, a humanized monoclonal antibody against TNF-α, is quickly emerging as the most potent self-administered biological agent for the treatment of psoriasis, with PASI 75 scores exceeding those of other comparable drugs. Only infliximab appears to be more effective, although with the disadvantage of requiring IV infusion.

Papoutsaki et al report on the results of an open study of 30 patients who were unresponsive to or who had contraindications to conventional systemic treatments as well as phototherapy, and who had failed to respond to other biological agents, including efalizumab, etanercept, and infliximab. These patients were treated with adalimumab, 40 mg subcutaneous weekly, often with dramatic results (Table 1).

In a study by Saurat et al,[1] the investigators present a rarity in the contemporary medical literature: a head-to-head comparison between 2 currently marketed drugs for a well-defined indication, in this case, psoriasis. Often drugs are compared by their response rates in uncontrolled or placebo-controlled studies, an inappropriate approach as protocols differ with respect to inclusion and exclusion criteria, drug dosing and administration, investigator assessment of patient response, data analysis, and so forth. In the Saurat et al study,[1] patients with moderate to severe psoriasis received either adalimumab (80 mg subcutaneously at baseline, then 40 mg every other week), methotrexate (7.5-25 mg weekly), or placebo for 16 weeks. The adalimumab-treated patients achieved peak PASI 75 significantly more frequently than did those treated with methotrexate or placebo (although the 19% PASI-75 rate for placebo might raise some eyebrows). Nevertheless, the data for these 2 studies suggest that adalimumab is a potent and important treatment for refractory plaque-type psoriasis.

B. H. Thiers, MD

Reference

1. Saurat J-H, Stingl G, Dubertret L, et al. Efficacy and safety results from the randomized controlled comparative study of adalimumab vs. methotrexate vs. placebo in patients with psoriasis (CHAMPION). *Br J Dermatol.* 2008;158:558-566.

Efficacy and safety results from the randomized controlled comparative study of adalimumab vs. methotrexate vs. placebo in patients with psoriasis (CHAMPION)

Saurat J-H, for the CHAMPION Study Investigators (Hôpital Cantonal Universitaire, Geneva; et al)
Br J Dermatol 158:558-566, 2007

Background.—Biologic therapies such as adalimumab, a tumour necrosis factor antagonist, are safe and effective in the treatment of moderate to severe chronic plaque psoriasis.

Objectives.—To compare a biologic agent with methotrexate, a traditional systemic agent, to define clearly the role of biologics in psoriasis.

Methods.—Patients with moderate to severe plaque psoriasis were randomized to adalimumab (80 mg subcutaneously at week 0, then 40 mg every other week, $n = 108$), methotrexate (7.5 mg orally, increased as needed and as tolerated to 25 mg weekly; $n = 110$) or placebo ($n = 53$) for 16 weeks. The primary efficacy endpoint was the proportion of patients achieving at least a 75% improvement in the Psoriasis Area and Severity Index (PASI 75) after 16 weeks. Safety was assessed at all visits through week 16.

Results.—After 16 weeks, 79.6% of adalimumab-treated patients achieved PASI 75, compared with 35.5% for methotrexate ($P < 0.001$ vs. adalimumab) and 18.9% for placebo ($P < 0.001$ vs. adalimumab). Statistically significantly more adalimumab-treated patients (16.7%) than methotrexate-treated patients (7.3%) or placebo-treated patients (1.9%) achieved complete clearance of disease. The response to adalimumab was rapid, with a 57% improvement in mean PASI observed at week 4. Adverse events were similar across treatment groups. Adverse events leading to study discontinuation were greatest in the methotrexate group, primarily because of hepatic-related adverse events.

Conclusions.—After 16 weeks, adalimumab demonstrated significantly superior efficacy and more rapid improvements in psoriasis compared with either methotrexate or placebo.

▶ Adalimumab, a humanized monoclonal antibody against TNF-α, is quickly emerging as the most potent self-administered biological agent for the treatment of psoriasis, with PASI 75 scores exceeding those of other comparable drugs. Only infliximab appears to be more effective, although with the disadvantage of requiring IV infusion. In a study by Papoutsaki et al,[1] the investigators report on the results of an open study of 30 patients who were unresponsive to or who had contraindications to conventional systemic treatments as well as phototherapy, and who had failed to respond to other biological agents, including efalizumab, etanercept, and infliximab. These patients were treated with adalimumab, 40 mg subcutaneous weekly, often with dramatic results. This current study by Saurat et al is a rarity in the contemporary medical literature: a head-to-head comparison between 2 currently marketed drugs for a well-defined indication, in this case, psoriasis. Often drugs are compared by their response rates in uncontrolled or placebo-controlled studies, an inappropriate approach as protocols differ with respect to inclusion and exclusion criteria, drug dosing and administration, investigator assessment of patient response, data analysis, and so forth. In this particular study, patients with moderate to severe psoriasis received either adalimumab (80 mg subcutaneously at baseline, then 40 mg every other week), methotrexate (7.5 mg-25 mg weekly), or placebo for 16 weeks. The adalimumab-treated patients achieved peak PASI 75 significantly more frequently than did those treated with methotrexate or placebo (although the 19% PASI-75 rate for placebo might raise some eyebrows). Nevertheless, the data for these 2 studies suggest that adalimumab is a potent and important treatment for refractory plaque-type psoriasis.

B. H. Thiers, MD

Reference

1. Papoutsaki M, Chimenti M-S, Costanzo A, et al. Adalimumab for severe psoriasis and psoriatic arthritis: an open-label study in 30 patients previously treated with other biologics. *J Am Acad Dermatol.* 2007;57:269-275.

Safety and Efficacy of Adalimumab in Treatment of Patients with Psoriatic Arthritis Who Had Failed Disease Modifying Antirheumatic Drug Therapy
Genovese MC, for the M02-570 Study Group (Stanford Univ Med Ctr, Palo Alto, Calif; et al)
J Rheumatol 34:1040-1050, 2007

Objective.—To demonstrate the safety and efficacy of adalimumab for the treatment of active psoriatic arthritis (PsA) in patients with an inadequate response to disease modifying antirheumatic drugs (DMARD).

Methods.—In a placebo controlled, double-blind, randomized, multicenter study, patients were treated for 12 weeks with subcutaneous injections of adalimumab 40 mg every other week (eow) or placebo, followed by a period of open-label treatment with adalimumab 40 mg eow. The primary efficacy endpoint was the percentage of patients who met the American College of Rheumatology (ACR20) core criteria at Week 12. Secondary efficacy measures included the modified Psoriatic Arthritis Response Criteria (PsARC) and assessments of disability, psoriatic lesions, and quality of life. For missing data, nonresponder imputation was used for ACR and PsARC scores and last observation carried forward for other measures.

Results.—A total of 100 patients received study drug (51 adalimumab, 49 placebo). At Week 12, an ACR20 response was achieved by 39% of adalimumab patients versus 16% of placebo patients (p = 0.012), and a PsARC response was achieved by 51% with adalimumab versus 24% with placebo (p = 0.007). At Week 12, measures of skin lesions and disability were statistically significantly improved with adalimumab. After Week 12, open-label adalimumab provided continued improvement for adalimumab patients and initiated rapid improvement for placebo patients, with ACR20 response rates of 65% and 57%, respectively, observed at Week 24. Serious adverse events had similar frequencies during therapy with placebo (4.1%), blinded adalimumab (2.0%), and open-label adalimumab (3.1%). No serious infections occurred during adalimumab therapy.

Conclusion.—In this study of patients who had active PsA and a previous, inadequate response to DMARD therapy, adalimumab was well tolerated and significantly reduced the signs, symptoms, and disability of PsA during 12 weeks of blinded and 12 weeks of open-label therapy. Adalimumab also improved psoriasis in these patients.

▶ The authors report the results of a 12-week randomized double-blind placebo controlled trial with a 12-week open label extension that evaluated adalimumab therapy in 100 adult patients with moderate to severe psoriatic arthritis. They show that the drug is effective and well tolerated in treating both psoriatic arthritis and the underlying psoriasis. Adalimumab is a human anti-TNF monoclonal antibody and the cautions associated with the use of other TNF inhibitors must be respected.

B. H. Thiers, MD

A randomized comparison of continuous vs. intermittent infliximab maintenance regimens over 1 year in the treatment of moderate-to-severe plaque psoriasis
Menter A, Feldman SR, Weinstein GD, et al (Baylor Univ Med Ctr, Dallas; Wake Forest Univ School of Medicine, Winston-Salem, NC; Univ of California, Irvine; et al)
J Am Acad Dermatol 56:31-44, 2007

Background.—Previous studies of infliximab in psoriasis have demonstrated rapid improvement with induction therapy and sustained response with regularly administered maintenance therapy.

Objective.—The efficacy and safety of continuous (every–8-week) and intermittent (as-needed) maintenance regimens were compared.

Methods.—Patients with moderate-to-severe psoriasis (n = 835) were randomized to induction therapy (weeks 0, 2, and 6) with infliximab 3 mg/kg or 5 mg/kg or placebo. Infliximab-treated patients were randomized again at week 14 to continuous or intermittent maintenance regimens at their induction dose.

Results.—At week 10, 75.5% and 70.3% of patients in the infliximab 5 mg/kg and 3 mg/kg groups, respectively, achieved PASI 75; 45.2% and 37.1% achieved PASI 90 (vs 1.9% [PASI 75] and 0.5% [PASI 90] for placebo; $P < .001$). Through week 50, PASI responses were better maintained with continuous compared with intermittent therapy within each dose, and with 5 mg/kg compared with 3 mg/kg continuous therapy.

Limitations.—Longer term (>1 year) maintenance therapy and further study of infliximab serum concentrations over this period, in both PASI 75 responders and non-responders, would be preferable.

Conclusions.—Through week 50, response was best maintained with continuous infliximab therapy. Infliximab was generally well-tolerated in most patients.

▶ This article by Menter et al and a study done by Poulalhon et al[1] confirm the high degree of efficacy of infliximab infusions in patients with moderate-to-severe psoriasis. Menter et al demonstrate that for sustained remission, every-8-week continuous maintenance therapy is superior to intermittent as-needed therapy. Poulalhon et al found a high frequency of infliximab-induced biologic autoimmunity without, in most cases, clinical evidence of autoimmunity. Nevertheless, especially considering the concomitant onset of polyarthritis in 3 cases, long-term prospective studies are warranted to accurately evaluate the clinical significance of the serologic abnormalities.

B. H. Thiers, MD

Reference

1. Poulalhon N, Begon E, Lebbé C, et al. A follow-up study in 28 patients treated with infliximab for severe recalcitrant psoriasis: evidence for efficacy and high incidence of biological autoimmunity. *Br J Dermatol.* 2007;156:329-336.

A follow-up study in 28 patients treated with infliximab for severe recalcitrant psoriasis: evidence for efficacy and high incidence of biological autoimmunity
Poulalhon N, Begon E, Lebbé C, et al (Université Paris 7; Université Médicine Paris 7)
Br J Dermatol 156:329-336, 2007

Background.—Infliximab, an antitumour necrosis factor-α chimeric monoclonal antibody, is effective for the treatment of severe psoriasis. While the induction of antinuclear antibodies (ANA) and antidouble-stranded-DNA antibodies (anti-dsDNA-ab) is frequently observed in patients with rheumatoid arthritis and Crohn disease receiving infliximab, the incidence of induced biological and clinical autoimmunity remains unknown in the context of psoriasis.

Objectives.—To investigate biological and clinical signs of autoimmunity in 28 patients receiving infliximab for severe, recalcitrant forms of psoriasis, and the clinical response to treatment.

Methods.—Twenty-eight patients, 15 men and 13 women (median age 39.4 years) with psoriasis refractory to three or more systemic treatments were included. Twenty presented with plaque-type psoriasis [median Psoriasis Area and Severity Index (PASI) score 25.9; range 7.2–48], five with psoriatic erythroderma (median PASI score 54; range 48–72) and three with generalized pustular psoriasis (GPP). Psoriatic arthritis was present in 13 patients (46.4%). Infliximab 5 mg kg^{-1} was given at week (W) 0, W2, W6 and every 8 weeks thereafter. Clinical data were assessed at baseline and before each infusion. Detection of ANA and of IgM and IgG anti dsDNA ab were performed at baseline and at W22 by immunofluorescence and enzyme-linked immunosorbent assay, respectively.

Results.—The mean number of infliximab infusions was 5.5 (range 2–15). Among patients with plaque-type and erythrodermic psoriasis, 17 of 25 (68%) and three of five reached a PASI improvement of 75% or more, respectively, while rapid improvement of clinical and biological signs was observed in all three patients with GPP. The prevalence of positive detection of ANA raised from 12% at baseline to 72% at W22 ($P = 0.0001$), an increase which was also observed for IgM anti-dsDNA-ab (68% vs. 0%, $P < 0.0001$), while no significant change was observed for the IgG isotype (16% vs. 0%, $P = 0.125$). Three patients developed nonerosive polyarthritis, without any other criteria for systemic lupus.

Conclusions.—The incidence of biological autoimmunity is high in patients with refractory psoriasis receiving infliximab. The concomitant onset of polyarthritis in three cases raises the need to investigate the incidence of autoimmune manifestations in psoriatic patients receiving infliximab in further large-scale studies.

▶ This article by Poulalhon et al and a study done by Menter et al[1] confirm the high degree of efficacy of infliximab infusions in patients with moderate-to-severe psoriasis. Menter et al demonstrate that for sustained remission, every 8-week continuous maintenance therapy is superior to intermittent as-needed therapy. Poulalhon et al found a high frequency of infliximab-induced biologic autoimmunity without, in most cases, clinical evidence of autoimmunity. Nevertheless, especially considering the concomittant onset of polyarthritis in 3 cases, long-term prospective studies are warranted to accurately evaluate the clinical significance of the serologic abnormalities.

B. H. Thiers, MD

Reference

1. Menter A, Feldman SR, Weinstein GD, et al. A randomized comparison of continuous vs. intermittent infliximab maintenance regimens over 1 year in the treatment of moderate-to-severe plaque psoriasis. *J Am Acad Dermatol.* 2007;56: 31-44.

Improved Survival in Psoriatic Arthritis With Calendar Time
Ali Y, Tom BDM, Schentag CT, et al (Univ of Toronto; Inst of Public Health, Cambridge, England)
Arthritis Rheum 56:2708-2714, 2007

Objective.—To determine whether there has been a change in mortality rates over the last 3 decades in patients with psoriatic arthritis (PsA) whose cases were followed prospectively.

Methods.—Patients receiving followup care according to a standard protocol at the University of Toronto PsA Clinic between 1978 and 2004 were included. Information on patient deaths was collected prospectively. Mortality data for the general population of Ontario, Canada, stratified by 5-year age bands, sex, and calendar year from 1978 to 2004, were used to calculate the reference rates. Standardized mortality ratios (SMRs) were calculated through use of Poisson regression models for the number of observed deaths. Time trend analyses were performed through the use of 10-year "rolling-average" SMRs and followup period–specific SMRs stratified by the period of entry into clinic.

Results.—Of 680 patients with PsA, 106 (15.6%) (55 women and 51 men) have died. Major causes of death were disease of the circulatory system, neoplasms, diseases of the respiratory system, diseases of the gastrointestinal system, injuries/poisoning, and unknown. The overall SMR for the period 1978–2004 was 1.36 (95% confidence interval 1.12, 1.64). The estimated number of life-years lost by the PsA patient cohort overall was 2.99 years (95% confidence interval 1.14, 4.77). For patients who entered the cohort during the years 1978–1986, the SMRs were 1.89, 1.83, and 1.21 for followup periods 1978–1986, 1987–1995, and 1996–2004, respectively. For patients who entered the cohort during the years 1987–1995, the SMRs were 0.55 and 0.82, while the SMR for those who entered during 1996–2004 was 0.56.

Conclusion.—The drop in SMRs in this PsA clinic population suggests that the mortality risk has improved over time. This improved survival may reflect disease severity at presentation in the earlier cohort as well as earlier diagnosis and more aggressive treatment in the more recent followup period.

▶ The authors show that the mortality risk for patients with PsA was higher in the 1970s and 1980s, and the more recent trend is toward improvement in survival. The reasons for this are uncertain but could indicate greater representation of patients with more severe disease in earlier years. Certainly, another important factor could be better control of the disease in more recent years, in which methotrexate has been given earlier during the disease course and in higher doses than previously. Other explanations cited by the authors include earlier referral of patients, more aggressive patient care (in addition to methotrexate), and more effective management of comorbid conditions. Interestingly, the same investigators previously showed that death in these patients does not appear to correlate with disease severity or proximity to medical care.[1]

B. H. Thiers, MD

Reference

1. Bond S, Farewell VT, Schentag CT, Lawless JF, Gladman DD. Reporting of mortality in a psoriatic arthritis clinic is primarily a function of the number of clinic contacts and not disease severity. *J Rheumatol.* 2005;32:2364-2367.

Psoriasis and Pustular Dermatitis Triggered by TNF-α Inhibitors in Patients With Rheumatologic Conditions

de Gannes GC, Ghoreishi M, Pope J, et al (Univ of British Columbia, Vancouver, Canada; Univ of Western Ontario, London; Univ of Alberta, Edmonton, Canada; et al)

Arch Dermatol 143:223-231, 2007

Background.—New onset or worsening of psoriasis has been reported in patients treated with tumor necrosis factor α (TNF-α) inhibitors for a variety of rheumatologic conditions. There is mounting evidence that a key innate immune pathway for triggering common human autoimmune disease, including psoriasis, involves plasmacytoid dendritic cell precursors (PDCs) and type 1 interferon (IFN) production. We present herein a case series with clinical and histopathologic evidence of psoriasis in patients with rheumatologic disease treated with TNF-α inhibitors. We propose that the cross regulation between TNF-α and IFN may have a role in the pathogenesis of this reaction.

Observations.—We observed new-onset psoriasis (n = 13) or severe exacerbation of psoriasis (n = 2) in 15 patients with a variety of rheumatologic conditions—rheumatoid arthritis (n = 13), psoriatic arthritis (n = 1), and seronegative arthritis (n = 1)—during treatment with etanercept (n = 6), infliximab (n = 5), and adalimumab (n = 4). Immunohistochemical staining of skin biopsy specimens for myxovirus-resistance protein A (MxA, a surrogate marker for lesional type 1 IFN activity) showed increased staining in TNF-α inhibitor–induced psoriasis compared with psoriasis vulgaris.

Conclusions.—New onset or severe exacerbation of psoriasis is a rare complication of TNF-α inhibitor therapy. The finding of increased production of IFN-α in TNF-α inhibitor–induced psoriasis is a possible pathophysiologic explanation for this reaction.

▶ The apparent paradox of a class of drugs that is highly effective for psoriasis actually inducing the disease is discussed in an accompanying editorial by Fiorentino.[1] He takes special note of the relative frequency of pustular lesions noted in such patients. Additionally, as noted by de Gannes et al, TNF-α inhibition is associated with IFN-α activation, and IFN-α has been associated with precipitation or reactivation of psoriasis. Clearly the cytokine milieu differs from patient to patient, as does the response to immunomodulatory therapies. A better understanding of the complex biological interactions involved in the pathogenesis of psoriasis will likely lead to even better therapies in the future.

B. H. Thiers, MD

Reference

1. Fiorentino DF. The yin and yang of TNF-α inhibition. *Arch Dermatol.* 2007;143: 233-236.

Oral R115866 in the treatment of moderate to severe plaque-type psoriasis

Verfaille CJ, Thissen CACB, Bovenschen HJ, et al (Maastricht Univ, The Netherlands; Univ Hosp Maastricht, The Netherlands; Radboud Univ, Nijmegen, The Netherlands; et al)

J Eur Acad Dermatol Venereol 21:1038-1046, 2007

Background.—R115866 (Rambazole®) is a new generation all-*trans* retinoic acid metabolism blocking agent, highly specific against the retinoic acid 4-hydroxylase. The drug alleviates hyperproliferation and normalizes differentiation of the epidermis in animal models of psoriasis.

Objective.—To explore the efficacy, safety and tolerability of systemic R115866 in patients with moderate to severe plaque-type psoriasis.

Patients and Methods.—In this open label, single-arm trial, patients were treated with R115866, 1 mg/day for 8 weeks, followed by a 2-week treatment-free follow-up period. Patients were monitored for efficacy and safety.

Results.—Nineteen patients (intent-to-treat population) were treated and 14 completed the entire study. Two patients discontinued due to lack of efficacy and three due to adverse events. At the end of the treatment, 26% of the patients showed at least 50% reduction in Psoriasis Area Severity Index (PASI) compared to baseline. Further improvement was observed at the end of the 2-week follow-up period where 47% of the patients showed a 50% or greater reduction in PASI. Kinetic data showed no evidence of accumulation of either R115866 or retinoic acid in plasma. The most common adverse events were pruritus, xerosis, cheilitis and an increase in blood triglycerides. The majority of adverse events were mild to moderate. No deaths or serious adverse events were reported.

Conclusion.—Eight-week daily treatment with 1 mg R115866 resulted in a significant reduction in PASI from baseline to end of therapy. Additional improvement was seen after the 2-week follow-up period. The drug was well tolerated. R115866 merits further evaluation to optimize its clinical efficacy and safety profile in moderate to severe plaque-type psoriasis.

▶ This same compound has also been tested for the treatment of acne.[1] It is an all-*trans* retinoic acid (RA) metabolism-blocking agent. The rationale behind its use is that it blocks the breakdown of the body's own all-*trans* RA, thereby augmenting endogenous intracellular all-*trans* RA levels. In animal models, a single oral dose of the drug transiently increases endogenous all-*trans* RA in rat skin. The current study suggests the possible efficacy of this drug in moderate to severe plaque-type psoriasis. In contrast to the aforementioned acne study, both male and female patients were included in the trial, although the issue of teratogenesis was not addressed. Higher doses and a treatment duration extending beyond 8 weeks might increase both the therapeutic efficacy and the potential side effects.

B. H. Thiers, MD

Reference

1. Verfaille CJ, Coel M, Boersma IH, Mertens J, Borgers M, Roseeuw D. Oral R115866 in the treatment of moderate to severe facial acne vulgaris: an exploratory study. 2007;157:122-126.

Loss-of-Function Variants of the Filaggrin Gene Are Not Major Susceptibility Factors for Psoriasis Vulgaris or Psoriatic Arthritis in German Patients

Hüffmeier U, Traupe H, Oji V, et al (Univ Erlangen-Nuremberg, Germany; Univ of Münster, Germany; Paulinenkrankenhaus, Bad Bentheim, Germany; et al)
J Invest Dermatol 127:1367-1370, 2007

Psoriasis vulgaris and atopic dermatitis share a number of features such as chronic cutaneous inflammation and disturbed epidermal barrier function. Genome-wide scans have revealed a conspicuous overlap of susceptibility loci for both diseases involving chromosomal regions 1q21, 3q21, 17q25, and 20p12. Recently, two loss-of-function variants in the gene encoding filaggrin at 1q21 were shown to be strongly associated with atopic dermatitis. In view of a possible genetic overlap of the two skin diseases, we investigated 375 patients suffering from psoriasis vulgaris, 375 patients with psoriatic arthritis, and 376 control probands. Moreover we directly studied expression of filaggrin in 10 patients suffering from psoriasis vulgaris. Our immunohistochemical analysis revealed a checkered pattern with alternating positive broadened or almost absent filaggrin expression. However, no association was found for the two variants of filaggrin (*FLG*). We conclude that despite a markedly altered filaggrin expression in psoriatic skin, loss-of-function variants of the *FLG* gene are neither associated with psoriasis vulgaris nor with psoriatic arthritis. The abnormal staining might reflect the altered epidermal differentiation. Our findings imply that the genetic background underlying the epidermal barrier defect in psoriasis is distinct from that found in atopic dermatitis.

▶ Loss-of-function mutations in the gene encoding filaggrin, which is an epidermal barrier protein, have been associated with ichthyosis vulgaris and atopic dermatitis.[1,2] Hüffmeier and colleagues failed to demonstrate a similar association for psoriasis or psoriatic arthritis, which is a not particularly surprising observation given the dissimilar pathogenetic mechanisms involved in psoriasis and psoriatic arthritis as compared with the other two diseases. Given the rarity of seeing both psoriasis and atopic dermatitis in the same individual, one would not expect to find that psoriasis and atopic dermatitis share a common genetic basis.

B. H. Thiers, MD

References

1. Smith FJ, Irvine AD, Terron-Kwiatkowski A, et al. Loss-of-function mutations in the gene encoding filaggrin cause ichthyosis vulgaris. *Nat Genet.* 2006;38:337-342.
2. Palmer CN, Irvine AD, Terron-Kwiatkowski A, et al. Common loss-of-function variants of the epidermal barrier protein filaggrin are a major predisposing factor for atopic dermatitis. *Nat Genet.* 2006;38:441-446.

Obesity, Waist Circumference, Weight Change, and the Risk of Psoriasis in Women: Nurses' Health Study II

Setty AR, Curhan G, Choi HK (Harvard Med School; Univ of British Columbia, Vancouver, Canada)
Arch Intern Med 167:1670-1675, 2007

Background.—Psoriasis is a common, chronic, inflammatory skin disorder. Higher adiposity may increase the risk of psoriasis, but, to our knowledge, no prospective data are available on this relationship.

Methods.—We prospectively examined the relationships between body mass index (BMI [calculated as weight in kilograms divided by height in meters squared]), weight change, waist circumference, hip circumference, waist-hip ratio, and incident psoriasis in 78,626 women over a 14-year period (1991-2005) in the Nurses' Health Study II. The primary outcome was incident, self-reported, physician-diagnosed psoriasis.

Results.—During the 14 years of follow-up, there were 892 self-reported incident cases of psoriasis. There was a graded positive association between BMI measured at multiple time points and the risk of incident psoriasis. When we analyzed BMI updated every 2 years, compared with a BMI of 21.0 through 22.9, the multivariate relative risks of psoriasis were 1.40 (95% confidence interval [CI], 1.13-1.73) for a BMI of 25.0 through 29.9; 1.48 (95% CI, 1.15-1.91) for a BMI of 30.0 through 34.9; and 2.69 (95% CI, 2.12-3.40) for a BMI of 35.0 or greater (P for trend, <.001). For BMI at the age of 18 years, the multivariate relative risk for the top BMI category ($\geq$30.0) was 1.73 (95% CI, 1.24-2.41) and that for a lower BMI category (<21.0) was 0.76 (95% CI, 0.65-0.90) (P for trend, <.001). Weight gain from the age of 18 years, higher waist circumference, hip circumference, and waist-hip ratio were all associated with a higher risk of incident psoriasis (all P values for trend, <.001).

Conclusion.—This large prospective study indicates that increased adiposity and weight gain are strong risk factors for incident psoriasis in women.

▶ The authors sought to prospectively evaluate the relationship between obesity and the incidence of psoriasis in a large prospective cohort of women. They found that measures such as the BMI, waist and hip circumference, waist:hip ratio, and factors such as weight gain since the age of 18 years were important risk factors for the development of the disease. The risk of psoriasis increased along with levels of adiposity, and a strong, consistent, dose–

response relationship was found. Conversely, a BMI of less than 21 correlated with a low risk of psoriasis. This study provides the first prospective evidence that obesity is a strong risk factor for the development of psoriasis and suggests that weight loss may be a potential target for the prevention and management of the disease.

B. H. Thiers, MD

Psoriasis: a possible risk factor for development of coronary artery calcification

Ludwig RJ, Herzog C, Rostock A, et al (Johann Wolfgang Goethe-Univ, Frankfurt am Main, Germany)
Br J Dermatol 156:271-276, 2007

Background.—Psoriasis is a chronic inflammatory skin disorder affecting about 2% of white-skinned individuals. Epidemiological data on the prevalence and degree of coronary artery calcification (CAC) as an indicator for cardiovascular diseases in patients with psoriasis are contradictory.

Objectives.—To study the prevalence and degree of CAC as an indicator for cardiovascular diseases in 32 patients with psoriasis matched for age, sex and risk factors to an equally sized control population.

Methods.—Noncontrast-enhanced 16-row spiral computed tomography was performed in patients and controls.

Results.—We found a significantly increased prevalence (59.4% vs. 28.1%, P = 0.015) and severity (CAC score according to Agatston 3.7 vs. 0.0, P = 0.019) of CAC in patients with psoriasis. Multiple linear regression calculations identified psoriasis as a likely independent risk factor for CAC.

Conclusions.—Our results point towards the potentially systemic nature of the inflammatory processes underlying the pathogenesis of psoriasis, which may therefore be considered a potentially severe systemic disease.

▶ Neimann et al[1] have previously shown that psoriasis is associated with multiple cardiovascular risk factors, with the association being strongest for patients with severe disease. Gelfand et al[2] reported that psoriasis confers an independent risk of myocardial infarction, with the relative risk being greatest for young patients with severe disease. The findings reported here by Ludwig et al are consistent with these previous observations. They show that psoriasis may be an independent risk factor for CAC and hypothesize that this results from a systemic inflammatory response associated with the skin disease. The importance of these findings is emphasized by evidence that CAC may be an accurate proxy for coronary atherosclerosis and a predictor of future atherosclerotic cardiovascular events.

B. H. Thiers, MD

References

1. Neimann AL, Shin DB, Wang X, Margolis DJ, Troxel AB, Gelfand JM. Prevalence of cardiovascular risk factors in patients with psoriasis. *J Am Acad Dermatol.* 2006;55:829-835.
2. Gelfand JM, Neimann AL, Shin DB, Wang X, Margolis DJ, Troxel AB. Risk of myocardial infarction in patients with psoriasis. *JAMA.* 2006;296:1735-1741.

High Prevalence of Thyroid Disease in Patients with Lichen Sclerosus
Birenbaum DL, Young RC (Dartmouth Hitchcock Med Ctr, Lebanon, NH)
J Reprod Med 52:28-30, 2007

Objective.—To investigate the association between lichen sclerosus and thyroid disease in our patient population.

Study Design.—This was a retrospective chart review of patients seen between January 1995 and September 2005 with biopsy-proven lichen sclerosus. Charts were reviewed to assess the patients' history of thyroid disease.

Results.—We identified 211 patients with biopsy-proven lichen sclerosus, 63 (29.9%) of whom had thyroid disease. In women < 55 years old, 25 of 74 (33.8%) had thyroid disease; in women $\geq$ 55 years old, 38 of 137 (27.7%) had thyroid disease.

Conclusion.—The prevalence of thyroid disease in our patients with biopsy-proven lichen sclerosus is almost 30% and is not dependent upon age. This prevalence is 5- to 30-fold greater than in the general population.

▶ Previous studies have suggested an autoimmune pathogenesis to lichen sclerosus; associated conditions have included thyroid disease, vitiligo, and alopecia. Birenbaum and Young sought to clarify the association between lichen sclerosus and thyroid disease by determining the prevalence of thyroid disease in their lichen sclerosus patients. Indeed, the prevalence was even higher than previously reported, with thyroid disease occurring 5 to 30 times more frequently in lichen sclerosus patients than in the general population. Admittedly, there may have been some selection bias, as often occurs with data reported from a tertiary care facility. The authors recommend that an assessment of thyroid function be performed in newly diagnosed patients with lichen sclerosus.

B. H. Thiers, MD

Topical testosterone versus clobetasol for vulvar lichen sclerosus
Ayhan A, Guven S, Guvendag Guven ES, et al (Hacettepe Univ, Ankara, Turkey)
Int J Gynecol Obstet 96:117-121, 2007

Objective.—To compare the effects of topical testosterone and clobetasol treatments on symptoms remission and recurrence rates in patients with vulvar lichen sclerosus (LS).

Methods.—A retrospective review of the records showed that, of 140 patients with biopsy-proven vulvar LS, 80 were treated with applications of testosterone propionate 2% in petrolatum and 60 with clobetasol 17-propionate 0.05%.

Results.—The response rates after 6 months were 77.5% for patients treated with testosterone and 91.7% for those treated with clobetasol ($P = 0.02$). The recurrence rates were 20% and 6.7% in the 2 groups, respectively ($P = 0.02$). Premenopausal patients had higher remission rates and lower recurrence rates than postmenopausal patients ($P > 0.05$). Considering whole patients, low remission rates and high recurrence rates were observed in patients who had had a hysterectomy ($P > 0.05$).

Conclusion.—Treatment of LS with a corticosteroid provided excellent remission rates. In this study, clobetasol 17-propionate 0.05% was superior to testosterone for both remission induction and maintenance therapy.

▶ The authors confirm previous reports documenting the efficacy of topical clobetasol in the treatment of vulvar lichen sclerosus. Their retrospective review also found that topical clobetasol was more effective than topical testosterone in the treatment of this condition and was associated with a lower recurrence rate. Premenopausal women appeared to respond better than postmenopausal women. No serious complications were reported.

B. H. Thiers, MD

A case-series of 29 patients with lichen planopilaris: The Cleveland Clinic Foundation experience on evaluation, diagnosis, and treatment
Cevasco NC, Bergfeld WF, Remzi BK, et al (Cleveland Clinic Found, Ohio)
J Am Acad Dermatol 57:47-53, 2007

Background.—Lichen planopilaris results in scaling, atrophy, and permanent alopecia with scarring and is thought to be autoimmune in origin.

Objective.—To evaluate the clinical findings of patients with LPP so as to aid in the evaluation and diagnosis of the disease and to review the current effective therapies.

Methods.—We reviewed the medical records of 29 patients with LPP that were seen in the Department of Dermatology at The Cleveland Clinic Foundation between 1992 and 2003.

Results.—Good responses in the active perimeter were seen with topical steroids, intralesional steroids, and tetracycline and in the inactive end-stage with hair transplants and scalp reductions.

Limitations.—This study was limited by being retrospective in nature.

Conclusion.—Although topical high-potency and intralesional corticosteroids remain the mainstay for treatment of LPP, the use of tetracycline in this disease may be more helpful than once thought.

▶ The provocative finding that the only treatment that provided a statistically significant number of good responses was tetracycline needs to be confirmed.

Other systemic treatments that have been anecdotally reported to be effective in LPP include griseofulvin, acitretin, hydroxychloroquine, cyclosporine, and thalidomide. These drugs have side effects that are by no means insignificant; however, neither should the disease be trivialized because of the associated scarring and the permanent nature of the alopecia.

B. H. Thiers, MD

3 Bacterial, Mycobacterial, and Fungal Infections

Antimicrobial Peptides Human β-Defensins Stimulate Epidermal Keratinocyte Migration, Proliferation and Production of Proinflammatory Cytokines and Chemokines
Niyonsaba F, Ushio H, Nakano N, et al (Juntendo Univ, Tokyo; Ehime Univ, Japan)
J Invest Dermatol 127:594-604, 2007

Besides their microbicidal functions, human β-defensins (hBD) and LL-37 activate different immune and inflammatory cells, and their expression is enhanced in inflamed skin and cutaneous wound sites. To protect against pathogens, the skin produces antimicrobial peptides including hBDs and LL-37. Therefore, the aim of our study was to investigate whether hBDs participate in cutaneous inflammation and wound healing by inducing keratinocyte migration, proliferation, and production of proinflammatory cytokines/chemokines. We found that hBD-2, -3, and -4 but not hBD-1 stimulated human keratinocytes to increase their gene expression and protein production of IL-6, IL-10, IP-10, monocyte chemoattractant protein-1, macrophage inflammatory protein-3α, and RANTES. This stimulatory effect was markedly suppressed by pertussis toxin and U-73122, inhibitors for G protein and phospholipase C, respectively. We also demonstrated that hBDs elicited intracellular Ca^{2+} mobilization, and increased keratinocyte migration, and proliferation. In addition, these peptides induced phosphorylation of EGFR, signal transducer and activator of transcription (STAT)1, and STAT3, which are intracellular signaling molecules involved in keratinocyte migration and proliferation. In our study, inhibition of these molecules significantly reduced hBD-mediated keratinocyte migration and proliferation. In conclusion, this study provides evidence that human antimicrobial peptides may be involved in skin immunity through stimulating cytokine/chemokine production, and participate in wound healing by promoting keratinocyte migration and proliferation.

► It is now recognized that certain players in the innate immune response at mucocutaneous surfaces are not limited to their efficient antimicrobial activities but can also assume complex roles that enhance both the innate and adaptive immune responses. Thus, peptides such as the β-defensins and cathelicidins are, at submicrobicidal concentrations, capable of chemoattraction for various immune effector cells and stimulation of cytokine and chemokine gene expression in a time frame appropriate to a rapid protective response. The term "alarmins" has been coined to aptly describe this behavior.[1] It had previously been shown that the chemoattractive effect of β-defensins on T lymphocytes is mediated by the G protein-linked chemokine receptor CCR6.[2]

In the current study, Niyonsaba et al showed that the activation of cytokine gene expression in keratinocytes by β-defensins and the human cathelicidin LL-37 also involved a G protein receptor. In contrast, stimulation of keratinocyte migration and proliferation appeared to be dependent upon epidermal growth factor receptor signaling. As the function of alarmins in immunity is clarified further, investigation into their therapeutic potential will surely follow.

G. M. P. Galbraith, MD

References

1. Oppenheim JJ, Yang D. Alarmins: chemotactic activators of immune responses. *Curr Opin Immunol.* 2005;17:359-365.
2. Yang D, Chertov O, Bykovskaia SN, et al. β-defensins: linking innate and adaptive immunity through dendritic and T cell CCR6. *Science.* 1999;286:525-528.

Fluoroquinolones vs β-Lactams for Empirical Treatment of Immunocompetent Patients With Skin and Soft Tissue Infections: A Meta-analysis of Randomized Controlled Trials
Falagas ME, Matthaiou DK, Vardakas KZ (Alfa Inst of Biomed Sciences, Athens, Greece; Henry Dunant Hosp, Athens, Greece; Tufts Univ, Boston)
Mayo Clin Proc 81:1553-1566, 2006

Objective.—To compare the effectiveness and safety of fluoroquinolones with β-lactams in the treatment of patients with skin and soft tissue infections (SSTIs).

Methods.—We searched the PubMed database, Cochrane Database of Controlled Trials, and references of relevant articles for study reports published between January 1980 and February 2006.

Results.—Twenty randomized controlled trials that enrolled 4817 patients were included in the analysis. Fluoroquinolones as empirical treatment of patients with SSTIs were more effective than β-lactams for the clinically evaluable patients (90.4% vs 88.2%; odds ratio [OR], 1.29; 95% confidence interval [CI], 1.00-1.66). This was also true in subset analyses of randomized controlled trials that studied ciprofloxacin (OR, 2.49; 95% CI,

1.45-4.26) and for patients with mild to moderate infections (OR, 1.83; 95% CI, 1.13-2.96). In contrast, no difference was found between the compared regimens for patients with moderate to severe infections (OR, 1.12; 95% CI, 0.80-1.55), for patients who did not receive third-generation cephalosporins as the comparator antibiotic (OR, 0.99; 95% CI, 0.73-1.34), or for the microbiologically evaluable patients (OR, 1.19; 95% CI, 0.89-1.59). Fluoroquinolones were also associated with more adverse effects (19.2% vs 15.2%; OR, 1.33; 95% CI, 1.13-1.57).

Conclusion.—The high proportion of successfully treated patients in the compared groups of antibiotics and the development of more adverse effects associated with fluoroquinolone use suggest that these antibiotics do not have substantial advantages compared with β-lactams for empirical treatment of patients with SSTIs.

▶ I have long wondered why physicians abandoned older, inexpensive, highly effective drugs for newer drugs that offer little advantage over existing therapies. Although one could argue that the fluoroquinolones offer a broader spectrum of activity than do the β-lactams, is this really relevant to the average immunocompetent patient that we see with SSTIs? Moreover, the overuse of these newer broad-spectrum agents creates a breeding ground for antibiotic resistance that inevitably will come back to haunt us.

B. H. Thiers, MD

Increasing rates of quinolone-resistant *Neisseria gonorrhoeae* in Paris, France

Farhi D, Gerhardt P, Falissard B, et al (Hôpital Cochin, Paris)
J Eur Acad Dermatol Venereol 21:818-821, 2007

Background.—Quinolone-resistant *Neisseria gonorrhoeae* (QRNG) rates are increasing worldwide.

Objectives.—(i) To assess the rate of QRNG among patients referred to a venereology clinic in Paris between 2000 and 2004; and (ii) to assess associated epidemiological factors.

Methods.—Retrospective study of consecutive cases over 2000–2004. Indications and techniques of swabbing and culture were constant over 2000–2004. Susceptibility of *N. gonorrhoeae* was tested to six antibiotics: ciprofloxacin, amoxicillin, cefotaxime, tetracycline, erythromycin, and spectinomycin. Epidemiological data and anatomical site of *N. gonorrhoeae* infection were collected.

Results.—Annual numbers of cases decreased ($P < 10^{-4}$) from 2000 ($n = 41$) to 2002 ($n = 12$), then increased ($P < 10^{-4}$) in 2004 ($n = 60$). Anorectal gonorrhoea was more frequent in 2003–2004 (22.0%, $n = 18/82$) than in 2000–2002 (3.9%, $n = 3/76$). QRNG rates increased from the period 2000–2002 (1.3%) to 2003 (22.7%, $P < 0.01$), and 2004 (30.2%, $P < 0.005$). All QRNG strains had a minimal inhibitory concentration of ciprofloxacin > 1.0 mg/L, thus fitting the international definition of quinolone resistance.

There were no significant changes in rates of *N. gonorrhoeae* resistance to the five other antibiotics. QRNG tended to be more frequent among men who have sex with men (MSM; 16.7% vs. 7.1%), HIV-infected patient (20.5% vs. 11.9%), and patients having more than five partners during the last year (24.4% vs. 17.1%), but statistical significance was not reached in multivariate analyses.

Conclusion.—We recommend (i) avoiding fluoroquinolones as first-line treatment for *N. gonorrhoeae* infections in Paris; (ii) that first-line treatment relies on third-generation cephalosporins or spectinomycin; and (iii) reinforcing targeted screening and prevention of gonorrhoea, especially among HIV-positive patients and MSM.

▶ This story has been played over and over in the history of medicine: overuse of antibiotics leads to antibiotic resistance. In 2004, the Centers for Disease Control and Prevention (CDC) modified its antimicrobial guidelines for the treatment of gonorrhea. They advised avoiding fluoroquinolones for gonorrhea in gay men and in all patients from Asia, the Pacific Islands (including Hawaii), and California, where fluoroquinolone resistance is especially prevalent. The data from this article would suggest the advisability of adding Paris to the list of locations where geographic factors may guide the choice of therapy.

B. H. Thiers, MD

Effect of antibiotic prescribing on antibiotic resistance in individual children in primary care: prospective cohort study
Chung A, Perera R, Brueggemann AB, et al (Univ of Oxford, England)
BMJ 335:429, 2007

Objective.—To assess the effect of community prescribing of an antibiotic for acute respiratory infection on the prevalence of antibiotic resistant bacteria in an individual child.

Study Design.—Observational cohort study with follow-up at two and 12 weeks.

Setting.—General practices in Oxfordshire.

Participants.—119 children with acute respiratory tract infection, of whom 71 received a β lactam antibiotic.

Main outcome measures.—Antibiotic resistance was assessed by the geometric mean minimum inhibitory concentration (MIC) for ampicillin and presence of the ICE*Hin1056* resistance element in up to four isolates of *Haemophilus* species recovered from throat swabs at recruitment, two weeks, and 12 weeks.

Results.—Prescribing amoxicillin to a child in general practice more than triples the mean minimum inhibitory concentration for ampicillin (9.2 μg/ml v 2.7 μg/ml, P=0.005) and doubles the risk of isolation of *Haemophilus* isolates possessing homologues of ICE*Hin1056* (67% v 36%; relative risk 1.9, 95% confidence interval 1.2 to 2.9) two weeks later. Although this increase is transient (by 12 weeks ampicillin resistance had fallen close to baseline), it is in the context of recovery of the element from 35% of children with *Haemophilus* isolates at recruitment and from 83% (76% to 89%) at some point in the study.

Conclusion.—The short term effect of amoxicillin prescribed in primary care is transitory in the individual child but sufficient to sustain a high level of antibiotic resistance in the population.

▶ Chung et al report that community prescribing of a β lactam antibiotic for acute respiratory infection doubles the prevalence of antibiotic-resistant bacteria in individual children. What do these results mean for dermatologists? As a group, dermatologists are heavy prescribers of antibiotics, mainly for acne. Indiscriminate prescribing of these drugs favors the development of antibiotic resistance, which will undoubtedly continue to appear by natural selection even as new antibiotics come to market. As suggested by Del Mar[1] in an accompanying editorial, antibiotics should be thought of like oil, a non-renewable resource to be carefully husbanded. Whether for acne or any other indication, antibiotics should only be prescribed when they are truly needed.

B. H. Thiers, MD

Reference

1. Del Mar C. Prescribing antibiotics in primary care. *BMJ*. 2007;335:407-408.

Invasive Methicillin-Resistant *Staphylococcus aureus* Infections in the United States
Klevens RM, for the Active Bacterial Core surveillance (ABCs) MRSA Investigators (Ctrs for Disease Control and Prevention, Atlanta, Ga; et al)
JAMA 298:1763-1771, 2007

Context.—As the epidemiology of infections with methicillin-resistant *Staphylococcus aureus* (MRSA) changes, accurate information on the scope and magnitude of MRSA infections in the US population is needed.

Objectives.—To describe the incidence and distribution of invasive MRSA disease in 9 US communities and to estimate the burden of invasive MRSA infections in the United States in 2005.

Design and Setting.—Active, population-based surveillance for invasive MRSA in 9 sites participating in the Active Bacterial Core surveillance (ABCs)/Emerging Infections Program Network from July 2004 through December 2005. Reports of MRSA were investigated and classified as either health care–associated (either hospital-onset or community-onset) or community-associated (patients without established health care risk factors for MRSA).

Main Outcome Measures.—Incidence rates and estimated number of invasive MRSA infections and in-hospital deaths among patients with MRSA in the United States in 2005; interval estimates of incidence excluding 1 site that appeared to be an outlier with the highest incidence; molecular characterization of infecting strains.

Results.—There were 8987 observed cases of invasive MRSA reported during the surveillance period. Most MRSA infections were health care–associated: 5250 (58.4%) were community-onset infections, 2389 (26.6%) were hospital-onset infections; 1234 (13.7%) were community-associated infections, and 114 (1.3%) could not be classified. In 2005, the standardized incidence rate of invasive MRSA was 31.8 per 100,000 (interval estimate, 24.4-35.2). Incidence rates were highest among persons 65 years and older (127.7 per 100,000; interval estimate, 92.6-156.9), blacks (66.5 per 100,000; interval estimate, 43.5-63.1), and males (37.5 per 100,000; interval estimate, 26.8-39.5). There were 1598 in-hospital deaths among patients with MRSA infection during the surveillance period. In 2005, the standardized mortality rate was 6.3 per 100,000 (interval estimate, 3.3-7.5). Molecular testing identified strains historically associated with community-associated disease outbreaks recovered from cultures in both hospital-onset and community-onset health care–associated infections in all surveillance areas.

Conclusions.—Invasive MRSA infection affects certain populations disproportionately. It is a major public health problem primarily related to health care but no longer confined to intensive care units, acute care hospitals, or any health care institution.

▶ The authors present data that demonstrate that MRSA infections are more prevalent than once believed and pose serious health risks not only in hospitals but also in the community at-large. While most such cases represent mild skin infections, the study by Klevens et al focused on more invasive disease. The overall incidence rate of such invasive infections was about 32 per 100,000 people, an "astounding" figure, according to an editorial that accompanied the article.[1] In fact, deaths tied to these infections may exceed those caused by AIDS. Interestingly, only about one quarter of the infections cited involved hospitalized patients, although more than half were in the health care system, including patients who had recently had surgery or were on kidney dialysis. Although the organism is often spread through open wounds or by exposure to medical equipment, in recent years, it has been noted to spread through prisons, gyms, locker rooms, and in poor urban neighborhoods.

B. H. Thiers, MD

Reference

1. Bancroft EA. Antimicrobial resistance: it's not just for hospitals. *JAMA.* 2007; 298:1803-1804.

Emergence of community-acquired methicillin-resistant *Staphylococcus aureus* soft tissue infections
Olesevich M, Kennedy A (Univ of Tennessee, Knoxville)
J Pediatr Surg 42:765-768, 2007

Purpose.—Our objective is to describe the changing incidence of community-acquired methicillin-resistant *Staphylococcus aureus* (CA-MRSA) and its treatment within East Tennessee.

Methods.—A retrospective chart review of 245 patients treated with incision and drainage of soft tissue infections from March 2000 to September 2005 was completed. Consent was obtained from our local institutional review board. Forty patients were excluded because no cultures were recorded or because they failed the criteria for the diagnosis of CA-MRSA. We examined our data using χ^2 analysis. *P* value of less than .05 was considered statistically significant.

Results.—The most common organism cultured was CA-MRSA (33%; 67 of 205). Non–CA-MRSA accounted for 4% (9 of 205). The age of patients ranged from 1 month to 21 years, with a mean age of 6.5 years. Stratified by year, the incidence of positive cultures for CA-MRSA has increased 159% since 2004 and 868% since 2003. In addition, the average age of patients has decreased from 8.3 years in 2000 to 6.1 years in 2005.

Conclusions.—Community-acquired MRSA has emerged as the dominant source of soft tissue infection requiring incision and drainage regardless of site in East Tennessee. This has caused a change in the choice of empiric antibiotic treatment of soft tissue abscesses in our region. These infections now account for the third most common reportable disease to the Department of Health in East Tennessee.

▶ MRSA infections have become ubiquitous in outpatient settings throughout the United States. They have been reported in adults and children. Although sulfonamides and fluoroquinolones often prove useful, resistance to antibiotics beyond the penicillin class, including sulfonamides and fluoroquinolones, has been reported.[1] Culture and sensitivity of infected lesions should guide the therapeutic plan.

B. H. Thiers, MD

Reference

1. Sattler CA, Mason EO Jr, Kaplan SL. Prospective comparison of risk factors and demographic and clinical characteristics of community-acquired, methicillin-resistant versus methicillin-susceptible *Staphylococcus aureus* infection in children. *Pediatr Infec Dis J.* 2002;21:910-917.

Community-Acquired Methicillin-Resistant *Staphylococcus aureus*: An Emerging Problem in the Athletic Population

Rihn JA, Michaels MG, Harner CD (Univ of Pittsburgh, Pa; Children's Hosp of Pittsburgh, Pa)

Am J Sports Med 33:1924-1929, 2005

Participants of contact sports are at risk for outbreaks of skin and soft tissue infection. Causes of reported outbreaks include *Staphylococcus aureus*, herpes simplex virus, *Streptococcus pyogenes*, and several fungi. Although once thought of solely as a nosocomial pathogen, methicillin-resistant *Staphylococcus aureus* has been identified as an emerging problem in the community, particularly in the athletic population. Despite a recent increase in reported outbreaks of community-acquired methicillin-resistant *Staphylococcus aureus* soft tissue infection in athletic teams, many sports medicine physicians are unfamiliar with the epidemiology of this pathogen. It is spread via person-to-person contact and is harbored within the anterior nares and on the skin of carriers. Outbreaks of community-acquired methicillin-resistant *Staphylococcus aureus* soft tissue infection are not treated by traditional β-lactam antibiotics, and they can be difficult to eradicate. Such infections have been associated with significant morbidity, with up to 70% of involved team members requiring hospitalization and intravenous antibiotics. A thorough understanding of community-acquired methicillin-resistant *Staphylococcus aureus* is essential for the sports medicine physician to properly identify, treat, and control infectious outbreaks.

▶ Uncomplicated SSTIs often present as furuncles, carbuncles, or abcesses that can be treated with simple incision and drainage. As shown by Rihn et al, complicating the management of these infections has been the recent emergence of MRSA outside the health care setting. Current guidelines still recommend incision and drainage of fluctuant lesions associated with uncomplicated MRSA SSTIs, with the role of additional antimicrobial therapy being much less established.[1-3] In a study by Ruhe et al,[4] the investigators show that although incision and drainage of any focal collection of fluids remain the mainstay of therapy, administration of active antimicrobial agents is associated with a statistically significant, but only moderate, impact on clinical outcome.

B. H. Thiers, MD

References

1. Stevens DL, Bisno AL, Chambers HF, et al. Practice guidelines for the diagnosis and management of skin and soft-tissue infections. *Clin Infect Dis.* 2005;41:1373-1406.
2. Chambers HF. Community-associated MRSA—resistance and virulence converge. *N Engl J Med.* 2005;352:1485-1487.
3. Moellering RC Jr. The growing menace of community-acquired methicillin-resistant *Staphylococcus aureus.* *Ann Intern Med.* 2006;144:368-369.
4. Ruhe JJ, Smith N, Bradsher RW, Menon A. Community-onset methicillin-resistant *Staphylococcus aureus* skin and soft-tissue infections: impact of antimicrobial therapy on outcome. *Clin Infect Dis.* 2007;44:777-784.

Community-Onset Methicillin-Resistant *Staphylococcus aureus* Skin and Soft-Tissue Infections: Impact of Antimicrobial Therapy on Outcome

Ruhe JJ, Smith N, Bradsher RW, et al (Univ of Arkansas, Little Rock; Central Arkansas Veterans Healthcare System, Little Rock; Arkansas Dept of Health and Human Services, Little Rock)
Clin Infect Dis 44:777-784, 2007

Background.—Conflicting data exist on the role of antimicrobial therapy for the treatment of uncomplicated community-onset methicillin-resistant *Staphylococcus aureus* (MRSA) skin and soft-tissue infections (SSTIs).

Methods.—We performed a retrospective cohort study of 492 adult patients with 531 independent episodes of community-onset MRSA SSTIs, which consisted of abscesses, furuncles/carbuncles, and cellulitis, at 2 tertiary care medical centers. The purpose of the study was to determine the impact of active antimicrobial therapy (i.e., the use of an agent to which the organism is susceptible) and other potential risk factors on the outcome for patients with uncomplicated community-onset MRSA SSTIs. Treatment failure was the primary outcome of interest and was defined as worsening signs of infection associated with microbiological and/or therapeutic indicators of an unsuccessful outcome. Bivariate analyses and logistic regression analyses were preformed to determine predictors of treatment failure.

Results.—An incision and drainage procedure was performed for the majority of patients. Treatment failure occurred in 45 (8%) of 531 episodes of community-onset MRSA SSTI. Therapy was successful for 296 (95%) of 312 patients who received an active antibiotic, compared with 190 (87%) of 219 of those who did not ($P = .001$ in bivariate analysis). Use of an inactive antimicrobial agent was an independent predictor of treatment failure on logistic regression analysis (adjusted odds ratio, 2.80; 95% confidence interval, 1.26–6.22; $P = .01$).

Conclusions.—Our findings suggest that certain patients with SSTIs that are likely caused by MRSA would benefit from treatment with an antimicrobial agent with activity against this organism.

▶ Uncomplicated SSTIs often present as furuncles, carbuncles, or abcesses that can be treated with simple incision and drainage. As shown by Rihn et al, complicating the management of these infections has been the recent emergence of MRSA outside the health care setting.[1] Current guidelines still recommend incision and drainage of fluctuant lesions associated with uncomplicated MRSA SSTIs, with the role of additional antimicrobial therapy being much less established.[2-4] Ruhe et al show that although incision and drainage of any focal collection of fluids remain the mainstay of therapy, administration of active antimicrobial agents is associated with a statistically significant, but only moderate, impact on clinical outcome.

B. H. Thiers, MD

References

1. Rihn JA, Michaels MG, Harner CD. Community-acquired methicillin-resistant *Staphylococcus aureus*: an emerging problem in the athletic population. *Am J Sports Med.* 2005;1924-1929.
2. Stevens DL, Bisno AL, Chambers HF, et al. Practice guidelines for the diagnosis and management of skin and soft-tissue infections. *Clin Infect Dis.* 2005;41:1373-1406.
3. Chambers HF. Community-associated MRSA—resistance and virulence converge. *N Engl J Med.* 2005;352:1485-1487.
4. Moellering RC Jr. The growing menace of community-acquired methicillin-resistant *Staphylococcus aureus. Ann Intern Med.* 2006;144:368-369.

Necrotizing Soft-Tissue Infections and Sepsis Caused by *Vibrio vulnificus* Compared with Those Caused by Aeromonas Species

Tsai Y-H, Hsu RW-W, Huang T-J, et al (Chang Gung Univ College of Medicine, Taiwan, Republic of China)

J Bone Joint Surg Am 89:631-636, 2007

Background.—Vibrio and Aeromonas species, which can cause necrotizing fasciitis and primary septicemia, are members of the Vibrionaceae family and thrive in aquatic environments. Because the clinical symptoms and signs of necrotizing fasciitis and sepsis caused by these two bacteria are similar, the purposes of this study were to describe the clinical characteristics of *Vibrio vulnificus* and Aeromonas infections, to analyze the risk factors for death, and to compare the effects of surgical treatment on the outcome.

Methods.—The cases of thirty-two patients with necrotizing soft-tissue infections and sepsis caused by *Vibrio vulnificus* (seventeen patients) and Aeromonas species (fifteen patients) were retrospectively reviewed over a four-year period. Surgical débridement or immediate limb amputation was initially performed in all patients. Demographic data, underlying diseases, laboratory results, and clinical outcome were analyzed for each patient in both groups.

Results.—Six patients in the *Vibrio vulnificus* group and four patients in the Aeromonas group died. The patients who died had significantly lower serum albumin levels than did the patients who survived ($p < 0.05$). The patients with a combination of hepatic dysfunction and diabetes mellitus had a higher mortality rate than those with either hepatic disease or diabetes mellitus alone ($p < 0.05$). The patients with *Vibrio vulnificus* infections had a significantly lower systolic blood pressure at presentation ($p = 0.006$). The patients with Aeromonas infections who died had significantly lower white blood-cell counts ($p = 0.03$) with significantly fewer numbers of segmented white blood cells than those who died in the *Vibrio vulnificus* group ($p = 0.01$).

Conclusions.—The contact history of patients with a rapid onset of cellulitis can alert clinicians to a differential diagnosis of soft-tissue infection with *Vibrio vulnificus* (contact with seawater or raw seafood) or Aeromonas species (contact with fresh or brackish water, soil, or wood). Early fasciotomy

ta h

and culture-directed antimicrobial therapy should be aggressively performed in those patients with hypotensive shock, leukopenia, severe hypoalbuminemia, and underlying chronic illness, especially a combination of hepatic dysfunction and diabetes mellitus.

▶ This is a rare but characteristic disease entity that is occasionally seen by those of us who practice in coastal settings. The authors emphasize the importance of early fasciotomy and culture-directed antimicrobial therapy. The prognosis is poor, because many infected patients have chronic underlying diseases such as hepatic insufficiency or diabetes. The rapid onset of cellulitis with blister formation, especially after contact with seawater, raw seafood, or fresh or brackish water, should lead the clinician to consider the possibility of this diagnosis, which is a true surgical emergency.

B. H. Thiers, MD

Bacteremia, Fever, and Splenomegaly Caused by a Newly Recognized Bartonella Species

Eremeeva ME, Gerns HL, Lydy SL, et al (Ctrs for Disease Control and Prevention, Atlanta, Ga; Univ of California at San Francisco; Harvard Med School)
N Engl J Med 356:2381-2387, 2007

Bartonella species cause serious human infections globally, including bacillary angiomatosis, Oroya fever, trench fever, and endocarditis. We describe a patient who had fever and splenomegaly after traveling to Peru and also had bacteremia from an organism that resembled *Bartonella bacilliformis*, the causative agent of Oroya fever, which is endemic to Peru. However, genetic analyses revealed that this fastidious bacterium represented a previously uncultured and unnamed bartonella species, closely related to *B. clarridgeiae* and more distantly related to *B. bacilliformis*. We characterized this isolate, including its ability to cause fever and sustained bacteremia in a rhesus macaque. The route of infection and burden of human disease associated with this newly described pathogen are currently unknown.

▶ The authors describe a new bartonella species that causes an illness with features similar to those observed in patients with Oroya fever. The reservoir and mechanism of human infections are uncertain, but it appears that the disease is transmitted by a vector other than the sand fly.[1] Bartonella is becoming an increasingly important pathogen in dermatology, with 9 species having been linked to human infections that yield clinical pictures as diverse as bacillary angiomatosis, cat scratch disease, and verruga peruana. It is likely that meticulous bedside-to-bench research will identify new pathogenetic species in the future.

B. H. Thiers, MD

Reference

1. Wormser GP. Discovery of new infectious diseases—bartonella species. *N Engl J Med.* 2007;356:2346-2347.

Five-Hour Diagnosis of Dermatophyte Nail Infections with Specific Detection of *Trichophyton rubrum*

Brillowska-Dąbrowska A, Saunte DM, Arendrup MC (Statens Serum Inst, Copenhagen)
J Clin Microbiol 45:1200-1204, 2007

A rapid two-step DNA extraction method and a multiplex PCR for the detection of dermatophytes in general and *Trichophyton rubrum* specifically were developed and evaluated with DNA extracted from pure cultures and from clinically diseased nails. DNA from the following dermatophytes was used: *Epidermophyton floccosum, Microsporum audouinii, Microsporum canis, Microsporum gypseum, Microsporum nanum, Trichophyton mentagrophytes, Trichophyton rubrum, Trichophyton schoenleinii, Trichophyton soudanense, Trichophyton terrestre, Trichophyton tonsurans, Trichophyton verrucosum,* and *Trichophyton violaceum.* Human DNA and DNA from the following nondermatophyte fungi were included as controls: *Alternaria, Aspergillus niger, Candida albicans, Candida glabrata, Candida krusei, Malassezia furfur, Saccharomyces cerevisiae,* and *Scopulariopsis brevicaulis.* A total of 118 nail samples received for routine microscopy and culture for dermatophytes were subsequently tested by the two PCRs separately and in a multiplex format. Using DNA extracted from pure cultures and the pan-dermatophyte PCR, the *T. rubrum*-specific PCR sequentially and in a multiplex format correctly detected all dermatophytes and additionally correctly identified *T. rubrum.* Comparison of the traditional diagnostic evaluation (microscopy and culture) of nail samples with PCR on DNA directly extracted from the nails showed excellent agreement between PCR and microscopy, but the number of samples with dermatophyte species identification was increased considerably from 22.9% to 41.5%, mainly due to the identification of *T. rubrum* by PCR in microscopy-positive but culture-negative samples. In conclusion, this 5-hour diagnostic test was shown to increase not only the speed but also the sensitivity of investigation for nail dermatophytosis.

▶ This article by Brillowska-Dąbrowska and colleagues and an article by Savin and colleagues[1] both describe new techniques for the more rapid diagnosis of dermatophyte nail infections. However, two questions come to mind: is the rapid diagnosis of onychomycosis really necessary, and what cost will be necessary to make it a reality? Brillowska-Dąbrowska and colleagues state that "rapid, specific, and low-cost diagnoses of onychomycosis may become broadly available in the near future." One can only hope that this is true.

B. H. Thiers, MD

Reference

1. Savin C, Huck S, Rolland C, et al. Multicenter evaluation of a commercial PCR–enzyme-linked immunosorbent assay diagnostic kit (Onychodiag) for diagnosis of dermatophytic onychomycosis. *J Clin Microbiol.* 2007;45:1205-1210.

Multicenter Evaluation of a Commercial PCR–Enzyme-Linked Immunosorbent Assay Diagnostic Kit (Onychodiag) for Diagnosis of Dermatophytic Onychomycosis

Savin C, Huck S, Rolland C, et al (Bio Advance, Bussy Saint Martin, France; Université Paris 7; Assistance Publique-Hôpitaux de Paris; et al)
J Clin Microbiol 45:1205-1210, 2007

We prospectively evaluated a new PCR–enzyme-linked immunosorbent assay kit (Onychodiag; BioAdvance, France) for the diagnosis of dermatophytic onychomycosis by testing nail samples from 438 patients with suspected onychomycosis and from 108 healthy controls in three independent laboratories. In two laboratories, samples were collected by trained mycologists as close as possible to the lesions (proximal samples). In one laboratory, samples were collected by other physicians. All samples were processed by conventional mycological techniques and by Onychodiag, blindly to the mycological results. An additional distal sample, collected by clipping the nail plate, was obtained from 75 patients and tested with Onychodiag alone. In patients with culture-proven dermatophytic onychomycosis, the sensitivity of Onychodiag was 83.6% (87.9% including the gray zone) and ranged from 75 to 100% according to the laboratory and the sampling conditions. The specificity was 100% when healthy subjects were considered true negative controls. Onychodiag was positive on 68 patient samples that were sterile or yielded nondermatophyte species in culture. Based on the results of Onychodiag for mycologically proven positive samples and true-negative samples, these results were considered true positives, and the poor performance of mycology on these samples was attributed to inconvenient sampling conditions or to contaminants. When tested on distal samples, Onychodiag was positive in 49/53 (92%) cases of proven dermatophytic onychomycosis. Finally, with either proximal or distal samples, Onychodiag provided a diagnosis of dermatophytic onychomycosis within 24 to 48 h after sampling, and its sensitivity was close to that of mycological techniques applied to proximal samples.

▶ This article by Savin and colleagues and an article by Brillowska-Dąbrowska and colleagues[1] both describe new techniques for the more rapid diagnosis of dermatophyte nail infections. However, two questions come to mind: is the rapid diagnosis of onychomycosis really necessary, and what cost will be necessary to make it a reality? Brillowska-Dąbrowska and colleagues state that "rapid, specific, and low-cost diagnoses of onychomycosis may become broadly available in the near future."[1(p1203)] One can only hope that this is true.

B. H. Thiers, MD

Reference

1. Brillowska-Dąbrowska A, Saunte DM, Arendrup MC. Five-hour diagnosis of dermatophyte nail infections with specific detection of *Trichophyton rubrum*. *J Clin Microbiol*. 2007;45:1200-1204.

Combination of surgical avulsion and topical therapy for single nail onychomycosis: a randomized controlled trial

Grover C, Bansal S, Nanda S, et al (Maulana Azad Med College, New Delhi, India)

Br J Dermatol 157:364-368, 2007

Background.—Conventional therapy of onychomycosis is prolonged and often frustrating, which is why combination therapy involving topical, oral and surgical measures has been advocated as the treatment of choice. There are no controlled studies evaluating the efficacy of nail avulsion followed by topical antifungal therapy.

Objectives.—To evaluate the efficacy of combined surgical and topical therapy for onychomycosis.

Methods.—Forty patients with single nail onychomycosis [28 with distal and lateral subungual onychomycosis, seven with total dystrophic onychomycosis (TDO) and five with proximal subungual onychomycosis] were randomly assigned to four treatment groups. Each group received avulsion of the involved nail, followed by ketoconazole 2% cream without (group I) or with occlusion (group II), or oxiconazole 1% cream without (group III) or with occlusion (group IV). Topical therapies were applied twice daily. The patients were reviewed monthly and treatment was continued until the regrowth of completely normal nail (mycologically negative). In cured cases, further monthly review was carried out for at least 6 months, without any form of therapy. At each visit direct microscopic examination was repeated.

Results.—There was a high dropout rate, with seven patients (group I), six patients (group II), six patients (group III) and eight patients (group IV) completing the treatment protocol. Out of these, mycological cure was achieved in three (43%) patients in group I, four (67%) in group II, two (33%) in group III and six (75%) in group IV. All the cases of TDO failed to respond to this therapy. Overall, 15 of 27 (56%) patients were cured with this approach. On further follow up, recurrence of onychomycosis was recorded in two patients in group I. No side-effects or long-term complications of the nail avulsion were encountered. Important limitations encountered in the present study included a small sample size, a high dropout rate (32%) and poor patient compliance.

Conclusions.—Contrary to earlier reports, surgical nail avulsion with topical antifungal agents was not found to be a very encouraging modality for the treatment of onychomycosis. Both oxiconazole and ketoconazole delivered comparable results. Occlusion improved the treatment outcome, although the difference was not statistically significant. As a subtype, TDO showed poorest response. Surgical nail avulsion followed by topical antifungal therapy cannot be generally recommended for the treatment of onychomycosis.

▶ The high dropout rate suggests caution in the interpretation of the results. Nevertheless, for patients with limited involvement of a single nail, this therapy may provide some benefits. For patients with total dystrophic onychomycosis, even systemic therapy is likely to fail.

B. H. Thiers, MD

Topical treatments for fungal infections of the skin and nails of the foot
Crawford F, Hollis S (Univ of Dundee, Edinburgh, Scotland)
Cochrane Database Syst Rev Issue 3 Art No:CD001434:1-123, 2007

Background.—Fungal infections of the feet normally occur in the outermost layer of the skin (epidermis). The skin between the toes is a frequent site of infection which can cause pain and itchiness. Fungal infections of the nail (onychomycosis) can affect the entire nail plate.

Objectives.—To assess the effects of topical treatments in successfully treating (rate of treatment failure) fungal infections of the skin of the feet and toenails and in preventing recurrence.

Search Strategy.—We searched the Cochrane Skin Group Specialised Register (January 2005), the Cochrane Central Register of Controlled Trials (*The Cochrane Library* Issue 1, 2005), MEDLINE and EMBASE (from inception to January 2005). We screened the Science Citation Index, BIOSIS, CAB - Health and Healthstar, CINAHL DARE, NHS Economic Evaluation Database and EconLit (March 2005). Bibliographies were searched.

Selection Criteria.—Randomised controlled trials (RCTs) using participants who had mycologically diagnosed fungal infections of the skin and nails of the foot.

Data Collection and Analysis.—Two authors independently summarised the included trials and appraised their quality of reporting using a structured data extraction tool.

Main Results.—Of the 144 identified papers, 67 trials met the inclusion criteria. Placebo-controlled trials yielded the following pooled risk ratios (RR) of treatment failure for skin infections: allylamines RR 0.33 (95% CI 0.24 to 0.44); azoles RR 0.30 (95% CI 0.20 to 0.45); ciclopiroxolamine RR 0.27 (95% CI 0.11 to 0.66); tolnaftate RR 0.19 (95% CI 0.08 to 0.44); butenafine RR 0.33 (95% CI 0.24 to 0.45); undecanoates RR 0.29 (95% CI 0.12 - 0.70). Meta-analysis of 11 trials comparing allylamines and azoles showed a risk ratio of treatment failure RR 0.63 (95% CI 0.42 to 0.94) in favour of allylamines. Evidence for the management of topical treatments for infections of the toenails is sparser. There is some evidence that ciclopiroxolamine and butenafine are both effective but they both need to be applied daily for prolonged periods (at least 1 year). The 6 trials of nail infections provided evidence that topical ciclopiroxolamine has poor cure rates and that amorolfine might be substantially more effective but more research is required.

Authors' Conclusions.—Placebo-controlled trials of allylamines and az-oles for athlete's foot consistently produce much higher percentages of cure than placebo. Allylamines cure slightly more infections than azoles and are now available OTC. Further research into the effectiveness of antifungal agents for nail infections is required.

▶ The Cochrane Collaboration publishes reviews that examine evidence-based data that are used to support therapeutic decision making. In the case of dermatophyte infections of the skin and toenails, uncertainty exists as to the less effective drugs and the optimal dose, frequency, and duration of treatment. As stated by the authors, the ideal topical antifungal cream should be fungicidal (allowing for a short duration of treatment), obtain high cure rates, minimize relapses, have minimal adverse effects, and be conducive to patient compliance. Crawford and Hollis found a great deal of evidence to support the efficacy of over-the-counter topical antifungal creams for the treatment of fungal skin infections. The most effective agent was terbinafine. For the topical treatment of onychomycosis, the evidence was much less convincing, although there was some evidence that cyclopirox olamine and butenafine might be effective if applied for prolonged periods (at least 1 year).

B. H. Thiers, MD

The Safety of Oral Antifungal Treatments for Superficial Dermatophytosis and Onychomycosis: A Meta-analysis
Chang C-H, Young-Xu Y, Kurth T, et al (Natl Taiwan Univ Hosp, Taipei; Harvard School of Public Health, Boston; EpiPatterns, Haverhill, NH; et al)
Am J Med 120:791-798, 2007

Purpose.—We estimated the absolute risks of treatment termination and incidence of adverse liver outcomes among all commonly used oral antifungal treatments for superficial dermatophytosis and onychomycosis.

Methods.—MEDLINE, EMBASE, and Cochrane Library were searched to identify randomized and nonrandomized controlled trials, case series, and cohort studies published before December 31, 2005. Two reviewers independently applied selection criteria, performed quality assessment, and extracted data. Treatment arms with the same regimen in terms of drug, type (continuous or intermittent), and dosage were combined to estimate the risk of an outcome of interest.

Results.—We identified 122 studies with approximately 20,000 enrolled patients for planned comparison. The pooled risks (95% confidence intervals) of treatment discontinuation resulting from adverse reactions for continuous therapy were 3.44% (95% confidence interval [CI], 2.28%-4.61%)

for terbinafine 250 mg/day; 1.96% (95% CI, 0.35%-3.57%) for itraconazole 100 mg/day; 4.21% (95% CI, 2.33%-6.09%) for itraconazole 200 mg/day; and 1.51% (95% CI, 0%-4.01%) for fluconazole 50 mg/day. For intermittent therapy, the pooled risks were as follows: pulse terbinafine: 2.09% (95% CI, 0%-4.42%); pulse itraconazole: 2.58% (95% CI, 1.15%-4.01%); intermittent fluconazole 150 mg/week: 1.98% (95% CI, 0.05%-3.92%); and intermittent fluconazole 300 to 450 mg/week: 5.76% (95% CI, 2.42%-9.10%). The risk of liver injury requiring termination of treatment ranged from 0.11% (continuous itraconazole 100 mg/day) to 1.22% (continuous fluconazole 50 mg/day). The risk of having asymptomatic elevation of serum transaminase but not requiring treatment discontinuation was less than 2.0% for all treatment regimens evaluated.

Conclusion.—Oral antifungal therapy against superficial dermatophytosis and onychomycosis, including intermittent and continuous terbinafine, itraconazole, and fluconazole, was associated with a low incidence of adverse events in an immunocompetent population.

▶ I was somewhat surprised (and disappointed) that this article appeared not in a dermatology journal but in a general medical journal. Nevertheless, the results are reassuring. Dermatologists know that oral antifungal agents, specifically oral terbinafine, itraconazole, and fluconazole, are associated with a low incidence of adverse events when used in the treatment of dermatophytosis and onychomycosis. In this study, Chang et al found that pulse therapy was associated with a lower risk of discontinuation because of adverse reactions than was continuous therapy. Overall, fluconazole seemed to have a lower risk of treatment discontinuation because of adverse events. In general, as the dosage of antifungal agents is increased, the incidence of adverse events is increased as well. The overall risk of adverse events was, however, quite low.

B. H. Thiers, MD

Posaconazole or Fluconazole for Prophylaxis in Severe Graft-versus-Host Disease
Ullmann AJ, Lipton JH, Vesole DH, et al (Johannes Gutenberg Univ, Mainz, Germany; Princess Margaret Hosp, Toronto; Med College of Wisconsin, Milwaukee; et al)
N Engl J Med 356:335-347, 2007

Background.—Invasive fungal infections are an important cause of morbidity and mortality after allogeneic hematopoietic stem-cell transplantation.

Methods.—In an international, randomized, double-blind trial, we compared oral posaconazole with oral fluconazole for prophylaxis against invasive fungal infections in patients with graft-versus-host disease (GVHD) who were receiving immunosuppressive therapy. The primary end point was the incidence of proven or probable invasive fungal infections from randomization to day 112 of the fixed treatment period of the study.

Results.—Of a total of 600 patients, 301 were assigned to posaconazole and 299 to fluconazole. At the end of the fixed 112-day treatment period, posaconazole was found to be as effective as fluconazole in preventing all invasive fungal infections (incidence, 5.3% and 9.0%, respectively; odds ratio, 0.56; 95 percent confidence interval [CI], 0.30 to 1.07; P=0.07) and was superior to fluconazole in preventing proven or probable invasive aspergillosis (2.3% vs. 7.0%; odds ratio, 0.31; 95% CI, 0.13 to 0.75; P=0.006). While patients were receiving study medications (exposure period), in the posaconazole group, as compared with the fluconazole group, there were fewer breakthrough invasive fungal infections (2.4% vs. 7.6%, P=0.004), particularly invasive aspergillosis (1.0% vs. 5.9%, P=0.001). Overall mortality was similar in the two groups, but the number of deaths from invasive fungal infections was lower in the posaconazole group (1%, vs. 4% in the fluconazole group; P=0.046). The incidence of treatment-related adverse events was similar in the two groups (36% in the posaconazole group and 38% in the fluconazole group), and the rates of treatment-related serious adverse events were 13% and 10%, respectively.

Conclusions.—Posaconazole was similar to fluconazole for prophylaxis against fungal infections among patients with GVHD. It was superior in preventing invasive aspergillosis and reducing the rate of deaths related to fungal infections.

▶ Ullmann et al present a randomized double-blind trial that showed posaconazole and fluconazole to be equally effective in preventing all invasive fungal diseases; posaconazole was more effective in preventing invasive aspergillosis. The patients studied were receiving immunosuppressive therapy for graft-versus-host disease (GVHD). Fewer deaths occurred in the posaconazole group, and the drug appeared to be safe and well-tolerated. Cornely et al,[1] in a prospective, randomized trial, compared the efficacy of posaconazole with either fluconazole or itraconazole for the prevention of invasive fungal disease in patients who were undergoing chemotherapy for acute leukemia or myelodysplastic syndromes. They found the incidence of proven and probable invasive fungal diseases to be significantly lower in the posaconazole group than in the fluconozole or itraconazole groups. Fewer cases of invasive aspergillosis occurred after posaconazole prophylaxis than after fluconazole or itraconazole prophylaxis. On the basis of currently available data, it now seems that posaconazole is the drug of choice for prophylaxis of invasive aspergillosis, whereas voriconazole remains the preferred treatment for proven or probable aspergillosis. Caspofungin and liposomal amphotericin B remain as options for empirical therapy.[2]

B. H. Thiers, MD

References

1. Cornely OA, Maertens J, Winston DJ, et al. Posaconazole vs. Fluconazole or Itraconazole Prophylaxis in Patients with Neutropenia. *N Engl J Med.* 2007;356:348-359.
2. DePauw BE, Donnelly JP. Prophylaxis and aspergillosis—has the principle been proven? *N Engl J Med.* 2007;356:409-411.

Posaconazole vs. Fluconazole or Itraconazole Prophylaxis in Patients with Neutropenia

Cornely OA, Maertens J, Winston DJ, et al (Univ of Cologne, Germany; Univ Hosp Gasthuisberg, Leuven, Belgium; Univ of California, Los Angeles; et al)
N Engl J Med 356:348-359, 2007

Background.—Patients with neutropenia resulting from chemotherapy for acute myelogenous leukemia or the myelodysplastic syndrome are at high risk for difficult-to-treat and often fatal invasive fungal infections.

Methods.—In this randomized, multicenter study involving evaluators who were unaware of treatment assignments, we compared the efficacy and safety of posaconazole with those of fluconazole or itraconazole as prophylaxis for patients with prolonged neutropenia. Patients received prophylaxis with each cycle of chemotherapy until recovery from neutropenia and complete remission, until occurrence of an invasive fungal infection, or for up to 12 weeks, whichever came first. We compared the incidence of proven or probable invasive fungal infections during treatment (the primary end point) between the posaconazole and fluconazole or itraconazole groups; death from any cause and time to death were secondary end points.

Results.—A total of 304 patients were randomly assigned to receive posaconazole, and 298 patients were randomly assigned to receive fluconazole (240) or itraconazole (58). Proven or probable invasive fungal infections were reported in 7 patients (2%) in the posaconazole group and 25 patients (8%) in the fluconazole or itraconazole group (absolute reduction in the posaconazole group, -6%; 95% confidence interval, -9.7 to -2.5%; $P<0.001$), fulfilling statistical criteria for superiority. Significantly fewer patients in the posaconazole group had invasive aspergillosis (2 [1%] vs. 20 [7%], $P<0.001$). Survival was significantly longer among recipients of posaconazole than among recipients of fluconazole or itraconazole ($P=0.04$). Serious adverse events possibly or probably related to treatment were reported by 19 patients (6%) in the posaconazole group and 6 patients (2%) in the fluconazole or itraconazole group ($P=0.01$). The most common treatment-related adverse events in both groups were gastrointestinal tract disturbances.

Conclusions.—In patients undergoing chemotherapy for acute myelogenous leukemia or the myelodysplastic syndrome, posaconazole prevented invasive fungal infections more effectively than did either fluconazole or itraconazole and improved overall survival. There were more serious adverse events possibly or probably related to treatment in the posaconazole group.

▶ Ullmann et al[1] present a randomized-double-blind trial that showed posaconazole and fluconazole to be equally effective in preventing all invasive fungal diseases; posaconazole was more effective in preventing invasive aspergillosis. The patients studied were receiving immunosuppressive therapy for graft-versus-host disease (GVHD). Fewer deaths occurred in the posaconazole group, and the drug appeared to be safe and well-tolerated. Cornely et al, in a prospective, randomized trial, compared the efficacy of posaconazole with either fluconazole or itraconazole for the prevention of invasive fungal disease in patients who were undergoing chemotherapy for acute leukemia or myelo-dysplastic syndromes. They found the incidence of proven and probable invasive fungal diseases to be significantly lower in the posaconazole group than in the fluconazole or itraconazole groups. Fewer cases of invasive aspergillosis occurred after posaconazole prophylaxis than after fluconazole or itraconazole prophylaxis. On the basis of currently available data, it now seems that posaconazole is the drug of choice for prophylaxis of invasive aspergillosis, whereas voriconazole remains the preferred treatment for proven or probable aspergillosis. Caspofungin and liposomal amphotericin B remain as options for empirical therapy.[2]

B. H. Thiers, MD

References

1. Ullmann AJ, Lipton JH, Vesole DH, et al. Posaconazole or fluconazole for prophylaxis in severe graft-versus-host disease. *N Engl J Med*. 2007;356:335-347.
2. DePauw BE, Donnelly JP. Prophylaxis of aspergillosis—has the principle been proven? *N Engl J Med*. 2007;356:409-411.

Anidulafungin versus Fluconazole for Invasive Candidiasis
Reboli AC, for the Anidulafungin Study Group (Univ of Medicine and Dentistry of New Jersey, Camden; et al)
N Engl J Med 356:2472-2482, 2007

Background.—Anidulafungin, a new echinocandin, has potent activity against candida species. We compared anidulafungin with fluconazole in a randomized, double-blind, noninferiority trial of treatment for invasive candidiasis.

Methods.—Adults with invasive candidiasis were randomly assigned to receive either intravenous anidulafungin or intravenous fluconazole. All patients could receive oral fluconazole after 10 days of intravenous therapy. The primary efficacy analysis assessed the global response (clinical and microbiologic) at the end of intravenous therapy in patients who had a positive baseline culture. Efficacy was also assessed at other time points.

Results.—Eighty-nine percent of the 245 patients in the primary analysis had candidemia only. *Candida albicans* was isolated in 62% of the 245 patients. In vitro fluconazole resistance was infrequent. Most of the patients (97%) did not have neutropenia. At the end of intravenous therapy, treatment was successful in 75.6% of patients treated with anidulafungin, as compared with 60.2% of those treated with fluconazole (difference, 15.4 percentage points; 95% confidence interval [CI], 3.9 to 27.0). The results were similar for other efficacy end points. The statistical analyses failed to show a "center effect"; when data from the site enrolling the largest number of patients were removed, success rates at the end of intravenous therapy were 73.2% in the anidulafungin group and 61.1% in the fluconazole group (difference, 12.1 percentage points; 95% CI, −1.1 to 25.3). The frequency and types of adverse events were similar in the two groups. The rate of death from all causes was 31% in the fluconazole group and 23% in the anidulafungin group (P=0.13).

Conclusions.—Anidulafungin was shown to be noninferior to fluconazole in the treatment of invasive candidiasis.

▶ The results of this study by Reboli and colleagues, which compared anidulafungin with fluconazole for the treatment of invasive candidiasis, fail to show a clear winner. Whether echinocandins are superior to azoles for the treatment of invasive candida infections is highly controversial. The new echinocandin antifungal agents provide practitioners with a broader choice for prophylaxis and therapy, but evidence is lacking to prove their superiority to older drugs.[1]

B. H. Thiers, MD

Reference

1. Sobel JD, Revankar SG. Echinocandins—first choice or first-line therapy for invasive candidiasis? *N Engl J Med.* 2007;356:2525-2526.

Micafungin versus liposomal amphotericin B for candidaemia and invasive candidosis: a phase III randomised double-blind trial
Kuse E-R, for the Micafungin Invasive Candidiasis Working Group (Klinik für Viszeral und Transplantationschirurgie, Hannover, Germany; et al)
Lancet 369:1519-1527, 2007

Background.—Invasive candidosis is increasingly prevalent in seriously ill patients. Our aim was to compare micafungin with liposomal amphotericin B for the treatment of adult patients with candidaemia or invasive candidosis.

Methods.—We did a double-blind, randomised, multinational non-inferiority study to compare micafungin (100 mg/day) with liposomal amphotericin B (3 mg/kg per day) as first-line treatment of candidaemia and invasive candidosis. The primary endpoint was treatment success, defined as both a clinical and a mycological response at the end of treatment. Primary analyses were done on a per-protocol basis.

Findings.—264 individuals were randomly assigned to treatment with micafungin; 267 were randomly assigned to receive liposomal amphotericin B. 202 individuals in the micafungin group and 190 in the liposomal amphotericin B group were included in the per-protocol analyses. Treatment success was observed for 181 (89.6%) patients treated with micafungin and 170 (89.5%) patients treated with liposomal amphotericin B. The difference in proportions, after stratification by neutropenic status at baseline, was 0.7% (95% CI −5.3 to 6.7). Efficacy was independent of the *Candida* spp and primary site of infection, as well as neutropenic status, APACHE II score, and whether a catheter was removed or replaced during the study. There were fewer treatment-related adverse events—including those that were serious or led to treatment discontinuation—with micafungin than there were with liposomal amphotericin B.

Interpretation.—Micafungin was as effective as—and caused fewer adverse events than—liposomal amphotericin B as first-line treatment of candidaemia and invasive candidosis.

▶ Serious infections caused by *Candida* species have in the past been treated with amphotericin B, which is well known for its potential toxicity, and fluconazole, which often has a limited spectrum of activity. Newer generation drugs such as liposomal amphotericin B, voriconazole, and the echinocandins caspofungin and anidulafungin have largely overcome these limitations. Micafungin, another echinocandin, has high success rates against candidemia in open-label studies. Kuse et al compared the efficacy of micafungin with liposomal amphotericin B in the treatment of adult patients with candidemia or invasive candidosis and found the drug to be as effective with fewer adverse events. Because micafungin appears to have broad spectrum activity against *Aspergillus* species, future studies should assess its efficacy in the treatment of invasive aspergillosis. The improved safety profile of micafungin likely results from its mechanism of action, which involves rather specific inhibition of fungal cell wall synthesis with little impact on human cells.

B. H. Thiers, MD

Treatment of actinomycetoma due to *Nocardia* spp. with amoxicillin–clavulanate
Bonifaz A, Flores P, Saúl A, et al (Gen Hosp of Mexico, Mexico DF)
Br J Dermatol 156:308-311, 2007

Background.—Actinomycetoma is a chronic occupational condition that occurs frequently in tropical regions. In Mexico 85% of cases are caused by *Nocardia brasiliensis*. There are two treatments of choice for these cases: a regimen of dapsone plus trimethoprim–sulfamethoxazole (co-trimoxazole) and, recently, amikacin, either alone or combined. However, not all cases respond properly to these therapies.

Objectives.—To report a retrospective, 11-year study of cases of actinomycetomas caused by *Nocardia* spp., treated with amoxicillin–clavulanate (co-amoxiclav).

Methods.—All cases were identified clinically and microbiologically and had previously failed standard therapies. Oral co-amoxiclav 875/125 mg was administered every 12 h. Clinical, microbiological and laboratory follow up was performed every 2 months during the treatment period.

Results.—Twenty-one cases of actinomycetoma were included, 19 caused by *N. brasiliensis* and one each by *N. asteroids* and *N. otitidiscaviarum*. Clinical and microbiological cure occurred in 15 of 21 cases (71%); two cases improved (10%) and four failed (19%). Mean treatment period was 9.6 months, during which neither side-effects nor laboratory test alterations were reported.

Conclusions.—Treatment with co-amoxiclav represents an alternative or rescue treatment for cases that have previously failed standard therapies.

▶ Although the overall mortality rate of actinomycetoma is not high, infection tends to be chronic with high morbidity and a tendency to disseminate to other organs. In Mexico, where it is an occupational hazard, the condition affects mainly the lower limbs, especially the foot, with the trunk being another common site of involvement. Bonifaz et al report their experience with 21 cases of actinomycetoma treated with amoxicillin–clavulanate, and showed it to be a reasonable alternative to existing therapies. One important drawback may be the relatively high cost of treatment, given that mycetoma is a disease that affects farmers and low-income people. The use of amoxicillin–clavulanate should also be restricted to infections caused by various *Nocardia* species, as this antibiotic may have little or no activity against mycetomas caused by *Actinomadura madure.*

B. H. Thiers, MD

4 Viral Infections (Excluding HIV Infection)

Cutaneous Human Papillomaviruses Persist on Healthy Skin
Hazard K, Karlsson A, Andersson K, et al (Lund Univ, Malmö, Sweden)
J Invest Dermatol 127:116-119, 2007

Cutaneous human papillomaviruses (HPVs) are frequently found in healthy skin and have also been implicated in non-melanoma skin cancer. For genital HPV types, a persistent infection with one of the high-risk types is a prerequisite for the development of cervical cancer. However, there is only limited data on whether infections with cutaneous HPV types persist over time. Serial forehead swab samples collected from 63 volunteers (42 healthy individuals and 31 renal transplant recipients (RTRs)), sampled 6.3 years (range: 5.0–7.0 years) apart, were analyzed for HPV using general primer PCR, cloning, and sequencing. Among the healthy individuals, the prevalences of HPV were 69% (29/42) at enrolment and 71% (30/42) at follow-up. Among the individuals positive at baseline, 48% (14/29) had a persistent infection. Among the RTRs, 71% (15/21) were positive for HPV at enrolment and 90% (19/21) at follow-up. A persistent infection was detected in 33% (5/15). In total, HPV was detected in 44 of the samples collected at baseline and the same virus was found at follow-up in 43% (19/44). Persistence was not significantly associated with age, sex, immunosuppressive treatment, history of warts, or genus of HPV. We conclude that cutaneous HPV infections commonly persist over several years on healthy skin.

▶ The authors sought to explore whether HPV types reported to be present on healthy skin persist after a lengthy time span and whether healthy subjects and immunosuppressed patients have different degrees of viral persistence. They found that cutaneous HPVs often persist for many years on healthy skin, with nearly half of healthy individuals being positive for the same HPV type 6 years later. Surprisingly, persistent HPV infections were not more common in immunosuppressed renal transplant recipients. There was no apparent correlation with the presence of warts or other skin diseases. Knowing that viral persistence is common helps us understand the biology of these viruses and may also aid in elucidating their role in the pathogenesis of various cutaneous disorders.

B. H. Thiers, MD

Duct Tape for the Treatment of Common Warts in Adults: A Double-blind Randomized Controlled Trial

Wenner R, Askari SK, Cham PMH, et al (Univ of Minnesota, Minneapolis; Saint Louis Univ; Minneapolis Veterans Affairs Med Ctr)
Arch Dermatol 143:309-313, 2007

Objective.—To evaluate the efficacy of duct tape occlusion therapy for the treatment of common warts in adults.

Design.—Double-blind controlled clinical intervention trial.

Setting.—Veterans Affairs medical center.

Participants.—A total of 90 immunocompetent adult volunteers with at least 1 wart measuring 2 to 15 mm were enrolled between October 1, 2004, and July 31, 2005. Eighty patients completed the study.

Intervention.—Patients were randomized by a computer-generated code to receive pads consisting of either moleskin with transparent duct tape (treatment group) or moleskin alone (control group). Patients were instructed to wear the pads for 7 consecutive days and leave the pad off on the seventh evening. This process was repeated for 2 months or until the wart resolved, whichever occurred first. Follow-up visits occurred at 1 and 2 months.

Main Outcome Measure.—Complete resolution of the target wart. Secondary outcomes included change in size of the target wart and recurrence rates at 6 months for warts with complete resolution.

Results.—There were no statistically significant differences in the proportions of patients with resolution of the target wart (8 [21%] of 39 patients in the treatment group vs 9 [22%] of 41 in the control group). Of patients with complete resolution, 6 (75%) in the treatment group and 3 (33%) in the control group had recurrence of the target wart by the sixth month.

Conclusion.—We found no statistically significant difference between duct tape and moleskin for the treatment of warts in an adult population.

▶ The results are in stark contrast to those reported by Focht et al, who found that duct tape occlusion was more effective than cryotherapy for treating warts.[1] Unfortunately, the patient population in the 2 studies differed (adults here vs primarily children in the earlier study) as did the methodologies and materials used. Unfortunately, there is still a lack of evidence-based data to declare any proposed wart treatment as the best.[2]

B. H. Thiers, MD

References

1. Focht DR 3rd, Spicer C, Fairchok MP. The efficacy of duct tape vs cryotherapy in the treatment of verruca vulgaris (the common wart). *Arch Pediatr Adolesc Med.* 2002;156:971-974.
2. Gibbs S, Harvey I, Sterling JC, Stark R. Local treatment for cutaneous warts. *Cochrane Database Syst Rev.* 2003;3:CD001781.

Comparative study of photodynamic therapy vs. CO₂ laser vaporization in treatment of condylomata acuminata, a randomized clinical trial

Chen K, Chang BZ, Ju M, et al (Chinese Academy of Med Sciences and Peking Union Med College, Nanjing, China)

Br J Dermatol 156:516-520, 2007

Background.—Most conventional therapies for condylomata acuminata (CA) are traumatic and have high recurrence rates.

Objectives.—To investigate the efficacy and safety of topical application of 5-aminolaevulinic acid (ALA) photodynamic therapy (PDT) for the treatment of CA.

Methods.—Sixty-five patients with CA were allocated into the treatment (ALA-PDT) group and treated with 20% ALA solution under occlusive dressing for 3 h followed by irradiation with the helium–neon laser at a dose of 100 J cm^{-2} and a power of 100 mW. Another 21 CA patients were allocated into the control group and treated with the CO_2 laser. The treatment was to be repeated 1 week later if the lesion was not completely removed after the first treatment.

Results.—After one treatment, the complete removal rate was 95% in the ALA-PDT group and 100% in the control group. After two treatments with ALA-PDT, the complete removal rate in the treatment group was 100%. The recurrence rate for ALA-PDT group was 6.3% which was significantly lower than that in control group (19.1%, $P < 0.05$). Moreover, the proportion of patients with adverse effects in the ALA-PDT group (13.9%) was also significantly lower than that in control group (100%, $P < 0.05$). The side-effects in patients treated with ALA-PDT mainly included mild burning and/or stinging restricted to the illuminated area.

Conclusions.—The present study shows that topical application of ALA-PDT is a simpler, more effective and safer therapy with a lower recurrence for treatment of CA compared with conventional CO_2 laser therapy.

▶ Genital warts are difficult to manage. The perfect treatment has yet to be developed. Physical modalities are often painful and can be associated with slow healing and scarring. Topical therapies often lack efficacy and are associated with a high recurrence rate. In this study, topical PDT using 20% 5-ALA in combination with a red laser light was compared with the CO_2 laser for the management of genital warts. Both modalities were equally effective but not surprisingly, the CO_2 laser was associated with slower healing, scarring, and more pain (only a topical anesthetic was used). Most importantly, a lower recurrence rate with PDT was noted. If these findings are confirmed, PDT could represent a new effective treatment modality, which is less painful, not associated with scarring, and relatively easy to perform.

P. G. Lang Jr, MD

Case–Control Study of Human Papillomavirus and Oropharyngeal Cancer

D'Souza G, Kreimer AR, Viscidi R, et al (Johns Hopkins Bloomberg School of Public Health, Baltimore, Md; Johns Hopkins Hosp, Baltimore, Md; Johns Hopkins Univ, Baltimore, Md; et al)
N Engl J Med 356:1944-1956, 2007

Background.—Substantial molecular evidence suggests a role for human papillomavirus (HPV) in the pathogenesis of oropharyngeal squamous-cell carcinoma, but epidemiologic data have been inconsistent.

Methods.—We performed a hospital-based, case–control study of 100 patients with newly diagnosed oropharyngeal cancer and 200 control patients without cancer to evaluate associations between HPV infection and oropharyngeal cancer. Multivariate logistic-regression models were used for case–control comparisons.

Results.—A high lifetime number of vaginal-sex partners (26 or more) was associated with oropharyngeal cancer (odds ratio, 3.1; 95% confidence interval [CI], 1.5 to 6.5), as was a high lifetime number of oral-sex partners (6 or more) (odds ratio, 3.4; 95% CI, 1.3 to 8.8). The degree of association increased with the number of vaginal-sex and oral-sex partners (P values for trend, 0.002 and 0.009, respectively). Oropharyngeal cancer was significantly associated with oral HPV type 16 (HPV-16) infection (odds ratio, 14.6; 95% CI, 6.3 to 36.6), oral infection with any of 37 types of HPV (odds ratio, 12.3; 95% CI, 5.4 to 26.4), and seropositivity for the HPV-16 L1 capsid protein (odds ratio, 32.2; 95% CI, 14.6 to 71.3). HPV-16 DNA was detected in 72% (95% CI, 62 to 81) of 100 paraffin-embedded tumor specimens, and 64% of patients with cancer were seropositive for the HPV-16 oncoprotein E6, E7, or both. HPV-16 L1 seropositivity was highly associated with oropharyngeal cancer among subjects with a history of heavy tobacco and alcohol use (odds ratio, 19.4; 95% CI, 3.3 to 113.9) and among those without such a history (odds ratio, 33.6; 95% CI, 13.3 to 84.8). The association was similarly increased among subjects with oral HPV-16 infection, regardless of their tobacco and alcohol use. By contrast, tobacco and alcohol use increased the association with oropharyngeal cancer primarily among subjects without exposure to HPV-16.

Conclusions.—Oral HPV infection is strongly associated with oropharyngeal cancer among subjects with or without the established risk factors of tobacco and alcohol use.

▶ Although it is widely accepted that HPV causes cervical cancer, the virus has also been associated with several other types of squamous cell carcinoma and a variety of precursor lesions at different sites, including the skin, vulva, vagina, penis, esophagus, conjunctiva, paranasal sinuses, and bronchus. However, the role of HPV in the pathogenesis of these lesions is less clear. The similar morphologic features of genital and oral HPV-associated lesions suggest that HPV may indeed be involved in oral and laryngeal squamous cell carcinoma. However, previous studies have shown highly variable detection rates of HPV DNA. D'Souza et al studied 100 patients with newly diagnosed oropharyngeal cancer and 200 control subjects who did not have cancer. A prevalent oral infection with HPV-16 and oral infection with any of 37 other HPV types were significantly associated with oropharyngeal cancer. In situ hybridization of paraffin-embedded specimens yielded HPV-16 in 72% of 60 sampled oropharyngeal cancers. The data also suggest that sexual behavior may be a risk factor for oropharyngeal cancer, as a high lifetime number of vaginal- or oral-sex partners was associated with its presence, with the degree of association increasing with the number of vaginal- or oral-sex partners. The relationship between smoking and alcohol use, which are known risk factors for oral cancer, and HPV-related pathways require further study. One interesting question brought up in an editorial that accompanied this study is whether some oral, oropharyngeal, and laryngeal cancers might be prevented by HPV vaccination.[1]

B. H. Thiers, MD

Reference

1. Syrjänen S. Human papillomaviruses in head and neck carcinomas. *N Engl J Med.* 2007;356:1993-1995.

Prevalence of HPV Infection Among Females in the United States
Dunne EF, Unger ER, Sternberg M, et al (Ctrs for Disease Control and Prevention, Atlanta, Ga; Ctrs for Disease Control and Prevention, Bethesda, Md)
JAMA 297:813-819, 2007

Context.—Human papillomavirus (HPV) infection is estimated to be the most common sexually transmitted infection. Baseline population prevalence data for HPV infection in the United States before widespread availability of a prophylactic HPV vaccine would be useful.

Objective.—To determine the prevalence of HPV among females in the United States.

Design, Setting, and Participants.—The National Health and Nutrition Examination Survey (NHANES) uses a representative sample of the US non-institutionalized civilian population. Females aged 14 to 59 years who were interviewed at home for NHANES 2003-2004 were examined in a mobile examination center and provided a self-collected vaginal swab specimen. Swabs were analyzed for HPV DNA by L1 consensus polymerase chain reaction followed by type-specific hybridization. Demographic and sexual behavior information was obtained from all participants.

Main Outcome Measures.—HPV prevalence by polymerase chain reaction.

Results.—The overall HPV prevalence was 26.8% (95% confidence interval [CI], 23.3%-30.9%) among US females aged 14 to 59 years (n = 1921). HPV prevalence was 24.5% (95% CI, 19.6%-30.5%) among females aged 14 to 19 years, 44.8% (95% CI, 36.3%-55.3%) among women aged 20 to 24 years, 27.4% (95% CI, 21.9%-34.2%) among women aged 25 to 29 years, 27.5% (95% CI, 20.8%-36.4%) among women aged 30 to 39 years, 25.2% (95% CI, 19.7%-32.2%) among women aged 40 to 49 years, and 19.6% (95% CI, 14.3%-26.8%) among women aged 50 to 59 years. There was a statistically significant trend for increasing HPV prevalence with each year of age from 14 to 24 years ($P<.001$), followed by a gradual decline in prevalence through 59 years ($P = .06$). HPV vaccine types 6 and 11 (low-risk types) and 16 and 18 (high-risk types) were detected in 3.4% of female participants; HPV-6 was detected in 1.3% (95% CI, 0.8%-2.3%), HPV-11 in 0.1% (95% CI, 0.03%-0.3%), HPV-16 in 1.5% (95% CI, 0.9%-2.6%), and HPV-18 in 0.8% (95% CI, 0.4%-1.5%) of female participants. Independent risk factors for HPV detection were age, marital status, and increasing numbers of lifetime and recent sex partners.

Conclusions.—HPV is common among females in the United States. Our data indicate that the burden of prevalent HPV infection among females was greater than previous estimates and was highest among those aged 20 to 24 years. However, the prevalence of HPV vaccine types was relatively low.

▶ The prevalence of HPV infection among females and the association of HPV infection with cervical cancer puts the importance of the recently developed HPV vaccine into perspective. Interestingly, the prevalence of HPV types associated with cervical cancer, and hence included in the vaccine, was relatively low.

B. H. Thiers, MD

Genital transmission of HPV in a mouse model is potentiated by nonoxynol-9 and inhibited by carrageenan
Roberts JN, Buck CB, Thompson CD, et al (NIH, Bethesda, Md; Science Applications International Corp (SAIC)-Frederick, Md)
Nat Med 13:857-861, 2007

Genital human papillomavirus (HPV) infection is the most common sexually transmitted infection, and virtually all cases of cervical cancer are attributable to infection by a subset of HPVs (reviewed in Trottier H, Franco EL. The epidemiology of genital human papillomavirus infection. *Vaccine.* 2006;24:S1-S15). Despite the high incidence of HPV infection and the recent development of a prophylactic vaccine that confers protection against some HPV types, many features of HPV infection are poorly understood. It remains worthwhile to consider other interventions against genital HPVs, particularly those that target infections not prevented by the current vaccine.

However, productive papillomavirus infection is species- and tissue-restricted, and traditional models use animal papillomaviruses that infect the skin or oral mucosa. Here we report the development of a mouse model of cervicovaginal infection with HPV16 that recapitulates the establishment phase of papillomavirus infection. Transduction of a reporter gene by an HPV16 pseudovirus was characterized by histology and quantified by whole-organ, multispectral imaging. Disruption of the integrity of the stratified or columnar genital epithelium was required for infection, which occurred after deposition of the virus on the basement membrane underlying basal keratinocytes. A widely used vaginal spermicide, nonoxynol-9 (N-9), greatly increased susceptibility to infection. In contrast, carrageenan, a polysaccharide present in some vaginal lubricants, prevented infection even in the presence of N-9, suggesting that carrageenan might serve as an effective topical HPV microbicide.

▶ The results suggest that that over-the-counter vaginal contraceptives containing N-9 might be a risk factor for a genital HPV infection in women. This increase in susceptibility to infection may result from N-9-mediated disruption and infection of the genital epithelium. Similar findings have been reported with HIV. Indeed, although N-9 has some inhibitory activity in vitro against the virus, its use in vaginal contraceptive has shown it either to be not protective or to actually increase the risk of HIV infection.[1] In contrast, carrageenan is well tolerated in the vaginal tract, and it is currently being studied as a possible topical microbicide against HIV.[2] Unfortunately, in most medical trials, AIDS gels have yielded disappointing results.

B. H. Thiers, MD

References

1. Wilkinson D, Tholandi M, Ramjee G, Rutherford GW. Nonoxynol-9 spermicide for prevention of vaginally acquired HIV and other sexually transmitted infections: systematic review and meta-analysis of randomized controlled trials including more than 5000 women. *Lancet Infec Dis.* 2002;2:613-617.
2. Coggins C, Blanchard K, Alvarez F, et al. Preliminary safety and acceptability of a carrageenan gel for possible use as a vaginal microbicide. *Sex Transm Infec.* 2000;76:480-483.

American Cancer Society Guideline for Human Papillomavirus (HPV) Vaccine Use to Prevent Cervical Cancer and Its Precursors
Saslow D, for the Gynecologic Cancer Advisory Group, Garcia F (American Cancer Society, Atlanta, Ga; et al)
CA Cancer J Clin 57:7-28, 2007

Background.—Cervical cancer screening has been successful in decreasing the incidence and mortality of squamous cell cervical cancer. The most recent (2002) update of the American Cancer Society (ACS) Guideline for the Early Detection of Cervical Cancer incorporated options that included liquid-based cytology and human papillomavirus (HPV) DNA testing. Since the publication of those guidelines, 2 vaccines against the most common cancer-causing HPV types have been developed and tested in clinical trials. This report reviews the ACS guidelines for use of the HPV vaccine and summarizes the policy and implementation issues and implications for screening associated with use of the HPV vaccine.

Overview.—Nearly all cervical cancers are causally related to HPV infections, and approximately 70% of cervical cancers are caused by HPV types 16 or 18. The most successful strategy for cervical cancer prevention has been the implementation of population-based organized and opportunistic screening programs that use exfoliative cervical cytology (Papanicolaou test). However, the imperfect sensitivity of cytology testing is estimated to be responsible for 30% of all cervical cancers, and provider error in the follow-up of abnormal results accounts for another 10%. The greatest burden of cervical cancer is found in underserved, resource-poor populations of women in whom at least 80% of all incident cervical cancer and related mortality occurs. Worldwide, HPV is typically the most common sexually transmitted infection. In the United States it is estimated that more than 6 million people are infected with genital HPV each year. Two prophylactic HPV vaccines—Gardasil and Cervarix—have been developed. The goal of prophylactic vaccination is to reduce the incidence of HPV-related genital disease, including cervical, penile, vulvar, vaginal, and anal cancers, and precancerous lesions. Efficacy studies for both vaccines have reported vaccine efficacy of 100% for prevention of HPV 16- and 18-related cervical intraepithelial neoplasia. Both Gardasil and Cervarix have had few safety issues during any clinical trials.

Conclusions.—If the duration of immunity is substantial or can be extended adequately through booster vaccinations, the high efficacy of the vaccines observed in Phase II and III studies suggested that female populations receiving prophylactic immunization will experience a reduction in the morbidity and mortality associated with HPV-related anogenital diseases. However, it is crucial that women undergo regular screening for cervical cancer, regardless of whether they have been vaccinated.

▶ Despite the life-saving potential of the HPV vaccine, its use has generated its fair share of controversy. These guidelines prepared by the American Cancer Society are based on available scientific evidence and are not meant to address moral and religious arguments that have proposed to restrict the use of the vaccine.

B. H. Thiers, MD

Quadrivalent Vaccine against Human Papillomavirus to Prevent High-Grade Cervical Lesions

Koutsky LA, for The FUTURE II Study Group (Univ of Washington, Seattle; et al)
N Engl J Med 356:1915-1927, 2007

Background.—Human papillomavirus types 16 (HPV-16) and 18 (HPV-18) cause approximately 70% of cervical cancers worldwide. A phase 3 trial was conducted to evaluate a quadrivalent vaccine against HPV types 6, 11, 16, and 18 (HPV-6/11/16/18) for the prevention of high-grade cervical lesions associated with HPV-16 and HPV-18.

Methods.—In this randomized, double-blind trial, we assigned 12,167 women between the ages of 15 and 26 years to receive three doses of either HPV-6/11/16/18 vaccine or placebo, administered at day 1, month 2, and month 6. The primary analysis was performed for a per-protocol susceptible population that included 5305 women in the vaccine group and 5260 in the placebo group who had no virologic evidence of infection with HPV-16 or HPV-18 through 1 month after the third dose (month 7). The primary composite end point was cervical intraepithelial neoplasia grade 2 or 3, adenocarcinoma in situ, or cervical cancer related to HPV-16 or HPV-18.

Results.—Subjects were followed for an average of 3 years after receiving the first dose of vaccine or placebo. Vaccine efficacy for the prevention of the primary composite end point was 98% (95.89% confidence interval [CI], 86 to 100) in the per-protocol susceptible population and 44% (95% CI, 26 to 58) in an intention-to-treat population of all women who had undergone randomization (those with or without previous infection). The estimated vaccine efficacy against all high-grade cervical lesions, regardless of causal HPV type, in this intention-to-treat population was 17% (95% CI, 1 to 31).

Conclusions.—In young women who had not been previously infected with HPV-16 or HPV-18, those in the vaccine group had a significantly lower occurrence of high-grade cervical intraepithelial neoplasia related to HPV-16 or HPV-18 than did those in the placebo group. (ClinicalTrials.gov number, NCT00092534.)

▶ The new quadrivalent vaccine marketed by Merck targets HPV serotypes 6, 11, 16, and 18. Types 6 and 11 are associated with anogenital warts and some low-grade neoplastic lesions, whereas types 16 and 18 cause most cervical cancers. This study and a study by Garland et al[1] show that the vaccine is highly effective against precancerous cervical lesions and anogenital warts. The vaccine efficacy was 90% to 100% in both trials over 3 years in young women not previously infected with the vaccine serotypes. However, it was considerably less effective in unselected women, some of whom either were already infected or had HPV-related diseases. The question of who should be vaccinated and when they should be vaccinated has been the source of considerable debate, with political, social, and religious factors clouding what should be a purely medical issue.[2] Moreover, the HPV vaccines are probably most needed in the developing world, where 80% of deaths from cervical cancer occur. However, in these countries the cost can be a deterrent.[3] Finally, the efficacy of the vaccine in preventing cervical cancer is limited by at least 2 factors. First, not all cervical cancer is caused by HPV-16 or HPV-18, and second, for the vaccine to be effective, young women must be vaccinated before they are infected with these 2 serotypes. Other questions that require answers are the durability of immune protection and whether young men should be vaccinated as well.[4,5]

B. H. Thiers, MD

References

1. Garland SM, Hernandez-Avila M, Wheeler CM, et al. Quadrivalent vaccine against human papillomavirus to prevent anogenital diseases. *N Engl J Med.* 2007;356: 1928-1943.
2. Charo RA. Politics, parents, and prophylaxis—mandating HPV vaccination in the United States. *N Engl J Med.* 2007;356:1905-1908.
3. Agosti JM, Goldie SJ. Introducing HPV vaccine in developing countries—key challenges and issues. *N Engl J Med.* 2007;356:1908-1910.
4. Baden LR, Curfman GD, Morrissey S, et al. Human papillomavirus vaccine—opportunity and challenge. *N Engl J Med.* 2007;356:1990-1991.
5. Sawaya GF, Smith-McCune K. HPV vaccination—more answers, more questions. *N Engl J Med.* 2007;356:1991-1993.

Quadrivalent Vaccine against Human Papillomavirus to Prevent Anogenital Diseases

Garland SM, for the Females United to Unilaterally Reduce Endo/Ectocervical Disease (FUTURE) I Investigators (Royal Women's Hosp, Carlton, Victoria, Australia; et al)

N Engl J Med 356:1928-1943, 2007

Background.—A phase 3 trial was conducted to evaluate the efficacy of a prophylactic quadrivalent vaccine in preventing anogenital diseases associated with human papillomavirus (HPV) types 6, 11, 16, and 18.

Methods.—In this randomized, placebo-controlled, double-blind trial involving 5455 women between the ages of 16 and 24 years, we assigned 2723 women to receive vaccine and 2732 to receive placebo at day 1, month 2, and month 6. The coprimary composite end points were the incidence of genital warts, vulvar or vaginal intraepithelial neoplasia, or cancer and the incidence of cervical intraepithelial neoplasia, adenocarcinoma in situ, or cancer associated with HPV type 6, 11, 16, or 18. Data for the primary analysis were collected for a per-protocol susceptible population of women who had no virologic evidence of HPV type 6, 11, 16, or 18 through 1 month after administration of the third dose.

Results.—The women were followed for an average of 3 years after administration of the first dose. In the per-protocol population, those followed for vulvar, vaginal, or perianal disease included 2261 women (83%) in the vaccine group and 2279 (83%) in the placebo group. Those followed for cervical disease included 2241 women (82%) in the vaccine group and 2258 (83%) in the placebo group. Vaccine efficacy was 100% for each of the coprimary end points. In an intention-to-treat analysis, including those with prevalent infection or disease caused by vaccine-type and non–vaccine-type HPV, vaccination reduced the rate of any vulvar or vaginal perianal lesions regardless of the causal HPV type by 34% (95% confidence interval [CI], 15 to 49), and the rate of cervical lesions regardless of the causal HPV type by 20% (95% CI, 8 to 31).

Conclusions.—The quadrivalent vaccine significantly reduced the incidence of HPV-associated anogenital diseases in young women. (ClinicalTrials.gov number, NCT00092521.)

▶ The new quadrivalent vaccine marketed by Merck targets HPV serotypes 6, 11, 16, and 18. Types 6 and 11 are associated with anogenital warts and some low-grade neoplastic lesions, whereas types 16 and 18 cause most cervical cancers. This study and a study by Koutsky et al[1] show that the vaccine is highly effective against precancerous cervical lesions and anogenital warts. The vaccine efficacy was 90% to 100% in both trials over 3 years in young women not previously infected with the vaccine serotypes. However, it was considerably less effective in unselected women, some of whom either were already infected or had HPV-related diseases. The question of who should be vaccinated and when they should be vaccinated has been the source of considerable debate, with political, social, and religious factors clouding what should be a purely medical issue.[2] Moreover, the HPV vaccines are probably most needed in the developing world, where 80% of deaths from cervical cancer occur. However, in these countries the cost can be a deterrent.[3] Finally, the efficacy of the vaccine in preventing cervical cancer is limited by at least 2 factors. First, not all cervical cancer is caused by HPV-16 or HPV-18, and second, for the vaccine to be effective, young women must be vaccinated before they are infected with these 2 serotypes. Other questions that require answers are the durability of immune protection and whether young men should be vaccinated as well.[4,5]

B. H. Thiers, MD

References

1. Koutsky LA, for the FUTURE II Study Group. Quadrivalent vaccine against human papillomavirus to prevent high-grade cervical lesions. *N Engl J Med*. 2007;356: 1915-1927.
2. Charo RA. Politics, parents, and prophylaxis—mandating HPV vaccination in the United States. *N Engl J Med*. 2007;356:1905-1908.
3. Agosti JM, Goldie SJ. Introducing HPV vaccine in developing countries—key challenges and issues. *N Engl J Med*. 2007;356:1908-1910.
4. Baden LR, Curfman GD, Morrissey S, et al. Human papillomavirus vaccine—opportunity and challenge. *N Engl J Med*. 2007;356:1990-1991.
5. Sawaya GF, Smith-McCune K. HPV vaccination—more answers, more questions. *N Engl J Med*. 2007;356:1991-1993.

Efficacy of a quadrivalent prophylactic human papillomavirus (types 6, 11, 16, and 18) L1 virus-like-particle vaccine against high-grade vulval and vaginal lesions: a combined analysis of three randomised clinical trials

Joura EA, Leodolter S, Hernandez-Avila M, et al (Med Univ of Vienna; Natl Inst of Public Health, Cuernavaca, Morelos, Mexico; et al)
Lancet 369:1693-1702, 2007

Background.—Vulval and vaginal cancers among younger women are often related to infection with human papillomavirus (HPV). These cancers are preceded by high-grade vulval intraepithelial neoplasia (VIN2–3) and vaginal intraepithelial neoplasia (VaIN2–3). Our aim was to do a combined analysis of three randomised clinical trials to assess the effect of a prophylactic quadrivalent HPV vaccine on the incidence of these diseases.

Methods.—18,174 women (16–26 years) were enrolled and randomised to receive either quadrivalent HPV6/11/16/18 L1 virus-like-particle vaccine or placebo at day 1, and months 2 and 6. Individuals underwent detailed anogenital examination at day 1, 1 month after dose three, and at 6–12-month intervals for up to 48 months. Suspect genital lesions were biopsied and read by a panel of pathologists and vaccine HPV type-specific DNA testing was done. The primary endpoint was the combined incidence of VIN2–3 or VaIN2–3 associated with HPV16 or HPV18. Primary efficacy analyses were done in a per-protocol population.

Findings.—The mean follow-up time was 3 years. Among women naive to HPV16 or HPV18 through 1 month after dose three (per-protocol population; vaccine n=7811; placebo n=7785), the vaccine was 100% effective (95% CI 72–100) against VIN2–3 or VaIN2–3 associated with HPV16 or HPV18. In the intention-to-treat population (which included 18,174 women who, at day 1, could have been infected with HPV16 or HPV18), vaccine efficacy against VIN2–3 or VaIN2–3 associated with HPV16 or HPV18 was 71% (37–88). The vaccine was 49% (18–69) effective against all VIN2–3 or VaIN2–3, irrespective of whether or not HPV DNA was detected in the lesion. The most common treatment-related adverse event was injection-site pain.

Interpretation.—Prophylactic administration of quadrivalent HPV vaccine was effective in preventing high-grade vulval and vaginal lesions associated with HPV16 or HPV18 infection in women who were naive to these types before vaccination. With time, such vaccination could result in reduced rates of HPV-related vulval and vaginal cancers.

▶ This article by Joura et al and an article by the Future II Study Group[1] present additional evidence documenting the efficacy of the Merck vaccine in preventing high-grade vulvar and vaginal lesions associated with HPV16 or HPV18. The maximum effect is achieved in girls who are vaccinated in early adolescence, and it is anticipated that widespread use of this vaccine will reduce morbidity, mortality, and health care costs associated with cervical cancer. Nevertheless, a number of important questions about the use of these vaccines remain, and are discussed explicitly in an accompanying commentary on the Future II Study Group article.[2] These include the duration of protection from HPV infection after immunization, the best age at which to vaccinate, the possible benefits of vaccinating boys and young men, the need for protection against infection by other virus types that might lead to cervical neoplasia, and the cost barrier to widespread use of the vaccine, especially in the developing world. Other important hurdles include the absence of a health-delivery infrastructure in many countries, the political debate surrounding the issue of voluntary versus mandatory vaccination, the unsubstantiated claims that HPV vaccination will encourage promiscuity, and the belief by some that vaccination may be unnecessary, given the effectiveness of cervical screening strategies.

B. H. Thiers, MD

References

1. Future II Study Group. Effect of prophylactic human papillomavirus L1 virus-like-particle vaccine on risk of cervical intraepithelial neoplasia grade 2, grade 3, and adenocarcinoma in situ: a combined analysis of four randomised clinical trials. *Lancet.* 2007;369:1861-1868.
2. Markman M. Human papillomavirus vaccines to prevent cervical cancer. *Lancet.* 2007;369:1837-1839.

Effect of prophylactic human papillomavirus L1 virus-like-particle vaccine on risk of cervical intraepithelial neoplasia grade 2, grade 3, and adenocarcinoma in situ: a combined analysis of four randomised clinical trials

The Future II Study Group (Emory Univ School of Medicine, Atlanta, Ga; et al)
Lancet 369:1861-1868, 2007

Background.—Cervical cancer and its obligate precursors, cervical intraepithelial neoplasia grades 2 and 3 (CIN2/3), and adenocarcinona in situ (AIS), are caused by oncogenic human papillomavirus (HPV). In this combined analysis of four clinical trials we assessed the effect of prophylactic HPV vaccination on these diseases.

Methods.—20,583 women aged 16–26 years were randomised to receive quadrivalent HPV6/11/16/18 vaccine (n=9087), its HPV16 vaccine component (n=1204), or placebo (n=10,292). They underwent periodic Papanicolaou testing, with colposcopy or biopsy for detected abnormalities. The primary composite endpoint was the combined incidence of HPV16/18-related CIN2/3, AIS, or cervical cancer.

Findings.—Mean follow-up was 3.0 years (SD 0.66) after first dose. In women negative for HPV16 or HPV18 infection during the vaccination regimen (n=17,129, per protocol), vaccine efficacy was 99% for the primary endpoint (95% CI 93–100), meeting the statistical criterion for success. In an intention-to-treat analysis of all randomised women (including those who were HPV16/18 naive or HPV16/18-infected at day 1), efficacy was

44% (95% CI 31–55); all but one case in vaccine recipients occurred in women infected with HPV16 or HPV18 before vaccination. In a second intention-to-treat analysis we noted an 18% reduction (95% CI 7–29) in the overall rate of CIN2/3 or AIS due to any HPV type.

Interpretation.—Administration of HPV vaccine to HPV-naive women, and women who are already sexually active, could substantially reduce the incidence of HPV16/18-related cervical precancers and cervical cancer.

▶ This article by the Future II Study Group and an article by Joura et al[1] present additional evidence documenting the efficacy of the Merck vaccine in preventing high-grade vulvar and vaginal lesions associated with HPV16 or HPV18. The maximum effect is achieved in girls who are vaccinated in early adolescence, and it is anticipated that widespread use of this vaccine will reduce morbidity, mortality, and health care costs associated with cervical cancer. Nevertheless, a number of important questions about the use of these vaccines remain and are discussed explicitly in an accompanying commentary.[2] These include the duration of protection from HPV infection after immunization, the best age at which to vaccinate, the possible benefits of vaccinating boys and young men, the need for protection against infection by other virus types that might lead to cervical neoplasia, and the cost barrier to widespread use of the vaccine, especially, in the developing world. Other important hurdles include the absence of a health-delivery infrastructure in many countries, the political debate surrounding the issue of voluntary versus mandatory vaccination, the unsubstantiated claims that HPV vaccination will encourage promiscuity, and the belief by some that vaccination may be unnecessary, given the effectiveness of cervical screening strategies.

B. H. Thiers, MD

References

1. Joura EA, Leodolter S, Hernandez-Avila M, et al. Efficacy of a quadrivalent prophylactic human papillomavirus (types 6, 11, 16, and 18) L1 virus-like-particle vaccine against high-grade vulval and vaginal lesions: a combined analysis of three randomised clinical trials. *Lancet.* 2007;369:1693-1702.
2. Markman M. Human papillomavirus vaccines to prevent cervical cancer. *Lancet.* 2007;369:1837-1839.

Efficacy of a prophylactic adjuvanted bivalent L1 virus-like-particle vaccine against infection with human papillomavirus types 16 and 18 in young women: an interim analysis of a phase III double-blind, randomised controlled trial
Paavonen J, for the HPV PATRICIA study group (Univ of Helsinki; et al)
Lancet 369:2161-2170, 2007

Background.—The aim of this interim analysis of a large, international phase III study was to assess the efficacy of an AS04 adjuvanted L1 virus-like-particle prophylactic candidate vaccine against infection with human papillomavirus (HPV) types 16 and 18 in young women.

Methods.—18,644 women aged 15–25 years were randomly assigned to receive either HPV16/18 vaccine (n=9319) or hepatitis A vaccine (n=9325) at 0, 1, and 6 months. Of these women, 88 were excluded because of high-grade cytology and 31 for missing cytology results. Thus, 9258 women received the HPV16/18 vaccine and 9267 received the control vaccine in the total vaccinated cohort for efficacy, which included women who had prevalent oncogenic HPV infections, often with several HPV types, as well as low-grade cytological abnormalities at study entry and who received at least one vaccine dose. We assessed cervical cytology and subsequent biopsy for 14 oncogenic HPV types by PCR. The primary endpoint—vaccine efficacy against cervical intraepithelial neoplasia (CIN) 2+ associated with HPV16 or HPV18—was assessed in women who were seronegative and DNA negative for the corresponding vaccine type at baseline (month 0) and allowed inclusion of lesions with several oncogenic HPV types. This interim event-defined analysis was triggered when at least 23 cases of CIN2+ with HPV16 or HPV18 DNA in the lesion were detected in the total vaccinated cohort for efficacy. Analyses were done on a modified intention-to-treat basis.

Findings.—Mean length of follow-up for women in the primary analysis for efficacy at the time of the interim analysis was 14.8 (SD 4.9) months. Two cases of CIN2+ associated with HPV16 or HPV18 DNA were seen in the HPV16/18 vaccine group; 21 were recorded in the control group. Of the 23 cases, 14 (two in the HPV16/18 vaccine group, 12 in the control group) contained several oncogenic HPV types. Vaccine efficacy against CIN2+ containing HPV16/18 DNA was 90.4% (97.9% CI 53.4–99.3; $p<0.0001$). No clinically meaningful differences were noted in safety outcomes between the study groups.

Interpretation.—The adjuvanted HPV16/18 vaccine showed prophylactic efficacy against CIN2+ associated with HPV16 or HPV18 and thus could be used for cervical cancer prevention.

▶ In this article, Paavonen et al present data from an international Phase III study assessing the efficacy of the GlaxoSmithKline HPV16/18 vaccine. The data are encouraging but their interpretation has limitations, as discussed in an accompanying editorial.[1] Given that cervical carcinogenesis often evolves over several decades, the follow-up was relatively brief. Moreover, it is uncertain whether the entry criteria for the clinical trials were truly representative of the general population. For example, the proportion of black and Hispanic participants was small; these women are at increased risk for cervical cancer. The effect of the vaccination on overall rates of CIN2/CIN3 was not reported, which limits the predictability of the potential public health impact of the vaccination. Certainly, vaccination is not a substitute for routine screening for cervical cancer, and women who are vaccinated must continue to have age-appropriate cervical cancer screening and appropriate follow-up.[2]

B. H. Thiers, MD

References

1. Kahn JA, Burk RD. Papillomavirus vaccines in perspective. *Lancet.* 2007;369: 2135-2137.
2. Markowitz LE, Dunne EF, Saraiya M, et al. Quadrivalent human papillomavirus vaccine: Recommendations of the Advisory Committee on Immunization Practices (ACIP). *MMWR Recomm Rep.* 2007;56:1-24.

Topical Resiquimod 0.01% Gel Decreases Herpes Simplex Virus Type 2 Genital Shedding: A Randomized, Controlled Trial

Mark KE, Corey L, Meng T-C, et al (Univ of Washington, Seattle; Fred Hutchinson Cancer Research Ctr, Seattle; 3M Pharmaceuticals, St Paul, Minn; et al)

J Infect Dis 195:1324-1331, 2007

Background.—Resiquimod, an investigational immune response modifier and Toll-like receptor (TLR) 7 and 8 agonist, stimulates production of cytokines that promote an antigen-specific T helper type 1 (Th1)–acquired immune response. In animal models, induction of Th1-specific responses modifies experimental herpes simplex virus (HSV) infection.

Methods.—We conducted a randomized, double-blind, vehicle-controlled trial to assess the efficacy of resiquimod 0.01% gel for reducing human anogenital HSV-2 mucosal reactivation. Adults with genital HSV-2 applied resiquimod or vehicle topically to herpes lesions 2 times weekly for 3 weeks and then collected daily anogenital swabs for 60 days for HSV DNA polymerase chain reaction. Recurrences during the subsequent 7 months were treated with study gel. During the final treatment-free 60 days, participants again collected daily swabs to assess shedding.

Results.—The median lesion and shedding rates were lower for resiquimod compared with vehicle recipients during the initial sampling period (10% vs. 16% [$P=.03$] and 10% vs. 17% [$P=.08$], respectively) and during the final sampling period (3% vs. 22% [$P<.001$] and 10% vs. 26% [$P=.009$], respectively). Resiquimod did not influence recurrence length.

Conclusions.—These findings suggest that the immunological control of HSV-2 reactivation and lesion clearance may differ and that TLR7 and TLR8 agonists can reduce the frequency of mucosal HSV-2 reactivation.

▶ Resiquimod, a cousin of imiquimod, induces the production of cytokines that activate the innate immune system, leading to a TH1 cell–mediated immune response. This influences immunological control of viral reactivation and clearance. Mark et al sought to determine whether application of topical resiquimod could inhibit reactivation of mucosal HSV-2 infection, and found some benefit in this regard. Unfortunately, this trial was stopped early by the sponsor when concurrent larger trials failed to show an effect. That decision was unfortunate, as the current study, because it is underpowered, only suggests efficacy rather than definitively demonstrating it, and data from larger trials might have produced more conclusive results.

B. H. Thiers, MD

The helicase primase inhibitor, BAY 57-1293 shows potent therapeutic antiviral activity superior to famciclovir in BALB/c mice infected with herpes simplex virus type 1

Biswas S, Jennens L, Field HJ (Cambridge Univ Veterinary School, England; Arrow Therapeutics Ltd, London)
Antiviral Res 75:30-35, 2007

BAY 57-1293 represents a new class of potent inhibitors of herpes simplex virus (HSV) that target the virus helicase primase complex. The present study was conducted using the zosteriform infection model in BALB/c mice. The helicase primase inhibitor, BAY 57-1293 was shown to be highly efficacious in this model. The beneficial effects of therapy were obtained rapidly (within 2 days) although the onset of treatment was delayed for 1 day after virus inoculation. The compound given orally, or intraperitoneally once per day at a dose of 15 mg/kg for 4 successive days was equally effective or superior to a much higher dose of famciclovir (1mg/ml, i.e. approximately 140–200mg/kg/day) given in the drinking water for 7 consecutive days, which, in our hands, is the most effective method for administering famciclovir to mice. In contrast to the vehicle-treated infected mice, all mice that received antiviral therapy looked normal and active with no mortality, no detectable loss of weight and no marked change in ear thickness. BAY 57-1293 and famciclovir reduced the virus titers in the skin to below the level of detection by days 3 and 7 post infection, respectively. In both BAY 57-1293 and famciclovir-treated mice, infectious virus titers in the ear pinna and brainstem remained below the level of detection. Consistent with these findings, BAY 57-1293 also showed a potent antiviral effect in an experiment involving a small number of severely immunocompromised athymic-nude BALB/c mice.

▶ Biswas et al provide a sneak preview of what likely will be the next generation of treatments for herpesvirus infections. Several important facts can be appreciated. First, the compound is rapidly and highly effective in a murine HSV-1 infection model, even when treatment is delayed for 1 day after virus inoculation. Second, the compound appears to be equally effective or superior to famciclovir given at a much higher dose. Third, the compound is quite effective even in severely immunocompromised athymic-nude BALB/c mice. Fourth, in this limited study, no evidence of drug resistance was noted. Clearly, a great deal of work still needs to be done before this compound can be considered clinically useful, but its promise is evident. Similarly, as more is learned about the viral life cycle, new approaches are also being investigated for the treatment of HIV infection.[1]

B. H. Thiers, MD

Reference

1. Esté JA, Telenti A. HIV entry inhibitors. *Lancet.* 2007;370:81-88.

Loss of Vaccine-Induced Immunity to Varicella over Time

Chaves SS, Gargiullo P, Zhang JX, et al (Ctrs for Disease Control and Prevention, Atlanta, Ga; Los Angeles County Dept of Health Services)
N Engl J Med 356:1121-1129, 2007

Background.—The introduction of universal varicella vaccination in 1995 has substantially reduced varicella-related morbidity and mortality in the United States. However, it remains unclear whether vaccine-induced immunity wanes over time, a condition that may result in increased susceptibility later in life, when the risk of serious complications may be greater than in childhood.

Methods.—We examined 10 years (1995 to 2004) of active surveillance data from a sentinel population of 350,000 subjects to determine whether the severity and incidence of breakthrough varicella (with an onset of rash >42 days after vaccination) increased with the time since vaccination. We used multivariate logistic regression to adjust for the year of disease onset (calendar year) and the subject's age at both disease onset and vaccination.

Results.—A total of 11,356 subjects were reported to have varicella during the surveillance period, of whom 1080 (9.5%) had breakthrough disease. Children between the ages of 8 and 12 years who had been vaccinated at least 5 years previously were significantly more likely to have moderate or severe disease than were those who had been vaccinated less than 5 years previously (risk ratio, 2.6; 95% confidence interval [CI], 1.2 to 5.8). The annual rate of breakthrough varicella significantly increased with the time since vaccination, from 1.6 cases per 1000 person-years (95% CI, 1.2 to 2.0) within 1 year after vaccination to 9.0 per 1000 person-years (95% CI, 6.9 to 11.7) at 5 years and 58.2 per 1000 person-years (95% CI, 36.0 to 94.0) at 9 years.

Conclusions.—A second dose of varicella vaccine, now recommended for all children, could improve protection from both primary vaccine failure and waning vaccine-induced immunity.

▶ Surveillance data collected from a sentinel population of subjects over a 10-year period after vaccination showed an increasing incidence of cases of varicella over time. These data were considered in 2006 by the Advisory Committee on Immunization Practices, and they recommended that children between 4 and 6 years of age receive a second dose of varicella vaccine. Continued surveillance will determine whether additional periodic vaccinations will be needed to prevent waning vaccine-induced immunity, particularly as the incidence of varicella decreases due to widespread vaccination of the population. Under this scenario, individuals would be less likely to periodically be exposed to the virus, which would naturally boost antibody titers; thus, persistence of vaccine-induced immunity to the varicella virus could theoretically decrease even more rapidly in the future.

S. Raimer, MD

Augmenting Immune Responses to Varicella Zoster Virus in Older Adults: A Randomized, Controlled Trial of Tai Chi

Irwin MR, Olmstead R, Oxman MN (Univ of California at Los Angeles; Univ of California at San Diego; San Diego Veterans Affairs Healthcare System, Calif)
J Am Geriatr Soc 55:511-517, 2007

Objectives.—To evaluate the effects of a behavioral intervention, Tai Chi, on resting and vaccine-stimulated levels of cell-mediated immunity (CMI) to varicella zoster virus (VZV) and on health functioning in older adults.

Design.—A prospective, randomized, controlled trial with allocation to two arms (Tai Chi and health education) for 25 weeks. After 16 weeks of intervention, subjects were vaccinated with VARIVAX, the live attenuated Oka/Merck VZV vaccine licensed to prevent varicella.

Setting.—Two urban U.S. communities between 2001 and 2005.

Participants.—A total of 112 healthy older adults aged 59 to 86.

Measurements.—The primary endpoint was a quantitative measure of VZV-CMI. Secondary outcomes were scores on the Medical Outcomes Study 36-item Short-Form Health Survey (SF-36).

Results.—The Tai Chi group showed higher levels of VZV-CMI than the health education group (P <.05), with a significant rate of increase (P <.001) that was nearly twice that found in the health education group. Tai Chi alone induced an increase in VZV-CMI that was comparable in magnitude with that induced by varicella vaccine, and the two were additive; Tai Chi, together with vaccine, produced a substantially higher level of VZV-CMI than vaccine alone. The Tai Chi group also showed significant improvements in SF-36 scores for physical functioning, bodily pain, vitality, and mental health (P <.05).

Conclusion.—Tai Chi augments resting levels of VZV-specific CMI and boosts VZV-CMI of the varicella vaccine.

▶ Much attention has been paid to the potential use of behavioral interventions to augment virus-specific immunity in older adults. Tai Chi incorporates aerobic activity, relaxation, and meditation, all of which have been reported to boost the CMI response. A previously reported small controlled pilot study found that a westernized, standardized version of Tai Chi, Tai Chi Chih (TCC) could boost CMI against the VZV. Irwin et al[1] sought to compare the effect of TCC with that of health education on baseline VZV-specific T-cell immunity in older adults and to determine whether TCC might augment the increase in immunity induced by the live attenuated varicella vaccine (the new high potent VZV vaccine was not available for use in this study). The authors found that TCC increased resting levels of VZV-specific CMI to a level comparable with that induced by the varicella vaccine. In addition, the combination of TCC and the varicella vaccine boosted VZV responder cell frequency nearly 40% to levels comparable to those reported in adults 30 years younger.

B. H. Thiers, MD

Reference

1. Irwin MR, Pike JL, Cole JC, Oxman MN. Effects of a behavioral intervention, Tai Chi Chih, on varicella-zoster virus specific immunity and health functioning in older adults. *Psychosom Med.* 2003;65:824-830.

A Cost-Effectiveness Comparison of Desipramine, Gabapentin, and Pregabalin for Treating Postherpetic Neuralgia

O'Connor AB, Noyes K, Holloway RG (Univ of Rochester, NY)
J Am Geriatr Soc 55:1176-1184, 2007

Objectives.—To compare the net health effects and costs resulting from treatment with different first-line postherpetic neuralgia (PHN) medications.

Design.—Cost–utility analysis using published literature.

Participants.—Hypothetical cohort of patients aged 60 to 80 with PHN.

Interventions.—Desipramine 100 mg/d, gabapentin 1,800 mg/d, and pregabalin 450 mg/d.

Measurements.—A decision model was designed to describe possible treatment outcomes, including different combinations of analgesia and side effects, during the first 3 months of therapy for moderate to severe PHN. The main outcome was cost per quality-adjusted life-year (QALY) gained. Costs were estimated using the perspective of a third-party payer. Multivariate, univariate, and probabilistic sensitivity analyses were performed, and the time frame of the model was varied to 1-month and 6-month horizons.

Results.—Desipramine was more effective and less expensive than gabapentin or pregabalin (dominant) under all conditions tested. Gabapentin was more effective than pregabalin but at an incremental cost of $216,000/QALY. Below $140/month, gabapentin became more cost-effective than pregabalin at a threshold of $50,000/QALY, and below $115/month gabapentin dominated pregabalin.

Conclusion.—Desipramine appears to be more effective and less expensive than gabapentin or pregabalin for the treatment of older patients with PHN in whom it is not contraindicated. After its price falls, generic gabapentin will likely be more cost-effective than pregabalin.

▶ Therapy of PHN is problematic, and good evidence-based data are difficult to obtain. Most authorities agree that tricyclic antidepressants are the most cost-effective drugs. Unfortunately, amitriptyline may be inappropriate for older persons because of the risk of serious side effects. In contrast, desipramine and nortriptyline appear to have equivalent efficacy but fewer anticholinergic and adrenergic side effects. An ECG has been recommended before initiation of a tricyclic antidepressant for patients 40 years and older.[1] Myriad other approaches have been suggested but none is entirely satisfactory because of either marginal efficacy or patient intolerance.

B. H. Thiers, MD

Reference

1. Dworkin RH, Backonja M, Rowbotham MC, et al. Advances in neuropathic pain: diagnosis, mechanisms, and treatment recommendations. *Arch Neurol.* 2003;63: 1524-1534.

Post-Herpetic Neuralgia in Older Adults: Evidence-Based Approaches to Clinical Management
Christo PJ, Hobelmann G, Maine DN (Johns Hopkins Univ School of Medicine, Baltimore, Md)
Drugs & Aging 24:1-19, 2007

Many individuals across the globe have been exposed to the varicella-zoster virus (VZV) that causes chickenpox. After chickenpox has resolved, the virus remains latent in the dorsal root ganglia where it can re-emerge later in life as herpes zoster, otherwise known as shingles. Herpes zoster is a transient disease characterised by a dermatomal rash that is usually associated with significant pain. Post-herpetic neuralgia (PHN) is the term used for the condition that exists if the pain persists after the rash has resolved. Advanced age and compromised cell-mediated immunity are significant risk factors for reactivation of herpes zoster and the subsequent development of PHN. Though the pathophysiology of PHN is unclear, studies suggest peripheral and central demyelination as well as neuronal destruction are involved.

Both the vaccine against VZV (Varivax®) and the newly released vaccine against herpes zoster (Zostavax®) may lead to substantial reductions in morbidity from herpes zoster and PHN. In addition, current evidence suggests that multiple medications are effective in reducing the pain associated with PHN. These include tricyclic antidepressants, antiepileptics, opioids, NMDA receptor antagonists as well as topical lidocaine (lignocaine) and capsaicin. Reasonable evidence supports the use of intrathecal corticosteroids, but the potential for neurological sequelae should prompt caution with their application. Epidural corticosteroids have not been shown to provide effective analgesia for PHN. Sympathetic blockade may assist in treating the pain of herpes zoster or PHN. For intractable PHN pain, practitioners have performed delicate surgeries and attempted novel therapies. Although such therapies may help reduce pain, they have been associated with disappointing results, with up to 50% of patients failing to receive acceptable pain relief. Hence, it is likely that the most effective future treatment for this disease will focus on prevention of VZV infection and immunisation against herpes zoster infection with a novel vaccine.

▶ Therapy of PHN is problematic, and good evidence-based data are difficult to obtain. Most authorities agree that tricyclic antidepressants are the most cost-effective drugs. Unfortunately, amitriptyline may be inappropriate for older persons because of the risk of serious side effects. In contrast, desipramine and nortriptyline appear to have equivalent efficacy but fewer anticholinergic and adrenergic side effects. An ECG has been recommended before initiation of a tricyclic antidepressant in patients 40 years and older.[1] Myriad other approaches have been suggested, but none is entirely satisfactory because of either marginal efficacy or patient intolerance. A reasonable algorithm for the treatment of post-herpetic neuralgia in older adults is given in Figure 1 of the original article.

B. H. Thiers, MD

Reference

1. Dworkin RH, Backonja M, Rowbotham MC, et al. Advances in neuropathic pain: diagnosis, mechanisms, and treatment recommendations. *Arch Neurol.* 2003;63: 1524-1534.

Agonistic Anti-CD40 Antibody Profoundly Suppresses the Immune Response to Infection with Lymphocytic Choriomeningitis Virus
Bartholdy C, Kauffmann SØ, Christensen JP, et al (Univ of Copenhagen)
J Immunol 178:1662-1670, 2007

Previous work has shown that agonistic Abs to CD40 (anti-CD40) can boost weak CD8 T cell responses as well as substitute for CD4 T cell function during chronic gammaherpes virus infection. Agonistic anti-CD40 treatment has, therefore, been suggested as a potential therapeutic strategy in immunocompromised patients. In this study, we investigated whether agonistic anti-CD40 could substitute for CD4 T cell help in generating a sustained CD8 T cell response and prevent viral recrudescence following infection with lymphocytic choriomeningitis virus (LCMV). Contrary to expectations, we found that anti-CD40 treatment of MHC class II-deficient mice infected with a moderate dose of LCMV resulted in severe suppression of the antiviral CD8 T cell response and uncontrolled virus spread, rather than improved CD8 T cell immune surveillance. In Ab-treated wild-type mice, the antiviral CD8 T cell response also collapsed prematurely, and virus clearance was delayed. Additional analysis revealed that, following anti-CD40 treatment, the virus-specific CD8 T cells initially proliferated normally, but an increased cell loss compared with that in untreated mice was observed. The anti-CD40-induced abortion of virus-specific CD8 T cells during LCMV infection was IL-12 independent, but depended partly on Fas expression. Notably, similar anti-CD40 treatment of vesicular stomatitis virus-infected mice resulted in an improved antiviral CD8 T cell response, demonstrating that the effect of anti-CD40 treatment varies with the virus infection studied. For this reason, we recommend further evaluation of the safety of this regimen before being applied to human patients.

▶ CD40 is an activating receptor expressed by antigen-presenting cells; engagement by its ligand (CD40L) present on the CD4+ T-lymphocyte membrane results in the induction of cytotoxic T cell and B cell responses. Much clinical interest in this receptor has been generated by the finding that antibodies to

CD40 can stimulate a vigorous immune response that is CD4⁺ T-cell independent, and such antibodies have been considered as potential vaccine adju-
vants. In addition, previous investigations have shown that treatment of MHC
class II-deficient mice with antibodies to CD40 prevented reactivation of latent
gammaherpes viruses.

In the current study, Bartholdy et al examined the effect of such antibodies
on the immune response to LCMV in a murine model in which CD4⁺ T-cell help
has been shown to be required for an effective and persistent cytotoxic T-cell
response and viral clearance. Their findings were both unexpected and of clinical significance, in that there was not only a marked reduction in number and
function of viral specific cytotoxic T cells, but also a dramatic increase in viral
load. Interestingly, Berner et al[1] recently reported a significant impairment of
the CD8⁺ T-cell response in a study of anti-CD40 effects in a mouse tumor
model. These findings add to the accumulating body of data describing the potential deleterious effects of immunotherapeutic antibodies to CD40, which
include the potential for autoimmune disease and systemic inflammatory
responses.

G. M. P. Galbraith, MD

Reference

1. Berner V, Liu H, Zhou Q, et al. IFN-mediates CD4+ T-cell loss and impairs
   secondary antitumor responses after successful initial immunotherapy. *Nat Med.*
   2007;13:354-360.

5 HIV Infection

Male circumcision for HIV prevention in young men in Kisumu, Kenya: a randomised controlled trial
Bailey RC, Moses S, Parker CB, et al (Univ of Illinois at Chicago; Univ of Manitoba, Winnipeg, Canada; NIH, Bethesda, Md; et al)
Lancet 369:643-656, 2007

Background.—Male circumcision could provide substantial protection against acquisition of HIV-1 infection. Our aim was to determine whether male circumcision had a protective effect against HIV infection, and to assess safety and changes in sexual behaviour related to this intervention.

Methods.—We did a randomised controlled trial of 2784 men aged 18–24 years in Kisumu, Kenya. Men were randomly assigned to an intervention group (circumcision; n=1391) or a control group (delayed circumcision, 1393), and assessed by HIV testing, medical examinations, and behavioural interviews during follow-ups at 1, 3, 6, 12, 18, and 24 months. HIV seroincidence was estimated in an intention-to-treat analysis. This trial is registered with ClinicalTrials.gov, with the number NCT00059371.

Findings.—The trial was stopped early on December 12, 2006, after a third interim analysis reviewed by the data and safety monitoring board. The median length of follow-up was 24 months. Follow-up for HIV status was incomplete for 240 (8.6%) participants. 22 men in the intervention group and 47 in the control group had tested positive for HIV when the study was stopped. The 2-year HIV incidence was 2.1% (95% CI 1.2–3.0) in the circumcision group and 4.2% (3.0–5.4) in the control group (p=0.0065); the relative risk of HIV infection in circumcised men was 0.47 (0.28–0.78), which corresponds to a reduction in the risk of acquiring an HIV infection of 53% (22–72). Adjusting for non-adherence to treatment and excluding four men found to be seropositive at enrollment, the protective effect of circumcision was 60% (32–77). Adverse events related to the intervention (21 events in 1.5% of those circumcised) resolved quickly. No behavioural risk compensation after circumcision was observed.

Interpretation.—Male circumcision significantly reduces the risk of HIV acquisition in young men in Africa. Where appropriate, voluntary, safe, and affordable circumcision services should be integrated with other HIV preventive interventions and provided as expeditiously as possible.

▶ This article by Bailey et al and an article by Gray et al[1] show that male circumcision halves the risk of adult males contracting HIV through heterosexual intercourse. One unanswered question is the effect of male circumcision on HIV transmission to women. A trial to test the hypothesis that male circumcision might also directly protect against male-female transmission of HIV is underway in Uganda, with results expected in 2008.

B. H. Thiers, MD

Reference

1. Gray RH, Kigozi G, Serwadda D, et al. Male circumcision for HIV prevention in men in Rakai, Uganda: a randomised trial. *Lancet*. 2007;369:657-666.

Male circumcision for HIV prevention in men in Rakai, Uganda: a randomised trial
Gray RH, Kigozi G, Serwadda D, et al (Johns Hopkins Univ, Baltimore, Md; Rakai Health Sciences Program, Entebbe, Uganda; Makerere Univ, Kampala, Uganda; et al)
Lancet 369:657-666, 2007

Background.—Ecological and observational studies suggest that male circumcision reduces the risk of HIV acquisition in men. Our aim was to investigate the effect of male circumcision on HIV incidence in men.

Methods.—4996 uncircumcised, HIV-negative men aged 15–49 years who agreed to HIV testing and counselling were enrolled in this randomised trial in rural Rakai district, Uganda. Men were randomly assigned to receive immediate circumcision (n=2474) or circumcision delayed for 24 months (2522). HIV testing, physical examination, and interviews were repeated at 6, 12, and 24 month follow-up visits. The primary outcome was HIV incidence. Analyses were done on a modified intention-to-treat basis. This trial is registered with ClinicalTrials.gov, with the number NCT00425984.

Findings.—Baseline characteristics of the men in the intervention and control groups were much the same at enrollment. Retention rates were much the same in the two groups, with 90–92% of participants retained at all time points. In the modified intention-to-treat analysis, HIV incidence over 24 months was 0.66 cases per 100 person-years in the intervention group and 1.33 cases per 100 person-years in the control group (estimated efficacy of intervention 51%, 95% CI 16–72; p=0.006). The as-treated efficacy was 55% (95% CI 22–75; p=0.002); efficacy from the Kaplan-Meier time-to-HIV-detection as-treated analysis was 60% (30–77; p=0.003). HIV incidence was lower in the intervention group than it was in the control group in all sociodemographic, behavioural, and sexually transmitted disease symptom subgroups. Moderate or severe adverse events occurred in 84

(3.6%) circumcisions; all resolved with treatment. Behaviours were much the same in both groups during follow-up.

Interpretation.—Male circumcision reduced HIV incidence in men without behavioural disinhibition. Circumcision can be recommended for HIV prevention in men.

▶ The article by Gray et al and an article by Bailey et al[1] show that male circumcision halves the risk of adult males contracting HIV through heterosexual intercourse. One unanswered question is the effect of male circumcision on HIV transmission to women. A trial to test the hypothesis that male circumcision might also directly protect against male-female transmission of HIV is underway in Uganda, with results expected in 2008.

B. H. Thiers, MD

Reference

1. Bailey RC, Moses S, Parker CB, et al. Male circumcision for HIV prevention in young men in Kisumu, Kenya: a randomised controlled trial. *Lancet.* 2007;369: 643-656.

Male and Female Circumcision Associated With Prevalent HIV Infection in Virgins and Adolescents in Kenya, Lesotho, and Tanzania

Brewer DD, Potterat JJ, Roberts JM Jr, et al (Interdisciplinary Scientific Research, Seattle; Colorado Springs, Colo; Univ of New Mexico, Albuquerque; et al)
Ann Epidemiol 17:217-226, 2007

Purpose.—Remarkable proportions of self-reported virgins and adolescents in eastern and southern Africa are infected with HIV, yet non-sexual routes of transmission have not been systematically investigated in such persons. Many observers in this region have recognized the potential for HIV transmission through unhygienic circumcision procedures. We assessed the relation between male and female circumcision (genital cutting) and prevalent HIV infection in Kenyan, Lesothoan, and Tanzanian virgins and adolescents.

Methods.—We analyzed data from recent cross-sectional national probability sample surveys of adolescents and adults in households, focusing on populations in which circumcision was common and usually occurred in puberty or later.

Results.—Circumcised male and female virgins were substantially more likely to be HIV infected than uncircumcised virgins (Kenyan females: 3.2% vs. 1.4%, odds ratio [OR] = 2.38; Kenyan males: 1.8% vs. 0%, OR undefined; Lesothoan males: 6.1% vs. 1.9%, OR 3.36; Tanzanian males: 2.9% vs. 1.0%, OR 2.99; weighted mean phi correlation = 0.07, 95% confidence interval, 0.03 to 0.11). Among adolescents, regardless of sexual experience, circumcision was just as strongly associated with prevalent HIV infection. However, uncircumcised adults were more likely to be HIV positive than cir cumcised adults. Self-reported sexual experience was independently related to HIV infection in adolescent Kenyan females, but was unrelated to HIV infection in adolescent Kenyan, Lesothoan, and Tanzanian males.

Conclusions.—HIV transmission may occur through circumcision-related blood exposures in eastern and southern Africa.

▶ In this article by Brewer et al, circumcision performed under unhygienic conditions could actually increase the transmission of HIV. They found that circumcised virgins and adolescents were more likely to carry HIV than their uncircumcised counterparts. This suggests that HIV is being transmitted nonsexually much more often than previously suspected, and that widespread male circumcision may not provide the much hoped for benefits. The truth may lie somewhere in the middle: circumcision may not be a "magic bullet," but when done under clean and safe conditions, it might be an important intervention.[1]

B. H. Thiers, MD

Reference

1. Karim QA. Prevention of HIV by male circumcision. *BMJ.* 2007;335:4-5.

Prognostic Significance of Immune Subset Measurement in Individuals With AIDS-Associated Kaposi's Sarcoma
Stebbing J, Sanitt A, Teague A, et al (Imperial College of Science, Medicine, and Technology, London)
J Clin Oncol 25:2230-2235, 2007

Purpose.—A prognostic index for AIDS-associated Kaposi's sarcoma (KS) diagnosed in the era of highly active antiretroviral therapy (HAART) was based on routine clinical and laboratory characteristics. Because immune subset measurement is often performed in HIV-positive individuals, we examined whether these were predictive of mortality independently of the prognostic index, or could predict time to progression of KS.

Patients and Methods.—We performed univariate and multivariate Cox regression analyses on a data set of 326 individuals with AIDS-associated KS to identify immune subset covariates predictive of overall survival and time to progression. Adaptive (CD8 T cell and CD19 B cell) and innate (CD16/56 natural-killer cell) immune parameters were studied by flow cytometry.

Results.—In univariate analyses, all three immune subsets had significant effects on overall survival ($P < .025$). In multivariate analyses including the prognostic index, only CD8 counts remained significant ($P = .026$), although its effect on the overall prognostic index is small. An increase of 100 cells/mm^3 in the CD8 count confers a 5% improvement in overall survival. Individuals with a higher CD8 count did not have an increased time to progression. Patients who were already on HAART at the time of KS diagnosis did not have a shorter time to progression than those who were antiretroviral naïve at KS diagnosis.

Conclusion.—The CD8 count appears to provide independent prognostic information in individuals with AIDS-associated KS. Measurement of the CD8 count is clinically useful in patients with KS.

▶ Although the role of factors such as HIV viral load and CD4 count in KS are well established, the clinical consequences of other routinely measured clinical laboratory variables have not been established. The authors investigated the role of routinely measured immune subset parameters in HAART-era patients with AIDS-associated KS. The data showed that the CD8 count, which measures cytotoxic T lymphocytes, has prognostic value, with increases in the CD8 count having favorable prognostic implications, presumably by virtue of better control of replication of both HIV- and KS-associated herpesvirus.

B. H. Thiers, MD

Normalisation of CD4 counts in patients with HIV-1 infection and maximum virological suppression who are taking combination antiretroviral therapy: an observational cohort study

Mocroft A, for the EuroSIDA study group (Royal Free and Univ College Med School, London; et al)
Lancet 370:407-413, 2007

Background.—Combination antiretroviral therapy (cART) has been shown to reduce mortality and morbidity in patients with HIV. As viral replication falls, the CD4 count increases, but whether the CD4 count returns to the level seen in HIV-negative people is unknown. We aimed to assess whether the CD4 count for patients with maximum virological suppression (viral load <50 copies per mL) continues to increase with long-term cART to reach levels seen in HIV-negative populations.

Methods.—We compared increases in CD4 counts in 1835 antiretroviral-naive patients who started cART from EuroSIDA, a pan-European observational cohort study. Rate of increase in CD4 count (per year) occurring between pairs of consecutive viral loads below 50 copies per mL was estimated using generalised linear models, accounting for multiple measurements for individual patients.

Findings.—The median CD4 count at starting cART was 204 cells per µL (IQR 85–330). The greatest mean yearly increase in CD4 count of 100 cells per µL was seen in the year after starting cART. Significant, but lower, yearly increases in CD4 count, around 50 cells per µL, were seen even at 5 years after starting cART in patients whose current CD4 count was less than 500 cells per µL. The only groups without significant increases in CD4 count were those where cART had been taken for more than 5 years with a current CD4 count of more than 500 cells per µL, (current mean CD4 count 774 cells per µL; 95% CI 764–783). Patients starting cART with low CD4 counts

(<200 cells per μL) had significant rises in CD4 counts even after 5 years of cART.

Interpretation.—Normalisation of CD4 counts in HIV-infected patients for all infected individuals might be achievable if viral suppression with cART can be maintained for a sufficiently long period of time.

▶ As discussed in an accompanying editorial, the observation by Mocroft et al that CD4 counts continue to increase on combination antiretroviral therapy (ART) until normal values are reached can only be generalized to patients on combination ART between periods of maximum virologic suppression.[1] Nevertheless, normalization of CD4 counts may be achievable even with low CD4 counts at baseline, at least for patients with ideal responses to combination ART. The practical value of these findings is uncertain. Most patients who need combination ART live in low-income countries, where monitoring of viral load may not be available. Thus, the ability to confer maximum virologic suppression under such circumstances is limited. Moreover, the CD4 count at the start of combination ART tends to be substantially lower in low-income countries than in high-income countries. Although the data may suggest that the average patient in a low-income country with advanced disease who starts ART may eventually be able to normalize his or her CD4 count (provided that maximum virological expression can be maintained), the reality of access to medical care and medical economics may mandate otherwise.

B. H. Thiers, MD

Reference

1. Maartens G, Boulle A. CD4 T-cell responses to combination antiretroviral therapy. *Lancet.* 2007;370:366-368.

Safety and efficacy of the HIV-1 integrase inhibitor raltegravir (MK-0518) in treatment-experienced patients with multidrug-resistant virus: a phase II randomised controlled trial
Grinsztejn B, for the Protocol 005 Team (Research Inst/Oswaldo Cruz Found, Rio de Janeiro, Brazil; et al)
Lancet 369:1261-1269, 2007

Background.—Raltegravir (MK-0518) is an HIV-1 integrase inhibitor with potent in-vitro activity against HIV-1 strains including those resistant to currently available antiretroviral drugs. The aim of this study was to assess the safety and efficacy of raltegravir when added to optimised background regimens in HIV-infected patients.

Methods.—HIV-infected patients with HIV-1 RNA viral load over 5000 copies per mL, CD4 cell counts over 50 cells per μL, and documented genotypic and phenotypic resistance to at least one nucleoside reverse transcriptase inhibitor, one non-nucleoside reverse transcriptase inhibitor, and one protease inhibitor were randomly assigned to receive raltegravir (200 mg, 400 mg, or 600 mg) or placebo orally twice daily in this multicentre, triple-blind, dose-ranging, randomised study. The primary endpoints were change in viral load from baseline at week 24 and safety. Analyses were done on a modified intention-to-treat basis.

Findings.—179 patients were eligible for randomisation. 44 patients were randomly assigned to receive 200 mg raltegravir, 45 to receive 400 mg raltegravir, and 45 to receive 600 mg raltegravir; 45 patients were randomly assigned to receive placebo. One patient in the 200 mg group did not receive treatment and was therefore excluded from the analyses. For all groups, the median duration of previous antiretroviral therapy was 9.9 years (range 0.4–17.3 years) and the mean baseline viral load was 4.7 (SD 0.5) $\log_{10}$ copies per mL. Four patients discontinued due to adverse experiences, three (2%) of the 133 patients across all raltegravir groups and one (2%) of the 45 patients on placebo. 41 patients discontinued due to lack of efficacy: 14 (11%) of the 133 patients across all raltegravir groups and 27 (60%) of the 45 patients on placebo. At week 24, mean change in viral load from baseline was -1.80 (95% CI -2.10 to -1.50) $\log_{10}$ copies per mL in the 200 mg group, -1.87 (-2.16 to -1.58) $\log_{10}$ copies per mL in the 400 mg group, -1.84 (-2.10 to -1.58) $\log_{10}$ copies per mL in the 600 mg group, and -0.35 (-0.61 to -0.09) $\log_{10}$ copies per mL for the placebo group. Raltegravir at all doses showed a safety profile much the same as placebo; there were no dose-related toxicities.

Interpretation.—In patients with few remaining treatment options, raltegravir at all doses studied provided better viral suppression than placebo when added to an optimised background regimen. The safety profile of raltegravir is comparable with that of placebo at all doses studied.

▶ Different therapies for HIV target different stages of the lifecycle of the virus. Existing therapies are limited by drug toxicity and the development of drug resistance. The existence of multidrug resistance strains and cross resistance to agents within a class has created a need for new classes of antiretroviral drugs.

Raltegravir is the first of a new class of antiretroviral drugs called integrase inhibitors. These agents target an essential enzyme for HIV that catalyzes the insertion of HIV DNA into the host cellular genome. The impressive results and good safety profile noted here in patients with advanced HIV-1 infection are indeed encouraging. If these results can be duplicated in larger studies and if no long-term unexpected side effects or resistance issues emerge, the drug will provide an exciting new option to include in initial regimens for highly active retroviral therapy.[1]

B. H. Thiers, MD

Reference

1. Cahn P, Sued O. Raltegravir: a new antiretroviral class for salvage therapy. *Lancet.* 2007;369:1235-1236.

C34, a Membrane Fusion Inhibitor, Blocks HIV Infection of Langerhans Cells and Viral Transmission to T Cells

Sugaya M, Hartley O, Root MJ, et al (Natl Cancer Inst, Bethesda, Md; Centre Médical Universitaire, Geneva; Thomas Jefferson Univ, Philadelphia)
J Invest Dermatol 127:1436-1443, 2007

Development of topical microbicides that prevent sexual transmission of HIV is an active area of investigation. The purpose of this study was to test the ability of the potent membrane fusion inhibitor C34, an HIV gp41 antagonist, to block HIV infection of human Langerhans cells (LCs) in an epithelial environment that mimics a major route of HIV infection. We incubated freshly isolated epidermal explants containing LCs with various doses of C34 before, during, and after exposing explants to HIV. Although C34 only partially blocked HIV infection of LCs when pre-incubated with skin, it displayed full, dose-dependent inhibition when present during and after viral exposure. The poor protection from HIV infectivity in pre-incubated samples is consistent with mechanism of C34 inhibition and starkly contrasts to the full protection provided by PSC-RANTES, an entry inhibitor that prevents HIV gp120 interaction with its co-receptor CCR5. Real-time PCR confirmed that C34 blocked HIV infection of LCs before reverse transcription and inhibited LC-mediated transfer of virus to T cells. We conclude that C34, if used topically at susceptible mucosal sites, and if continually present, has the potential to block sexual transmission of HIV.

▶ Sugaya and colleagues studied the ability of the membrane fusion inhibitor C34, which is an antagonist of HIV gp41 (the transmembrane subunit of the viral envelope glycoprotein Env), to block HIV infection of human LCs. Although the results appear promising, history has taught us that, when attempting to block the transmission of this virus, in vitro activity does not always correlate with in vivo efficacy.[1] Better agents for the decreasing of HIV transmission are badly needed.[2]

B. H. Thiers, MD

References

1. Van Damme L, Ramjee G, Alary M, et al. Effectiveness of COL-1492, a nonoxynol-9 vaginal gel, on HIV-1 transmission in female sex workers: a randomised controlled trial. *Lancet.* 2002;360:971-977.
2. Imrie J, Elford J, Kippax S, Hart GJ. Biomedical HIV prevention—and social science. *Lancet.* 2007;370:10-11.

Reduction of HIV-1 RNA Levels with Therapy to Suppress Herpes Simplex Virus
Nagot N, for the ANRS 1285 Study Group (London School of Hygiene and Tropical Medicine; et al)
N Engl J Med 356:790-799, 2007

Background.—Epidemiologic data suggest that infection with herpes simplex virus type 2 (HSV-2) is associated with increased genital shedding of human immunodeficiency virus type 1 (HIV-1) RNA and HIV-1 transmissibility.

Methods.—We conducted a randomized, double-blind, placebo-controlled trial of HSV suppressive therapy with valacyclovir (at a dose of 500 mg twice daily) in Burkina Faso among women who were seropositive for HIV-1 and HSV-2; all were ineligible for highly active antiretroviral therapy. The patients were followed for 24 weeks (12 weeks before and 12 weeks after randomization). Regression models were used to assess the effect of valacyclovir on the presence and quantity of genital and plasma HIV-1 RNA and genital HSV-2 DNA during treatment, adjusting for baseline values, and to evaluate the effect over time.

Results.—A total of 140 women were randomly assigned to treatment groups; 136 were included in the analyses. At enrollment, the median CD4 cell count was 446 cells per cubic millimeter, and the mean plasma viral load was $4.44 \log_{10}$ copies per milliliter. With the use of summary-measures analysis, valacyclovir therapy was found to be associated with a significant decrease in the frequency of genital HIV-1 RNA (odds ratio, 0.41; 95% confidence interval [CI], 0.21 to 0.80) and in the mean quantity of the virus ($\log_{10}$ copies per milliliter, −0.29; 95% CI, −0.44 to −0.15). However, there was no significant decrease in detection of HIV (risk ratio, 0.93; 95% CI, 0.81 to 1.07). HSV suppressive therapy also reduced the mean plasma HIV-1 RNA level by $0.53 \log_{10}$ copy per milliliter (95% CI, −0.72 to −0.35). Repeated-measures analysis showed that these effects became significantly stronger during the 3 months of follow-up.

Conclusions.—HSV suppressive therapy significantly reduces genital and plasma HIV-1 RNA levels in dually infected women. This finding may have important implications for HIV control.

▶ Nagot et al note the association of HSV-2 with significantly higher amounts of HIV-1 in women with sexually acquired HIV-1 infection. This suggests that HIV-1 replication can be reduced with antiviral therapy directed at HSV-2, even though acyclovir has no direct activity against HIV. The findings highlight the potential benefit of screening and treating subclinical HSV-2 infection in patients with HIV. The interconnection between the 2 organisms is well documented and clinically relevant, as the vast majority of patients with sexually acquired HIV also have HSV-2 infection. The bottom line is that routine HSV-2 testing should be incorporated into the initial evaluation of HIV-seropositive patients.[1]

B. H. Thiers, MD

Reference

1. Corey L. Synergistic copathogens—HIV-1 and HSV-2. *N Engl J Med.* 2007;356: 854-856.

Class of Antiretroviral Drugs and the Risk of Myocardial Infarction
Lundgren LD, for The DAD Study Group (Univ of Copenhagen; et al)
N Engl J Med 356:1723-1735, 2007

Background.—We have previously demonstrated an association between combination antiretroviral therapy and the risk of myocardial infarction. It is not clear whether this association differs according to the class of antiretroviral drugs. We conducted a study to investigate the association of cumulative exposure to protease inhibitors and nonnucleoside reverse-transcriptase inhibitors with the risk of myocardial infarction.

Methods.—We analyzed data collected through February 2005 from our prospective observational study of 23,437 patients infected with the human immunodeficiency virus. The incidence rates of myocardial infarction during the follow-up period were calculated, and the associations between myocardial infarction and exposure to protease inhibitors or nonnucleoside reverse-transcriptase inhibitors were determined.

Results.—Three hundred forty-five patients had a myocardial infarction during 94,469 person-years of observation. The incidence of myocardial infarction increased from 1.53 per 1000 person-years in those not exposed to protease inhibitors to 6.01 per 1000 person-years in those exposed to protease inhibitors for more than 6 years. After adjustment for exposure to the other drug class and established cardiovascular risk factors (excluding lipid levels), the relative rate of myocardial infarction per year of protease-inhibitor exposure was 1.16 (95% confidence interval [CI], 1.10 to 1.23), whereas the relative rate per year of exposure to nonnucleoside reverse-transcriptase inhibitors was 1.05 (95% CI, 0.98 to 1.13). Adjustment for serum lipid levels further reduced the effect of exposure to each drug class to 1.10 (95% CI, 1.04 to 1.18) and 1.00 (95% CI, 0.93 to 1.09), respectively.

Conclusions.—Increased exposure to protease inhibitors is associated with an increased risk of myocardial infarction, which is partly explained by dyslipidemia. We found no evidence of such an association for nonnucleoside reverse-transcriptase inhibitors; however, the number of person-years of observation for exposure to this class of drug was less than that for exposure to protease inhibitors.

▶ The authors found that increased exposure to protease inhibitors was associated with drug-induced dyslipidemia; no such association was seen with the non-nucleoside reverse transcriptase inhibitors. The magnitude of increased cardiovascular risk with the protease inhibitors was not high, with the relative risk per year of exposure to the drugs being 1.16. Less certain is whether the use of non-nucleoside reverse transcriptase inhibitors is associated with a lower risk of myocardial infarction. Similarly, the incidence of myocardial infarction among patients exposed to protease inhibitors for more than 6 years was only 0.6% per year. This risk certainly appears to be manageable and pales in comparison to the cardiovascular risks associated with diabetes and smoking.[1,2] Clearly, the benefits of antiretroviral therapy outweigh the risks, particularly if the risks are managed appropriately.

B. H. Thiers, MD

References

1. Stein JH. Cardiovascular risks of antiretroviral therapy. *N Engl J Med.* 2007;356: 1773-1775.
2. Hughes MD, Williams PL. Challenges in using observational studies to evaluate adverse effects of treatment. *N Engl J Med.* 2007;356:1705-1707.

Incidence of cancers in people with HIV/AIDS compared with immuno-suppressed transplant recipients: a meta-analysis
Grulich AE, van Leeuwen MT, Falster MO, et al (Univ of New South Wales, Sydney, Australia)
Lancet 370:59-67, 2007

Background.—Only a few types of cancer are recognised as being directly related to immune deficiency in people with HIV/AIDS. Large population-based studies in transplant recipients have shown that a wider range of cancers could be associated with immune deficiency. Our aim was to compare cancer incidence in population-based cohort studies of people with HIV/AIDS and people immunosuppressed after solid organ transplantation.

Methods.—Two investigators independently identified eligible studies through searches of PubMed and reference lists. Random-effects meta-analyses of log standardised incidence ratios (SIRs) were calculated by type of cancer for both immune deficient populations.

Findings.—Seven studies of people with HIV/AIDS (n=444,172) and five of transplant recipients (n=31,977) were included. For 20 of the 28 types of cancer examined, there was a significantly increased incidence in both populations. Most of these were cancers with a known infectious cause, including all three types of AIDS-defining cancer, all HPV-related cancers, as well as Hodgkin's lymphoma (HIV/AIDS meta-analysis SIR 11.03, 95% CI 8.43–14.4; transplant 3.89, 2.42–6.26), liver cancer (HIV/AIDS 5.22, 3.32–8.20; transplant 2.13, 1.16–3.91), and stomach cancer (HIV/AIDS 1.90, 1.53–2.36; transplant 2.04, 1.49–2.79). Most common epithelial cancers did not occur at increased rates.

Interpretation.—The similarity of the pattern of increased risk of cancer in the two populations suggests that it is immune deficiency, rather than other risk factors for cancer, that is responsible for the increased risk.

Infection-related cancer will probably become an increasingly important complication of long-term HIV infection.

▶ The authors used meta-analyses to examine cancer incidence in published population-based studies of organ transplant recipients and patients with HIV/AIDS, and compared the findings. The data showed an increased incidence of an extensive range of cancers in both groups, with the pattern of increased risk being much the same in both populations. Many, but not all, of these cancers are associated with a known or suspected infectious cause. The authors concluded that the range of infection-related cancers associated with immune deficiencies is much wider than previously appreciated and that a range of infectious organisms, such as Epstein-Barr virus (EBV) and human papillomavirus (HPV), appears to be implicated. The high rate of cancer at a broad range of sites suggests a critical role for the immune system in the prevention of cancers related to infection. With an increasing number of patients being iatrogenically immunosuppressed (eg, for transplants) or living longer with diseases associated with immunosuppression (eg, HIV/AIDS), cancer is likely to become an increasingly important cause of morbidity in these individuals. Unfortunately, the most important markers of immune function with respect to tumor surveillance are unknown. The CD4 count may not explain all of the effects of HIV on cancer susceptibility, and no corresponding marker for immune deficiency in transplant patients is available.[1]

B. H. Thiers, MD

Reference

1. Clifford G, Franceschi S. Immunity, infection, and cancer. *Lancet.* 2007;370:6-7.

6 Parasitic Infections, Bites, and Infestations

Accuracy of standard dermoscopy for diagnosing scabies
Dupuy A, Dehen L, Bourrat E, et al (Hôpital Saint-Louis, Paris)
J Am Acad Dermatol 56:53-62, 2007

Background.—Scabies is a contagious skin infestation caused by the human mite *Sarcoptes scabiei*. The usual reference method for definitive diagnosis is ex vivo identification of the mite with microscopic examination of skin scrapings. We compared diagnostic accuracy of in vivo dermoscopic (DS) mite identification using a pocket handheld low-magnification DS with the reference method.

Methods.—We conducted a prospective, nonrandomized, evaluator-blinded, noninferiority study to compare sensitivities (main outcome) and other diagnostic properties of DS and microscopic examination of skin scrapings. Among 756 patients with a presumptive diagnosis of scabies consulting in one center, 238 were sequentially submitted to the two diagnostic procedures. Three dermoscopists (one expert, two inexperienced) were involved. Diagnostic strategies using clinical skills only, DS results, and a combination of both were compared.

Results.—Sensitivities were 91% (95% confidence interval: 86-96) for DS and 90% (95% confidence interval: 85-96) for microscopic examination of skin scrapings ($P = .005$ for noninferiority). Specificities were 86% (95% confidence interval: 80-92) for DS and 100% (by definition) for microscopic examination of skin scrapings. DS sensitivities were similar for the expert and inexperienced dermoscopists, whereas differences were observed in specificities. However, diagnostic accuracy of inexperienced dermoscopists steadily increased during the study. Compared with clinical-based, DS-based treatment decision rule minimized the number of false-positive and false-negative findings, whereas a treatment decision rule based on combination of clinical presumption and DS result drastically reduced the number of patients with scabies left untreated.

Limitations.—There is no definitive standard for ruling out the diagnosis of scabies.

Conclusions.—Standard DS with a handheld DS is a useful tool for diagnosing scabies, with high sensitivity, even in inexperienced hands. It greatly enhances clinical skills for making treatment decisions.

► Dupuy et al show that dermoscopy can be a valuable tool for the diagnosis of scabies. The procedure requires a degree of expertise for maximal accuracy, but the authors do show that the performance of inexperienced dermoscopists improved steadily during the study. Clearly, dermoscopy is less time-consuming and is associated with better patient acceptance than skin scrapings. The use of dermoscopy for the diagnosis of scabies appears to be particularly suitable for screening large patient populations, such as schools or nursing homes, or communities, especially in underdeveloped countries.

B. H. Thiers, MD

Multifunctional T$_H$1 cells define a correlate of vaccine-mediated protection against *Leishmania major*
Darrah PA, Patel DT, De Luca PM, et al (NIH, Bethesda, Md; Statens Serum Inst, Copenhagen; Infectious Disease Research Inst, Seattle; et al)
Nature Med 13:843-850, 2007

CD4$^+$ T cells have a crucial role in mediating protection against a variety of pathogens through production of specific cytokines. However, substantial heterogeneity in CD4$^+$ T-cell cytokine responses has limited the ability to define an immune correlate of protection after vaccination. Here, using multiparameter flow cytometry to assess the immune responses after immunization, we show that the degree of protection against *Leishmania major* infection in mice is predicted by the frequency of CD4$^+$ T cells simultaneously producing interferon-γ, interleukin-2 and tumor necrosis factor. Notably, multifunctional effector cells generated by all vaccines tested are unique in their capacity to produce high amounts of interferon-γ. These data show that the quality of a CD4$^+$ T-cell cytokine response can be a crucial determinant in whether a vaccine is protective, and may provide a new and useful prospective immune correlate of protection for vaccines based on T-helper type 1 (T$_H$1) cells.

► This article reports significant progress in the prevention and treatment of a disease that represents a significant world health problem. Darrah and colleagues note that effector memory cells enhance the production of interferon-γ for mediating protection against *L major*. Vaccines that target specific CD4$^+$ T-cell cytokine responses will help determine the success of preventive vaccines for the disorder. Another artible by von Stebut[1] discusses the possible role for dendritic cell-based vaccines, especially in the light of new data demonstrating the role of dendritic cells in the induction of the T$_H$1 helper cell response.

B. H. Thiers, MD

Reference

1. von Stebut. Cutaneous *Leishmania* infection: progress in pathogenesis research and experimental therapy. *Exp Dermatol.* 2007;16:340-346.

Cutaneous *Leishmania* infection: progress in pathogenesis research and experimental therapy

von Stebut (Johannes Gutenberg-Univ Mainz, Germany)
Exp Dermatol 16:340-346, 2007

Studies in murine experimental *Leishmania major* infection have helped to understand the requirements for efficient development of T helper (Th)1/ cytotoxic T (Tc)1-mediated protection against the parasite. As such they have revealed that Fcγ receptor (FcγR)I and FcγRIII-mediated uptake of *L. major* amastigotes by dendritic cells (DC) is an important prerequisite for Th1 development. In addition, DC-derived cytokines contribute to adequate T-cell education. DC-based vaccines may thus provide an important tool for both the development of a prophylactic vaccine against leishmaniasis and— together with leishmanicidal drugs—for eliciting immune-deviating functions towards protective immunity in non-healing leishmaniasis. This review highlights recent advances in the understanding of the role of DC for the induction of Th1/Tc1-predominant immunity against *L. major* and how this knowledge may translate into clinical approaches.

▶ This article by von Stebut reports significant progress in the prevention and treatment of a disease that represents a significant world health problem. The article discusses the possible role for dendritic cell-based vaccines, especially in the light of new data demonstrating the role of dendritic cells in the induction of the T_H1 helper cell response. In another article by Darrah et al,[1] the authors note that effector memory cells enhance the production of interferon-γ for mediating protection against *L major.* Vaccines that target specific CD4+ T-cell cytokine responses will help determine the success of preventive vaccines for the disorder.

B. H. Thiers, MD

Reference

1. Darrah PA, Patel DT, De Luca PM, et al. Multifunctional T_H1 cells define a correlate of vaccine-mediated protection against *Leishmania major. Nature Med.* 2007;13:843-850.

Role of Imiquimod and Parenteral Meglumine Antimoniate in the Initial Treatment of Cutaneous Leishmaniasis

Arevalo I, Tulliano G, Quispe A, et al (New York Univ School of Medicine; Universidad Peruana Cayetano Heredia, Lima, Peru; Pasteur Inst, Paris; et al)
Clin Infect Dis 44:1549-1554, 2007

Background.—Cutaneous leishmaniasis is a serious public health problem in the developing world. The main therapeutic agent—pentavalent antimony, developed >50 years ago—is expensive, often accompanied by severe adverse effects, and complicated by the emergence of drug resistance. Better therapies are urgently needed. In the present pilot study, we compared the use of imiquimod, an immunomodulatory molecule, to the use of meglumine antimoniate alone and in combination for the initial treatment of cutaneous leishmaniasis.

Materials and Methods.—Patients with newly diagnosed cutaneous leishmaniasis were enrolled from a single referral center in Lima, Peru, from August 2005 through October 2005. Patients were randomly assigned to 1 of 3 treatment groups and received either imiquimod 7.5% cream administered topically every other day for 20 days, intravenous meglumine antimoniate administered at a dosage of 20 mg/kg per day every day for 20 days, or combination therapy with both intravenous meglumine antimoniate and imiquimod 7.5% cream. Patients were evaluated weekly and at 1 and 3 months after treatment. Patients who had healed lesions at 3 months were considered to be clinically cured.

Results.—Although several patients showed initial resolution of symptoms with imiquimod treatment alone, all of these patients experienced relapse after treatment discontinuation. Four (57%) of 7 patients treated with meglumine antimoniate alone and 7 (100%) of 7 patients treated with combination therapy were cured. Combination therapy was not only more effective than the other 2 treatments ($P<.05$) but also led to faster healing and better cosmetic results.

Conclusion.—Combination therapy with imiquimod and meglumine antimoniate is a promising regimen for the initial treatment of cutaneous leishmaniasis that warrants additional larger studies.

▶ Arevalo et al suggest that topical imiquimod may be a useful adjunct to conventional therapy for the treatment of cutaneous leishmaniasis. In this study, when used in combination with meglumine antimoniate, it was associated with a higher rate of cure, an increased rate of healing, and an improved cosmetic outcome. When used alone, imiquimod appeared to have some initial effect but failed to achieve a response that was maintained after treatment was stopped. Larger studies are needed to confirm the benefits of combination therapy reported here and to assess various other combination regimens.

B. H. Thiers, MD

Transgenic malaria-resistant mosquitoes have a fitness advantage when feeding on *Plasmodium*-infected blood
Marrelli MT, Li C, Rasgon JL, et al (Johns Hopkins Univ, Baltimore, Md)
Proc Natl Acad Sci U S A 104:5580-5583, 2007

The introduction of genes that impair *Plasmodium* development into mosquito populations is a strategy being considered for malaria control. The effect of the transgene on mosquito fitness is a crucial parameter influencing the success of this approach. We have previously shown that anopheline mosquitoes expressing the SM1 peptide in the midgut lumen are impaired for transmission of *Plasmodium berghei*. Moreover, the transgenic mosquitoes had no noticeable fitness load compared with nontransgenic mosquitoes when fed on noninfected mice. Here we show that when fed on mice infected with *P. berghei*, these transgenic mosquitoes are more fit (higher fecundity and lower mortality) than sibling nontransgenic mosquitoes. In cage experiments, transgenic mosquitoes gradually replaced nontransgenics when mosquitoes were maintained on mice infected with gametocyte-producing parasites (strain ANKA 2.34) but not when maintained on mice infected with gametocyte-deficient parasites (strain ANKA 2.33). These findings suggest that when feeding on *Plasmodium*-infected blood, transgenic malaria-resistant mosquitoes have a selective advantage over nontransgenic mosquitoes. This fitness advantage has important implications for devising malaria control strategies by means of genetic modification of mosquitoes.

▶ New strategies to control malaria target novel components of the vector–pathogen interaction. Marrelli and colleagues studied the small peptide molecule SM1, which has been shown to bind to mosquito salivary and mid gut cells and to impair plasmodium development and its subsequent transmission from this insect vector. Mosquitoes expressing the plasmodium-resistant SM1 replaced wild-type, disease-transmitting mosquitoes in mixed cage populations, thereby suggesting that a genetically altered, malaria-resistant mosquito could be used to reduce transmission of the disease.[1]

B. H. Thiers, MD

Reference

1. Klempner MS, Unnasch TR, Hu LT. Taking a bite out of vector-transmitted infectious diseases. *N Engl J Med.* 2007;356:2567-2569.

A Molecular Link between Malaria and Epstein–Barr Virus Reactivation

Chêne A, Donati D, Guerreiro-Cacais AO, et al (Karolinska Institutet, Stockholm; Swedish Inst for Infectious Disease Control; Uganda Cancer Inst, Kampala; et al)

PLoS Path 3:826-834, 2007

Although malaria and Epstein–Barr (EBV) infection are recognized cofactors in the genesis of endemic Burkitt lymphoma (BL), their relative contribution is not understood. BL, the most common paediatric cancer in equatorial Africa, is a high-grade B cell lymphoma characterized by *c-myc* translocation. EBV is a ubiquitous B lymphotropic virus that persists in a latent state after primary infection, and in Africa, most children have seroconverted by 3 y of age. Malaria infection profoundly affects the B cell compartment, inducing polyclonal activation and hyper-gammaglobulinemia. We recently identified the cystein-rich inter-domain region 1α (CIDR1α) of the *Plasmodium falciparum* membrane protein 1 as a polyclonal B cell activator that preferentially activates the memory compartment, where EBV is known to persist. Here, we have addressed the mechanisms of interaction between CIDR1α and EBV in the context of B cells. We show that CIDR1α binds to the EBV-positive B cell line Akata and increases the number of cells switching to the viral lytic cycle as measured by green fluorescent protein (GFP) expression driven by a lytic promoter. The virus production in CIDR1α-exposed cultures was directly proportional to the number of GFP-positive Akata cells (lytic EBV) and to the increased expression of the EBV lytic promoter BZLF1. Furthermore, CIDR1α stimulated the production of EBV in peripheral blood mononuclear cells derived from healthy donors and children with BL. Our results suggest that *P. falciparum* antigens such as CIDR1α can directly induce EBV reactivation during malaria infection that may increase the risk of BL development for children living in malaria-endemic areas. To our knowledge, this is the first report to show that a microbial protein can drive a latently infected B cell into EBV replication.

▶ Chêne et al suggest that two pathogens, the malaria parasite and EBV, may interact in the pathogenesis of Burkitt lymphoma.[1] Latent EBV infection is found in >90% of the world's population. This persistent infection is generally lifelong but harmless, unless the equilibrium between the host and the virus is upset, as appears to be the case with coincident malaria infection, which seems to increase viral replication. Chêne et al propose a mechanism that may underlie this interaction. It is worth remembering that EBV is a herpesvirus, and some of the lessons learned in studying the interplay between the malaria parasite and EBV may help unlock the mysteries regarding the reactivation of other herpesviruses. For example, very often recurrent herpes labialis (or "cold sores") becomes manifest when an individual has a upper respiratory tract infection. Is this another example of interaction between two pathogens causing activation of a latent herpesvirus infection?

B. H. Thiers, MD

Reference

1. Thorley-Lawson DA, Duca KA. Pathogens cooperate in lymphomagenesis. *Nat Med.* 2007;13:906-907.

Maltreatment of *Strongyloides* Infection: Case Series and Worldwide Physicians-in-Training Survey

Boulware DR, Stauffer WM, Hendel-Paterson BR, et al (Univ of Minnesota, Minneapolis; Regions Hosp/HealthPartners, St Paul, Minn; Universidade Federal do Paraná, Curitiba PR, Brazil; et al)
Am J Med 120:545-551, 2007

Background.—Strongyloidiasis infects hundreds of millions of people worldwide and is an important cause of mortality from intestinal helminth infection in developed countries. The persistence of infection, increasing international travel, lack of familiarity by health care providers, and potential for iatrogenic hyperinfection all make strongyloidiasis an important emerging infection.

Methods.—Two studies were performed. A retrospective chart review of *Strongyloides stercoralis* cases identified through microbiology laboratory records from 1993-2002 was conducted. Subsequently, 363 resident physicians in 15 training programs worldwide were queried with a case scenario of strongyloidiasis, presenting an immigrant with wheezing and eosinophilia. The evaluation focused on resident recognition and diagnostic recommendations.

Results.—In 151 strongyloidiasis cases, stool ova and parasite sensitivity is poor (51%), and eosinophilia (>5% or >400 cells/µL) commonly present (84%). Diagnosis averaged 56 months (intra-quartile range: 4-72 months) after immigration. Presenting complaints were nonspecific, although 10% presented with wheezing. Hyperinfection occurred in 5 patients prescribed corticosteroids, with 2 deaths. Treatment errors occurred more often among providers unfamiliar with immigrant health (relative risk of error: 8.4; 95% confidence interval, 3.4-21.0; $P <.001$). When presented with a hypothetical case scenario, US physicians-in-training had poor recognition (9%) of the need for parasite screening and frequently advocated empiric corticosteroids (23%). International trainees had superior recognition at 56% ($P <.001$). Among US trainees, 41% were unable to choose any parasite causing pulmonary symptoms.

Conclusions.—Strongyloidiasis is present in US patients. Diagnostic consideration should occur with appropriate exposure, nonspecific symptoms including wheezing, or eosinophilia (>5% relative or >400 eosinophils/µL). US residents' helminth knowledge is limited and places immigrants in iatrogenic danger. Information about *Strongyloides* should be included in US training and continuing medical education programs.

▶ *Strongyloides* infection should be considered in patients with history of travel to developing countries regardless of the time since potential exposure. Clues to the diagnosis include wheezing, abdominal distress, and eosinophilia. Stool examinations are insensitive, although immunoglobulin G serology is available. Physicians need to be aware that infection persists indefinitely. Most deaths associated with *Strongyloides* are iatrogenic. For example, steroids given to a patient with chronic, asymptomatic *Strongyloides* infection can lead to life-threatening hyperinfection that has an approximately 50% mortality rate because of gram-negative sepsis resulting from penetration of larvae through the gut wall.

B. H. Thiers, MD

Chitin induces accumulation in tissue of innate immune cells associated with allergy

Reese TA, Liang H-E, Tager AM, et al (Univ of California San Francisco; Harvard Med School; Vrije Universiteit, Amsterdam)
Nature 447:92-96, 2007

Allergic and parasitic worm immunity is characterized by infiltration of tissues with interleukin (IL)-4- and IL-13-expressing cells, including T-helper-2 cells, eosinophils and basophils. Tissue macrophages assume a distinct phenotype, designated alternatively activated macrophages. Relatively little is known about the factors that trigger these host responses. Chitin, a widespread environmental biopolymer of N-acetyl-β-D-glucosamine, provides structural rigidity to fungi, crustaceans, helminths and insects. Here, we show that chitin induces the accumulation in tissue of IL-4-expressing innate immune cells, including eosinophils and basophils, when given to mice. Tissue infiltration was unaffected by the absence of Toll-like-receptor-mediated lipopolysaccharide recognition but did not occur if the injected chitin was pre-treated with the IL-4- and IL-13-inducible mammalian chitinase, AMCase, or if the chitin was injected into mice that overexpressed AMCase. Chitin mediated alternative macrophage activation in vivo and the production of leukotriene B_4, which was required for optimal immune cell recruitment. Chitin is a recognition element for tissue infiltration by innate cells implicated in allergic and helminth immunity and this process can be negatively regulated by a vertebrate chitinase.

▶ Chitin is a structural component of fungi, arthropods, and helminths and, as such, is ubiquitous in the environment. Humans and other mammals are therefore commonly exposed to this substance either directly, when it may result in allergy in a susceptible individual, or, in the case of parasitic helminths, by infection. The immune response to such infection bears many similarities to that which occurs in an allergic response. Interestingly, mammals, which do not possess chitin, nevertheless are capable of producing several chitinase-like enzymes, which are strongly induced in mice infected with a parasitic helminth.

In the current study, Reese et al showed that mice exposed to purified chitin mounted an early immune response characterized by tissue infiltration by basophils and eosinophils similar to that induced by infection and that this response did not occur in transgenic mice that constitutively expressed high levels of chitinase. Given that under physiologic circumstances, the expression of chitinase does not peak until day 9 of helminth infection, it is likely that these enzymes play an important role in regulation of the response to chitin.

G. M. P. Galbraith, MD

7 Disorders of the Pilosebaceous Apparatus

Loss-of-Function Mutations in the *Filaggrin* Gene and Alopecia Areata: Strong Risk Factor for a Severe Course of Disease in Patients Comorbid for Atopic Disease
Betz RC, Pforr J, Flaquer A, et al (Univ of Bonn, Germany; Univ of Düsseldorf, Germany; Univ of Antwerp, Belgium; et al)
J Invest Dermatol 127:2539-2453, 2007

Alopecia areata (AA) is a common dermatological disease, which affects nearly 2% of the general population. Association of AA with atopic disease has been repeatedly reported. Loss-of-function mutations in the *filaggrin* gene (*FLG*) may be considered as promising candidates in AA, as they have been observed to be a strong risk factor in atopic dermatitis. The *FLG* mutations R501X and 2282del4 were genotyped in a large sample of AA patients ($n=449$) and controls ($n=473$). Although no significant association was observed in the patient sample overall, *FLG* mutations were significantly associated with the presence of atopic dermatitis among AA patients. Furthermore, the presence of *FLG* mutations had a strong impact on the clinical course of AA in comorbid patients. For example, 19 of the 22 mutation carriers among AA patients with atopic dermatitis showed a severe form of the disease ($P=0.003$; odds ratio (OR)$=5.47$ (95% confidence interval (CI): 1.59–18.76)). In conclusion, our data suggest that when AA occurs in conjunction with FLG-associated atopic disorder, the clinical presentation of AA may be more severe.

▶ FLG protein is required for keratinization of the skin and normal dermal barrier function. The *FLG* gene located on chromosome 1q21 encodes profilaggrin, the precursor protein. *FLG* mutations have been shown to be major susceptibility determinants of atopic dermatitis and ichthyosis vulgaris. In this study, Betz et al examined the frequency of 2 null *FLG* mutations in patients with AA alone and those with a history of atopy. No differences were seen between the total patient group and healthy control subjects. However, an increase of null allele frequency was seen in patients with associated atopy, and within that group, the possession of the null allele was seen more frequently in those patients with alopecia totalis or universalis. These results, although interesting, must be viewed with some caution. For example, the designation of atopy in the patient group was based on history alone. The null allele frequency of both mutations studied was very low (1.5% and 2.5% in the control population), and the data for both mutations were combined for analysis. Furthermore, in the statistical analysis of data, no corrections were made for multiple comparisons. The authors state that these investigations were exploratory; further studies of a well characterized patient population will be required for confirmation of these findings.

G. M. P. Galbraith, MD

A low-glycemic-load diet improves symptoms in acne vulgaris patients: a randomized controlled trial
Smith RN, Mann NJ, Braue A, et al (RMIT Univ, Melbourne, Australia; Royal Melbourne Hosp, Parkville, Australia; Turku Univ, Finland; et al)
Am J Clin Nutr 86:107-115, 2007

Background.—Although the pathogenesis of acne is currently unknown, recent epidemiologic studies of non-Westernized populations suggest that dietary factors, including the glycemic load, may be involved.

Objective.—The objective was to determine whether a low-glycemic-load diet improves acne lesion counts in young males.

Design.—Forty-three male acne patients aged 15-25 y were recruited for a 12-wk, parallel design, dietary intervention incorporating investigator-blinded dermatology assessments. The experimental treatment was a low-glycemic-load diet composed of 25% energy from protein and 45% from low-glycemic-index carbohydrates. In contrast, the control situation emphasized carbohydrate-dense foods without reference to the glycemic index. Acne lesion counts and severity were assessed during monthly visits, and insulin sensitivity (using the homeostasis model assessment) was measured at baseline and 12 wk.

Results.—At 12 wk, mean (SEM) total lesion counts had decreased more ($P=0.03$) in the low-glycemic-load group (-23.5 ± 3.9) than in the control group (-12.0 ± 3.5). The experimental diet also resulted in a greater reduction in weight (-2.9 ± 0.8 compared with 0.5 ± 0.3 kg; $P<0.001$) and body mass index (in kg/m²; -0.92 ± 0.25 compared with 0.01 ± 0.11; $P=0.001$) and a greater improvement in insulin sensitivity (-0.22 ± 0.12 compared with 0.47 ± 0.31; $P=0.026$) than did the control diet.

Conclusion.—The improvement in acne and insulin sensitivity after a low-glycemic-load diet suggests that nutrition-related lifestyle factors may play a role in the pathogenesis of acne. However, further studies are needed to isolate the independent effects of weight loss and dietary intervention and to further elucidate the underlying pathophysiologic mechanisms.

▶ In the middle part of the last century, acne was considered to be aggravated by eating excessive amounts of carbohydrates and high-sugar foods. This diet-acne connection fell from favor in 1969 when a clinical study found no exacerbation of acne lesions with intake of chocolate, although the chocolate and placebo bars were evidently of similar nutritional composition.[1] It recently has again been postulated that high-glycemic load diets may contribute to the prevalence of acne seen in Western countries.[2] This was a rather small study that relied on self reporting of dietary intakes, which is not ideal, but it did show a decrease in the number of pustules in the group on the low-glycemic diet as compared to the control group. Individuals on the low-glycemic diet also had improved insulin sensitivity compared with those with a high-glycemic intake. A much larger study would be needed to determine whether a low-glycemic diet is of any benefit in improving acne. Nevertheless, it would not appear unreasonable to attempt dietary manipulation as a part of a therapeutic regimen, especially as the diet does appear to have health benefits beyond acne.

S. Raimer, MD

References

1. Fulton JE, Plewig G, Kligman A. Effect of chocolate on acne vulgaris. *JAMA.* 1969;210:2071-2074.
2. Cordain L, Lindeberg S, Hurtado M, Hill K, Eaton SB, Brand-Miller J. Acne vulgaris: a disease of Western civilization. *Arch Dermatol.* 2002;138:1584-1590.

Is minocycline therapy in acne associated with antineutrophil cytoplasmic antibody positivity? A cross-sectional study
Marzo-Ortega H, Baxter K, Strauss RM, et al (Univ of Leeds, England; Churchill Hosp, Oxford, England)
Br J Dermatol 156:1005-1009, 2007

Background.—Minocycline (MN), one of the commonly prescribed therapies for acne, is known to be associated with autoimmune disorders including drug-induced lupus. However, data are sparse regarding the prevalence of autoimmune disease in acne or in patients with acne treated with MN.

Objectives.—To establish the prevalence of antinuclear antibodies (ANA), antineutrophil cytoplasmic antibodies (ANCA) and new autoimmune syndromes in an MN-exposed and unexposed population with acne.

Methods.—In a cross-sectional study, 252 patients with acne vulgaris were assessed. Sixty-nine per cent had been exposed to MN at some point or were taking the drug at the time of the interview. Data recorded included duration of disease (acne) and drug history as well as possible side-effects of drugs, in particular joint symptoms (pain and swelling). In addition, blood was taken for ANA, ANCA, liver function tests and HLA analysis.

Results.—There was no statistical difference in the prevalence of ANA positivity between patients exposed (13%) or not exposed (11%) to MN. However, higher titres of ANA (1/160 or higher) were found in the MN-exposed group (45% compared with 12% in the unexposed group). ANCA positivity was found in 7% of the MN-exposed group but no positivity was found in the unexposed cohort ($P = 0.022$). In 58% of cases, the ANCA detected were of the perinuclear pattern (p-ANCA) with myeloperoxidase specificity, and this finding was associated with clinical symptoms in the majority of cases. Two p-ANCA-positive patients were thought in retrospect to have developed a drug-induced lupus syndrome.

Conclusions.—ANA positivity is seen in patients with acne irrespective of exposure to MN; however, p-ANCA appear to be a serological marker for developing autoimmune disease in patients receiving MN.

▶ The results are somewhat muddied by the inclusion of both currently exposed and previously exposed patients in the MN group. Nevertheless, the finding of ANCA-positivity in the exposed but not the unexposed group does imply a drug-induced phenomenon. Many earlier signs of autoimmune disease are nonspecific, and if these results are confirmed, the finding of ANCA-positivity could prove to be a useful marker for detecting drug-induced autoimmune disease in MN-treated patients.

B. H. Thiers, MD

Association or lack of association between tetracycline class antibiotics used for acne vulgaris and lupus erythematosus

Margolis DJ, Hoffstad O, Bilker W (Univ of Pennsylvania, Philadelphia)
Br J Dermatol 157:540-546, 2007

Background.—Previous studies have associated tetracyclines and, perhaps more specifically, minocycline use for the treatment of acne with onset of drug-induced lupus erythematosus (LE).

Objectives.—To determine the frequency of LE among those with acne who used antibiotics from the tetracycline class of antibiotics.

Methods.—A retrospective cohort study of individuals aged 15–35 years with acne within the practices of the general practice physicians in the U.K. who participate in The Health Information Network (THIN). Our outcome measure was physician reports of LE.

Results.—We identified 97,694 subjects with acne who were followed for about 520,000 person-years. They were on average about 22 years old and 57.5% were female. Minocycline exposure was noted in 24.8% of our subjects, doxycycline exposure in 15.6%, other tetracyclines in 42.3%, and 17.3% had not received a tetracycline antibiotic. The overall hazard ratio for the association of minocycline to LE was 2.64 (95% confidence interval 1.51–4.66) and when adjusted for age and gender was 3.11 (1.77–5.48). Those affected were often treated for LE. No association was noted for doxycycline and the other tetracyclines.

Conclusions.—The use of minocycline and not the other tetracyclines is associated with LE. LE as reported in THIN often required systemic therapy.

Overall, the event is uncommon but the risk and benefit of minocycline therapy must be carefully considered.

▶ The authors sought to determine whether any of the various tetracycline class antibiotics is associated with lupus erythematosus. They found a modest risk with minocycline exposure, with the risk increasing with duration of exposure. Nevertheless, the risk was still increased with exposures of less than 6 months. Many of their subjects had relatively severe disease and required systemic therapy. Increased risk was not seen with other antibiotics in the tetracycline family. As with all drugs, physicians need to weigh the benefit-risk ratio before prescribing minocycline, which is an important treatment alternative for patients with acne.

B. H. Thiers, MD

Anti-androgenic Therapy Using Oral Spironolactone for Acne Vulgaris in Asians
Sato K, Matsumoto D, Iizuka F, et al (Univ of Tokyo; Ritz Med Clinic, Tokyo)
Aesthetic Plast Surg 30:689-694, 2006

Background.—Few studies have addressed anti-androgenic therapy using oral spironolactone for acne in Asians. Obtaining this race-specific information is important because Westerners and Asians respond differently to hormone therapy. This study aimed to examine the efficacy and safety of oral spironolactone used to treat acne in Asians.

Methods.—Spironolactone (initial dose, 200 mg/day) was administered orally to 139 Japanese patients (116 females and 23 males) with acne. Serum laboratory data, including various hormones and electrolytes, were examined for 25 of the subjects.

Results.—Most of the female patients who completed the 20-week regimen exhibited excellent improvement (evaluated by a photographic grading scale), although some discontinued treatment because of menstrual disturbances or other reasons. The treatment was less efficacious for the males than for the females, and because gynecomastia developed in three male patients, spironolactone treatment for males was stopped. Examination of the serum of 25 patients did not identify any toxicity associated with the treatment. Drug eruptions and edema in the lower extremities were each seen in three patients.

Conclusion.—Oral spironolactone is effective and safe for the treatment of acne in Asian females, and can be a good option for severe, recurring, and widespread types of the condition.

▶ Several anecdotal reports have supported the efficacy of oral spironolactone for treating acne vulgaris in women; however, experience in large numbers of patients has not been documented. Unfortunately, as a generic drug that has been around for decades, there is little motivation for any pharmaceutical company to invest the large sums of money that would be necessary to perform a double-blind, randomized, placebo-controlled trial involving substantial numbers of patients. My own experience with the drug is similar to that reported by Sato et al; it can be effective in selected individuals, although menstrual irregularities in women and gynecomastia in men can be troublesome adverse events. Nevertheless, anti-androgen therapy may be a reasonable option in patients with recalcitrant acne who decline isotretinoin therapy.

B. H. Thiers, MD

Isotretinoin therapy and the incidence of acne relapse: a nested case-control study

Azoulay L, Oraichi D, Bérard A (Univ of Montreal; CHU Sainte-Justine, Montreal)
Br J Dermatol 157:1240-1248, 2007

Background.—Previous studies on predictors of acne relapse in patients treated with isotretinoin had either small sample sizes, short follow-up periods, or lacked population-based data.

Objectives.—To identify and quantify predictors of acne relapse, and predictors of receiving a second isotretinoin treatment.

Methods.—Using the Régie de l'Assurance Maladie du Québec (RAMQ) and Quebec's hospital discharge (Med-Écho) administrative databases, a population-based cohort of 17,351 first-time isotretinoin users was assembled between 1984 and 2003. A nested case–control analysis was performed to determine predictors of acne relapse (as defined by receiving an antiacne medication). A second nested case–control analysis was performed to determine predictors of receiving a second isotretinoin treatment. The index date of cases was the calendar date of dispensing an antiacne medication (isotretinoin or other). Five controls were matched to each case on follow-up time. Rate ratios were estimated using conditional logistic regression.

Results.—A total of 7100 (41%) subjects experienced an acne relapse. These were matched to 35,500 controls. Being male, under 16 years of age and living in an urban area, and receiving isotretinoin cumulative doses greater than 2450 mg and an isotretinoin treatment longer than 121 days were statistically associated ($P < 0.05$) with acne relapse. The publishing of the different Canadian acne guidelines had no impact on the incidence of acne relapse ($P > 0.05$). A total of 4443 (26%) subjects required a second isotretinoin treatment. These were matched to 22 215 controls. There was a greater probability of receiving a second isotretinoin treatment after the publishing of the Canadian acne guidelines ($P < 0.05$).

Conclusion.—A relatively high rate of subjects experienced an acne relapse after an isotretinoin treatment.

▶ This article addresses the question of how "permanent" is the response of acne to isotretinoin. Although dermatologists initially were hopeful that isotretinoin might represent a true "cure" for acne, many years of experience has taught us that while the drug is clearly quite potent and useful, many responding patients do eventually require further therapy. From personal experience and confirmed by the authors, such patients often are young males. It is interesting that Azoulay et al also found that acne relapse also correlated with higher doses of isotretinoin and a more prolonged duration of treatment, suggesting that these individuals had more severe acne before the initiation of treatment. Another interesting correlate to the need for further therapy was living in an urban area, a finding that might reflect the fact that these individuals had greater access to physicians and, thus, were more likely to consult them to receive additional treatment.

B. H. Thiers, MD

Patient Receipt and Understanding of Written Information Provided with Isotretinoin and Estrogen Prescriptions
LaPointe NMA, Pappas P, Deverka P, et al (Duke Clin Research Inst, Durham, NC; Duke Univ, Durham, NC)
J Gen Intern Med 22:98-101, 2007

Background.—Medication guides (MG) and mandatory patient package inserts (MPPI) are required with some prescription medications.

Objective.—We sought to determine how many patients receive, read, and understand these mandated materials.

Design and Participants.—A total of 3,620 patients were identified as filling prescriptions for isotretinoin or selected estrogen products from February 2004 to January 2005. Patients were surveyed to gauge receipt and understanding of the MG for isotretinoin and the MPPI for estrogen.

Measurements and Main Results.—A total of 500 patients completed the survey, with 186 (93%) of the 200 isotretinoin patients and 258 (86%) of the 300 estrogen patients reporting receipt of the MG/MPPI with their most recent prescription. The majority of respondents reported confidence in their knowledge of their medication (86% for isotretinoin and 75% for estrogen). However, the mean score on 5 questions assessing recognition of medication risks was only slightly better than the score expected from guessing (3.1 vs 2.5, $P<.01$ for both isotretinoin and estrogen).

Conclusions.—Despite receiving the information and reporting confidence in medication knowledge, patients' understanding of major risks with these medications was poor. This finding highlights the need to develop better risk communication strategies to improve the safe and effective use of prescription medications.

▶ Although I agree with the overall conclusions of the study, ie, that the content, presentation, and distribution of medication information to the patient needs to be done in an understandable and practical manner, ultimately the patient must take responsibility for reading and understanding the material given to him. It is shocking that so many patients thought isotretinoin could cause bleeding, heart attacks, and abnormal heart rhythms. Nevertheless, leaving aside the controversy regarding mental problems or suicide, I personally am reassured that 96% of those questioned knew that it may cause birth defects, although obviously I would have been happier if this number was 100%.

B. H. Thiers, MD

Oral R115866 in the treatment of moderate to severe facial acne vulgaris: an exploratory study
Verfaille CJ, Coel M, Boersma IH, et al (Maastricht Univ, The Netherlands; Barrier Therapeutics NV, Geel, Belgium; private practice in Dermatology, Vilvoorde, Belgium; et al)
Br J Dermatol 157:122-126, 2007

Background.—R115866 (Rambazole™; Barrier Therapeutics NV, Geel, Belgium), a new-generation retinoic acid metabolism-blocking agent, is a nonretinoid compound enhancing intracellularly the endogenous levels of all-*trans*-retinoic acid by blocking its catabolism. By virtue of this property, and the proven positive effects of retinoids in the treatment of acne, R115866 could potentially be a useful drug for acne.

Objectives.—To explore the efficacy, safety and tolerability of systemic R115866 in male patients with moderate to severe facial acne vulgaris (at least 15 papules and/or pustules and at least two nodulocystic lesions).

Methods.—In this exploratory trial, 17 patients were treated with oral R115866 1 mg once daily for 12 weeks, followed by a 4-week treatment-free period.

Results.—At the end of treatment (week 12, n = 16) a mean reduction in inflammatory lesion count of 77.4% (P < 0.001), in noninflammatory lesion count of 58.3% (P < 0.001) and in total lesion count of 76.0% (P < 0.001) was observed as compared with baseline. All lesion counts were significantly reduced from week 4 onwards. Mild side-effects were reported occasionally.

Conclusions.—The current data indicate that treatment with oral R115866 1 mg once daily for 12 weeks in patients with moderate to severe facial acne vulgaris is efficacious and well tolerated and merits further investigation.

▶ The authors report their experience with a new-generation, non-retinoid retinoic acid metabolism-blocking agent in the treatment of acne. They state that the compound appears to be as effective as oral tazarotene in treating noninflammatory lesions but may be more effective than tazarotene in improving inflammatory lesions. Such comparisons using historical tazarotene data may not be entirely appropriate. Increased triglyceride levels, a known side effect of oral isotretinoin, were observed in 3 of 17 patients, but were not reported as an adverse event. Surprisingly, the authors do not address the teratogenic potential of the compound, although only males were included in the study.

B. H. Thiers, MD

Increased serine protease activity and cathelicidin promotes skin inflammation in rosacea

Yamasaki K, di Nardo A, Bardan A, et al (Univ of California, San Diego; Asahikawa Med College, Japan; INSERM U563, Toulouse, France; et al)
Nat Med 13:975-980, 2007

Acne rosacea is an inflammatory skin disease that affects 3% of the US population over 30 years of age and is characterized by erythema, papulopustules and telangiectasia. The etiology of this disorder is unknown, although symptoms are exacerbated by factors that trigger innate immune responses, such as the release of cathelicidin antimicrobial peptides. Here we show that individuals with rosacea express abnormally high levels of cathelicidin in their facial skin and that the proteolytically processed forms of cathelicidin peptides found in rosacea are different from those present in normal individuals. These cathelicidin peptides are a result of a post-translational processing abnormality associated with an increase in stratum corneum tryptic enzyme (SCTE) in the epidermis. In mice, injection of the cathelicidin peptides found in rosacea, addition of SCTE, and increasing protease activity by targeted deletion of the serine protease inhibitor gene *Spink5* each increases inflammation in mouse skin. The role of cathelicidin in enabling SCTE-mediated inflammation is verified in mice with a targeted deletion of *Camp*, the gene encoding cathelicidin. These findings confirm the role of cathelicidin in skin inflammatory responses and suggest an explanation for the pathogenesis of rosacea by demonstrating that an exacerbated innate immune response can reproduce elements of this disease.

▶ It's always nice to see dermatology and dermatologists featured in a well-respected, high–impact factor journal like *Nature Medicine*. Cathelicidins are peptides that protect against infection by gram-positive and gram-negative bacteria and some viruses. They may have direct microbicidal activity in addition to an ability to stimulate host defenses against these organisms. Yamasaki et al present an interesting new hypothesis about the pathogenesis of rosacea. They found increased levels of proteolytically processed cathelicidins and a related serine protease in the skin of patients affected with the disorder. The trigger for the abnormal cathelicidin processing, which suggests compromise of the innate immune system, remains uncertain. Nevertheless, the findings, if confirmed, suggest that targeting cathelicidins or serine protease may represent a future treatment strategy for rosacea.[1]

Some antibiotics may do just that. Although antibiotic therapy is acknowledged as effective in rosacea, the findings imply that simply targeting bacteria may not be the optimal approach. For example, tetracycline therapy often remains effective despite the development of tetracycline resistance. Interestingly, tetracycline-class antibiotics inhibit the production of enzymes that change the form of cathelicidin and accelerate the production of the altered protein, which may explain their real mechanism of action in this disease.

B. H. Thiers, MD

Reference

1. Bevins CL, Liu F-T. Rosacea: skin innate immunity gone awry? *Nat Med.* 2007; 13:904-906.

Pimecrolimus cream 1% for papulopustular rosacea: a randomized vehicle-controlled double-blind trial
Weissenbacher S, Merkl J, Hildebrandt B, et al (Technical Univ of Munich; Ludwig-Maximilian-Univ of Munich; Novartis Pharma, Nuremberg, Germany)
Br J Dermatol 156:728-732, 2007

Background.—Rosacea remains difficult to treat, despite many therapeutic options.

Objectives.—To investigate the effect of pimecrolimus cream 1% (Elidel®; Novartis Pharma, Nuremberg, Germany) in the treatment of papulopustular rosacea.

Methods.—Forty patients with rosacea (25 men and 15 women, mean age 58 years) were enrolled in a randomized, vehicle-controlled, double-blind study. For 4–8 weeks, patients applied pimecrolimus cream or vehicle twice daily to the involved areas on the face. Rosacea severity score, subjective severity assessment and quality of life assessment were obtained, along with photographic documentation.

Results.—Both treatment groups of 20 patients showed an improvement after 4 weeks. The differences were not significant ($P > 0.05$) with regard to mean absolute values, mean percentage changes from baseline, or mean absolute values as differences from baseline for the total score or scores of the different clinical signs (erythema, population, scaling and pustules). In the subjective severity score and the quality of life assessment, there was also no significant difference between pimecrolimus and the vehicle ($P > 0.05$).

Conclusions.—Treatment of rosacea for 4–8 weeks with the topical calcineurin inhibitor pimecrolimus cream 1% was not more efficacious than treatment with the vehicle cream.

▶ The results are certainly disappointing. Despite previous hopeful anecdotal reports, Weissenbacher et al found little evidence to support the efficacy of pimecrolimus cream in their randomized, vehicle-controlled, double-blind study of patients with rosacea. Perhaps some rosacea subtypes will prove more responsive to pimecrolimus therapy than others. It is also possible that a longer treatment period might have shown some benefit from the drug. Nevertheless, the results emphasize the importance of high-quality studies to assess the efficacy of any purported new "paradigm" for treating skin diseases.

B. H. Thiers, MD

Infliximab for severe hidradenitis suppurativa: Transient clinical efficacy in 7 consecutive patients

Fardet L, Dupuy A, Kerob D, et al (Hosp Saint-Louis, Paris; Hosp Saint-Antoine, Paris)

J Am Acad Dermatol 56:624-628, 2007

Background.—Hidradenitis suppurativa (HS) is a chronic and debilitating disorder. Despite its significant prevalence, few reports of therapeutic studies are available. Recent case studies have reported the efficacy of antitumor necrosis factor monoclonal antibodies in treating the condition. In the study presented here, we assessed the safety and efficacy of infliximab in a series of patients with severe HS.

Methods.—We reviewed all consecutive patients with severe HS and treated with infliximab between October 2004 and December 2005. They were evaluated using the Sartorius severity score, a physician and patient overall assessment, and the Skindex-29 quality-of-life index. A substantive response was defined as marked or moderate overall improvement assessed by both physician and patient.

Results.—Seven patients were reviewed. All received at least 3 infusions of infliximab (5 mg/kg) in weeks 0, 2, and 6, and 5 patients received a fourth infusion at week 10. At week 6, a substantive improvement was seen in 5 patients. With the other 2 patients, any improvement was minimal or nonexistent. At week 10, there was a substantive response in 2 of the 5 patients. Adverse events occurred in 3 patients: abdominal pain caused by colon cancer, a multifocal motor neuropathy with conduction block, and a severe allergic reaction.

Limitations.—We have reported on only 7 patients. All had severe and chronic disease.

Conclusion.—The efficacy of infliximab in patients with severe HS seems transient and is associated with significant toxicity. Prospective randomized studies are required to better assess the benefit-risk ratio of antitumor necrosis factor agents for this indication.

▶ In contrast with previous anecdotal reports, this article by Fardet and colleagues suggests significant caution and skepticism regarding the use of infliximab for the treatment of HS. Certainly it is possible that their unimpressive results reflect the severity of the underlying disease in a selected group of patients. The frequency of adverse events is also troublesome, although the relationship of some of these to the infliximab treatment is uncertain. Larger randomized, double-blind, controlled trials will be necessary to establish the role of infliximab in the control of this characteristically treatment-resistant disease.

B. H. Thiers, MD

Long-term efficacy of a single course of infliximab in hidradenitis suppurativa

Mekkes JR, Bos JD (Univ of Amsterdam)
Br J Dermatol 158:370-374, 2008

Background.—Hidradenitis suppurativa is a chronic inflammatory skin disease characterized by abscess formation, predominantly in the axillae and groins. The disease is difficult to treat and has a severe impact on quality of life. Recently, several case reports have been published describing successful treatment of hidradenitis suppurativa with infliximab and other tumour necrosis factor α inhibitors.

Objectives.—To evaluate the long-term efficacy of a single course of infliximab.

Methods.—Ten patients with severe, recalcitrant hidradenitis were treated with infliximab (three infusions of 5 mg kg^{-1} at weeks 0, 2 and 6) and followed up for at least 1 year. The disease activity was measured using laboratory parameters and a recently developed acne score. The patients rated the efficacy of infliximab on a 10-point scale at regular intervals. Quality of life was measured before and after treatment using the Dermatology Quality of Life Index (DQLI).

Results.—All patients improved within 2–6 weeks. The average acne score diminished from 164 ± 50 (mean ± SD) before treatment to 89 ± 49 after 1 year ($P = 0.002$). The mean CRP (C-reactive protein) was reduced from 31.7 mg mL^{-1} to 5.5 mg mL^{-1} after 1 month ($P = 0.015$). Patients judged the efficacy with a score of 7.9. The mean DQLI was reduced from 18.4 ± 7.9 before treatment to 9.3 ± 9.1 after 1 year ($P = 0.007$). In three patients long-lasting improvement was observed, with no recurrence of lesions in a 2-year follow-up period. The other patients showed recurrence of lesions after 8.5 months (range 4.3–13.4 months).

Conclusions.—Infliximab is an effective treatment in severe hidradenitis suppurativa, leading to reduction of symptoms for a prolonged period.

▶ These results are somewhat better than those reported by Fardet et al.[1] In this report by Mekkes and Bos, 10 patients with unresponsive, severe hidradenitis suppurativa were given 3 infusions of infliximab 5 mg/kg at baseline and at weeks 2 and 6. All improved initially, with 3 showing long-lasting improvement and 7 relapsing an average of 8.5 months after treatment. Adverse reactions were observed in 3 patients. There are many obstacles to the use of infliximab for this indication, including the need for IV administration and the cost. Given that the number of patients with severe hidradenitis is relatively small compared with those who have, for example, rheumatoid arthritis, psoriasis, and inflammatory bowel disease, it is unlikely that any pharmaceutical company will invest the time, money, and effort to perform the large-scale studies necessary to assess its true place in the treatment of this condition and to achieve FDA blessing for its use. This is unfortunate as hidradenitis has a severe impact on quality of life.

B. H. Thiers, MD

Reference

1. Fardet L, Dupuy A, Kerob D. Infliximab for severe hidradenitis suppurativa: transient clinical efficacy in 7 consecutive patients. *J Am Acad Dermatol.* 2007;56: 624-628.

8 Photobiology

Solar UV Forecasts: A Randomized Trial Assessing Their Impact on Adults' Sun-Protection Behavior
Dixon HG, Hill DJ, Karoly DJ, et al (Cancer Council Victoria, Australia; Univ of Oklahoma, Norman; Deakin Univ, Victoria, Australia)
Health Ed Behav 34:486-502, 2007

This study examined the effectiveness of solar UV forecasts and supporting communications in assisting adults to protect themselves from excessive weekend sun exposure. The study was conducted in Australia, where 557 adult participants with workplace e-mail and Internet access were randomly allocated to one of three weather forecast conditions: standard forecast (no UV), standard forecast + UV, standard forecast + UV + sun-protection messages. From late spring through summer and early autumn, they were e-mailed weekend weather forecasts late in the working week. Each Monday they were e-mailed a prompt to complete a Web-based questionnaire to report sun-related behavior and any sunburn experienced during the previous weekend. There were no significant differences between weather forecast conditions in reported hat use, sunscreen use, sun avoidance, or sunburn. Results indicate that provision of solar-UV forecasts in weather forecasts did not promote markedly enhanced personal sun-protection practices among the adults surveyed.

▶ The UV index has become a standard part of weather forecasts in many areas. Dixon et al sought to determine how well forecasts of weather conditions impacted sun-protection behavior. The results were disappointing. They found that UV forecasts that promoted the effectiveness and importance of sun protection did not reduce sun exposure or enhance sun protection among their sample of Australian adults. A similar randomized control trial in Sweden found that a UV Index informational brochure and personal UV radiation intensity indicators were not as effective at promoting sun protection as that of a general brochure on sun protection.[1] The data suggest that behavioral studies should be undertaken before investing significantly in interventions that are presumed to be health promoting.

B. H. Thiers, MD

Reference

1. Bränström R, Ullén H, Brandberg Y. A randomized population-based intervention to examine the effects of the ultraviolet index on tanning behaviour. *Eur J Cancer.* 2003;39:968-974.

The relation between sun protection factor and amount of sunscreen applied *in vivo*

Faurschou A, Wulf HC (Bispebjerg Hosp, Copenhagen)
Br J Dermatol 156:716-719, 2007

Background.—The declared sun protection factor (SPF) is based on the use of a sunscreen layer of 2 mg cm^{-2}. However, only around a quarter (0.5 mg cm^{-2}) of this amount is applied by sunbathers. Theoretical calculations have suggested that the effective SPF is related to sunscreen quantity in an exponential way but this was not confirmed *in vitro* and has not been studied *in vivo*.

Objectives.—To investigate the relation between SPF and sunscreen amount *in vivo*.

Subjects and Methods.—On the backs of 20 healthy volunteers, five areas of 34 cm^2 each were marked. One area was phototested to determine the ultraviolet (UV) sensitivity. Four areas were treated with a sunscreen SPF 4 in different amounts: 0.5, 1, 2 and 4 mg cm^{-2}. Thirty minutes after sunscreen application a phototest was conducted on each area. The effective SPF was calculated 22–26 h after irradiation using the UV dose needed to produce just perceptible erythema (minimal erythema dose) on protected and unprotected skin.

Results.—In all areas the mean SPF was significantly different from an SPF of 1 (no protection) ($P \leq 0.0001$) and the SPFs of the areas with the various amounts of sunscreen differed significantly from each other ($P \leq 0.0008$). The relation between the sunscreen amount applied and the SPF provided was most likely to follow exponential growth ($r^2 = 0.903$).

Conclusions.—This study indicates that the relation between SPF and sunscreen quantity follows exponential growth. Application of 1 mg cm^{-2} or 0.5 mg cm^{-2} makes the SPF fall as the square or fourth root, respectively, and 4 mg cm^{-2} results in an almost squared SPF.

▶ Dermatologists know that patients generally do not apply sunscreen in a quantity sufficient to achieve the SPF factor listed on the label. Faurschou and Wulf showed that this relationship is even more dramatic than previously may have been assumed, with the measured SPF increasing exponentially as the amount of sunscreen applied is increased. Of course, the reverse is also true, with small amounts of sunscreen providing even less protection than would be assumed using a linear model. Patients need to be reminded to apply sunscreen thickly and frequently to obtain the maximum benefit.

B. H. Thiers, MD

Depletion of CD4+ Cells Exacerbates the Cutaneous Response to Acute and Chronic UVB Exposure

Hatton JL, Parent A, Tober KL, et al (Ohio State Univ, Columbus)
J Invest Dermatol 127:1507-1515, 2007

Solid organ transplant recipients have a 60–250-fold increased likelihood of developing sunlight-induced squamous cell carcinoma (SCC) compared with the general population. This increased risk is linked to the immunosuppressive drugs taken by these patients to modulate T cell function, thus preventing organ rejection. To determine the importance of T cells in the development of cutaneous SCC, we examined the effects of selectively depleting Skh-1 mice of systemic CD4+ or CD8+ T cells, using monoclonal antibodies, on ultraviolet B (UVB) radiation-induced inflammation and tumor development. Decreases in systemic CD4+ but not CD8+ T cells significantly increased and prolonged the acute UVB-induced cutaneous inflammatory response, as measured by neutrophil influx, myeloperoxidase activity, and prostaglandin E_2 levels. Significantly more p53+ keratinocytes were observed in UVB-exposed CD4-depleted than in CD4-replete mice, and this difference was abrogated in mice depleted of neutrophils before UVB exposure. Increased acute inflammation was associated with significantly increased tumor numbers in CD4-depleted mice chronically exposed to UVB. Furthermore, topical treatment with the anti-inflammatory drug celecoxib significantly decreased tumor numbers in both CD4-replete and CD4-depleted mice. Our findings suggest that CD4+ T cells play an important role in modulating both the acute inflammatory and the chronic carcinogenic response of the skin to UVB.

▶ Hatton and colleagues used a murine model of UVB-induced nonmelanoma skin cancer to show that the specific depletion of CD4+ cells enhances susceptibility to UVB-induced SCC. The authors hypothesized that both increased UVB-induced cutaneous inflammation and decreased tumor immunosurveillance contribute to the enhanced skin tumor development observed in CD-4–depleted mice. This report suggests an important role for CD4+ cells in maintaining cutaneous homeostasis and in modulating information. Although the role of CD8+ cells remains uncertain, the data presented support the possibility that a balance between the two cell types may be necessary to regulate cutaneous inflammation.

B. H. Thiers, MD

Protection from photodamage by topical application of caffeine after ultraviolet irradiation

Koo S-W, Hirakawa S, Fujii S, et al (Harvard Med School, Boston; Ehime Univ, Japan; Univ of Washington, Seattle)
Br J Dermatol 156:957-964, 2007

Background.—Characterization of mechanisms that can reverse residual damage from prior skin exposure to ultraviolet (UV) would be of considerable biological and therapeutic interest. Topical caffeine application to mouse skin that had previously been treated with UV has been shown to inhibit the subsequent development of squamous cell carcinomas.

Objectives.—We used an established mouse photodamage model to investigate other possible effects of topical caffeine application after UV.

Methods.—SKH-1 hairless mice were treated with ultraviolet B (UVB) followed immediately by topical application of caffeine or vehicle three times weekly for 11 weeks.

Results.—Caffeine applied topically after UV treatment resulted in a significant decrease in UV-induced skin roughness/transverse rhytides as assessed by treatment-blinded examiners. Histologically, topical caffeine application after a single dose of UVB more than doubled the number of apoptotic keratinocytes as evaluated by sunburn cell formation, caspase 3 cleavage and terminal deoxynucleotidyl transferase-mediated dUTP-biotin nick-end labelling (TUNEL) staining. A trend towards decreased solar elastosis was noted in the caffeine-treated group although this was not statistically significant. Other histological parameters including epidermal hyperplasia, solar elastosis and angiogenesis were increased in mice treated with UV but topical application of caffeine did not alter these particular UV effects.

Conclusions.—These findings support the concept that topical application of caffeine to mouse skin after UV irradiation promotes the deletion of DNA-damaged keratinocytes and may partially diminish photodamage as well as photocarcinogenesis.

▶ A previous study has shown that caffeine can prevent UVB-induced skin cancer in an "at risk" mouse model. Koo et al examined the role of caffeine in protection from chronic photodamage after UVB exposure. They found that mice in whom caffeine was applied topically after UVB exposure showed decreased visual evidence of photodamage and increased numbers of apoptotic keratinocytes, a proxy for deletion of DNA-damaged cells. Not only does caffeine have an apparent reparative effect on photodamaged skin, but it also absorbs light in the UV spectrum and can have a sunscreen-like photoprotective effect as well. Should studies like this one be confirmed in human beings, one can foresee the day when caffeine is added to sunscreen products, both for its photoprotective effects and for its postexposure reparative effects, which might have a preventative influence on photodamage and photocarcinogenesis. Then again, why not just have a cup of coffee after a long day at the beach?

B. H. Thiers, MD

Effects of polyphenols on skin damage due to ultraviolet A rays: an experimental study on rats

Sevin A, Öztaş P, Senen D, et al (Ankara Numune Education and Research Hosp, Turkey; Ankara Dişkapi Education and Research Hosp, Turkey; Ankara Univ, Turkey)

J Eur Acad Dermatol Venereol 21:650-656, 2007

Background.—Ultraviolet (UV) radiation causes many acute and chronic conditions such as oedema of the skin, sunburn, immunosuppression, photo-ageing and skin cancer. The use of antioxidants has become of paramount importance in prevention of the damage caused by ultraviolet radiation. Epigallocatechin-3-gallate (EGCG), one of the main components of green tea, has been reported to have anti-inflammatory, antioxidant and anticarcinogenic properties.

Aim.—The aim of this experimental study was to investigate to what extent EGCG prevented acute skin damage caused by UVA.

Material and Method.—The sample contained 2% EGCG, which was prepared in hydrophilic ointment (USP XXIV) as the vehicle. Twenty-four 12-week-old Wistar albino rats are included in the study and divided into four groups, each containing six rats. Group I was formed to be the control group, which was not applied any topical medication or exposed to UV radiation. Group II was formed to observe acute effects of UVA on the skin, Group III was formed to observe effectiveness of topical EGCG on the skin applied 30 min after exposure to UVA, and Group IV was formed to observe topical EGCG applied 30 min before exposure to UVA. All groups were examined for sunburn cells, leucocyte infiltration, dermo-epidermal activity, collagen changes and elastic fibre pathologies on 24 and 72 h. Statistical analysis was performed using SPSS 11.5, and chi-squared test was used for the evaluation of parameters.

Results.—Group IV showed a statistically significant decrease in sunburn cells and dermo-epidermal activation compared with Group II. Group II showed significant increase in all parameters compared with Group I, showing the effects of UV exposure alone, and no difference was detected in Group II and III.

Conclusion.—These results show a protective effect of EGCG when applied topically before UVA exposure. No benefit was detected when EGCG was applied after UV exposure.

▶ Sevin et al attempted to determine to what extent EGCG, a primary component of green tea, could prevent acute skin damage after UVA exposure. Using a Wistar albino rat model, they found that topical EGCG could prevent acute UVA damage by reducing sunburn cell formation and damage at the dermal-epidermal junction. These findings suggest that EGCG may be useful as a protective agent against UVA radiation.

B. H. Thiers, MD

Green tea and skin cancer: photoimmunology, angiogenesis and DNA repair

Katiyar S, Elmets CA, Katiyar SK (Univ of Alabama at Birmingham; Birmingham VA Med Ctr, Ala)
J Nutr Biochem 18:287-296, 2007

Human skin is constantly exposed to numerous noxious physical, chemical and environmental agents. Some of these agents directly or indirectly adversely affect the skin. Cutaneous overexposure to environmental solar ultraviolet (UV) radiation (290–400 nm) has a variety of adverse effects on human health, including the development of melanoma and nonmelanoma skin cancers. Therefore, there is a need to develop measures or strategies, and nutritional components are increasingly being explored for this purpose. The polyphenols present in green tea (*Camellia sinensis*) have been shown to have numerous health benefits, including protection from UV carcinogenesis. (–)-Epigallocatechin-3-gallate (EGCG) is the major and most photoprotective polyphenolic component of green tea. In this review article, we have discussed the most recent investigations and mechanistic studies that define and support the photoprotective efficacy of green tea polyphenols (GTPs) against UV carcinogenesis. The oral administration of GTPs in drinking water or the topical application of EGCG prevents UVB-induced skin tumor development in mice, and this prevention is mediated through: (a) the induction of immunoregulatory cytokine interleukin (IL) 12; (b) IL-12-dependent DNA repair following nucleotide excision repair mechanism; (c) the inhibition of UV-induced immunosuppression through IL-12-dependent DNA repair; (d) the inhibition of angiogenic factors; and (e) the stimulation of cytotoxic T cells in a tumor microenvironment. New mechanistic information strongly supports and explains the chemopreventive activity of GTPs against photocarcinogenesis (Fig 3).

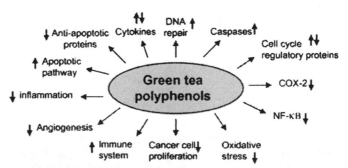

FIGURE 3.—Molecular targets of GTPs. (↑) Up-regulation; (↓) down-regulation. (Courtesy Katiyar S, Elmets CA, Katiyar SK. Green tea and skin cancer: photoimmunology, angiogenesis and DNA repair. *J Nutr Biochem.* 2007;18:287-296. Copyright Elsevier, 2007.)

▶ Katiyar et al present a comprehensive view of state-of-the-art knowledge of the preventative effects of green tea against skin cancer. The body of knowledge accumulated by these investigators and others is impressive, and we look forward to the day when the antiphotocarcinogenic potential of green tea becomes harnessed for human benefit. Remarkably, green tea appears to be effective either through oral administration or topical application on the skin and may be used in combinations with sunscreens or skin care lotions. It is safe and nontoxic. Clinical trials in high-risk human populations that assess the usefulness of green tea polyphenols or EGCG in preventing skin cancer are eagerly awaited.

B. H. Thiers, MD

Sulforaphane mobilizes cellular defenses that protect skin against damage by UV radiation
Talalay P, Fahey JW, Healy ZR, et al (Johns Hopkins Univ, Baltimore, Md)
Proc Natl Acad Sci U S A 104:17500-17505, 2007

UV radiation (UVR) is a complete carcinogen that elicits a constellation of pathological events, including direct DNA damage, generation of reactive oxidants that peroxidize lipids and damage other cellular components, initiation of inflammation, and suppression of the immune response. Recent dramatic increases in the incidence of nonmelanoma skin cancers are largely attributable to higher exposure of an aging population to UVR. Therefore, the development of cellular strategies for intrinsic protection of the skin against the deleterious effects of UVR is imperative. Here we show that erythema resulting from UVR is a comprehensive and noninvasive biomarker for assessing UVR damage and can be precisely and easily quantified in human skin. Topical application of sulforaphane-rich extracts of 3-day-old broccoli sprouts up-regulated phase 2 enzymes in the mouse and human skin, protected against UVR-induced inflammation and edema in mice, and reduced susceptibility to erythema arising from narrow-band 311-nm UVR in humans. In six human subjects (three males and three females, 28–53 years of age), the mean reduction in erythema across six doses of UVR (300–800 mJ/cm² in 100 mJ/cm² increments) was 37.7% (range 8.37–78.1%; $P = 0.025$). This protection against a carcinogen in humans is catalytic and long lasting.

▶ Talalay et al show that application of sulforaphane, an isothiocyanate derived from broccoli, can reduce UV-induced erythema, edema, and inflammation, presumably through induction of cytoprotective proteins. A more convincing argument that this compound might protect against skin cancer will require studies that also unequivocally demonstrate a reduction in DNA damage. This may, in fact, be the case, at least in certain murine models, in which topical application of broccoli sprout extracts containing sulforaphane strongly suppresses tumor development.[1] It should be recognized that sulforaphane is not a sunscreen and does not absorb UV light; it simply may protect against

UV-induced damage. Nevertheless, your mother may have been right: broccoli is good for you!

The same group has shown that sulforaphane may reduce blistering in certain types of epidermolysis bullosa simplex.[1]

B. H. Thiers, MD

Reference

1. Kerns ML, DePianto D, Dinkova-Kostova AT, Talalay P, Coulombe PA. Reprogramming of keratin biosynthesis by sulforaphane restores skin integrity in epidermolysis bullosa simplex. *Proc Natl Acad Sci U S A*. 2007;104:14460-14465.

A porphomethene inhibitor of uroporphyrinogen decarboxylase causes porphyria cutanea tarda
Phillips JD, Bergonia HA, Reilly CA, et al (Univ of Utah School of Medicine, Salt Lake City)
Proc Natl Acad Sci U S A 104:5079-5084, 2007

Porphyria cutanea tarda (PCT), the most common form of porphyria in humans, is due to reduced activity of uroporphyrinogen decarboxylase (URO-D) in the liver. Previous studies have demonstrated that protein levels of URO-D do not change when catalytic activity is reduced, suggesting that an inhibitor of URO-D is generated in hepatocytes. Here, we describe the identification and characterization of an inhibitor of URO-D in liver cytosolic extracts from two murine models of PCT: wild-type mice treated with iron, δ-aminolevulinic acid, and polychlorinated biphenyls; and mice with one null allele of *Uro-d* and two null alleles of the hemochromatosis gene (*Uro-d$^{+/-}$, Hfe$^{-/-}$*) that develop PCT with no treatments. In both models, we identified an inhibitor of recombinant human URO-D (rhURO-D). The inhibitor was characterized by solid-phase extraction, chromatography, UV-visible spectroscopy, and mass spectroscopy and proved to be uroporphomethene, a compound in which one bridge carbon in the uroporphyrinogen macrocycle is oxidized. We synthesized uroporphomethene by photooxidation of enzymatically generated uroporphyrinogen I or III. Both uroporphomethenes inhibited rhURO-D, but the III isomer porphomethene was a more potent inhibitor. Finally, we detected an inhibitor of rhURO-D in cytosolic extracts of liver biopsy samples of patients with PCT. These studies define the mechanism underlying clinical expression of the PCT phenotype, namely oxidation of uroporphyrinogen to uroporphomethene, a competitive inhibitor of URO-D. The oxidation reaction is iron-dependent.

▶ Previous studies have shown that a common mechanism likely underlies the PCT phenotype (specifically a reduction in the activity of the hepatic uroporphyrinogen decarboxylase enzyme). It has been speculated that this occurs through the generation of an inhibitor of that enzyme by an iron-dependent pathway. Phillips and colleagues identify this inhibitor to be a porphomethene that is formed by the partial oxidation of uroporphyrinogen. The authors suggest that CYP1A2 converts uroporphyrinogen to uroporpho-methene in an oxidative, iron-dependent reaction. How this occurs and the precise interactions of the genetic and environmental factors involved remain to be determined.

B. H. Thiers, MD

Narrowband UVB therapy for vitiligo: does the repigmentation last?
Sitek JC, Loeb M, Ronnevig JR (Ulleval Univ Hosp, Oslo, Norway; SINTEF Health Research, Oslo, Norway; Natl Hosp, Oslo, Norway)
J Eur Acad Dermatol Venereol 21:891-896, 2007

Background.—Since 1997, a number of trials have shown promising re-sults in treating generalized vitiligo with narrowband ultraviolet B (UVB) both in adults and children. However, there is little knowledge concerning the duration and permanency of the treatment-induced repigmentation.

Objective.—Our main objective was to perform a follow-up trial of suc-cessfully treated patients receiving narrowband UVB for generalized vitiligo.

Methods.—We have investigated to what degree the treatment-induced repigmentation remains stable for up to 2 years post-treatment. We per-formed an initial open trial including 31 patients with generalized vitiligo. They received narrowband UVB thrice weekly for up to 12 months. Patients experiencing > 75% repigmentation were defined responders and were in-cluded in the follow-up trial. Responders were followed every 6 months for up to 2 years after cessation of treatment. We observed the pigmentation sta-tus and registered any changes indicating loss of pigmentation and relapse.

Results.—Eleven of the 31 treated patients were included in the follow-up trial. Six patients had relapse and five patients had stable response 24 months after cessation of treatment. Four out of six relapses were within 6 months post-treatment.

Conclusion.—In our study population of 31 patients with generalized vitiligo, five patients (16%) experienced > 75% stable repigmentation 2 years after cessation of a treatment programme of up to 1 years narrowband UVB therapy.

▶ Sitek et al found the repigmentation after NBUVB to be quite durable, al-though their data were compromised by the small number of patients who re-ported for follow-up examination. In another article, Casacci et al[1] suggest that 308-nm monochromatic excimer light might be more effective than conven-tional NBUVB phototherapy in the treatment of vitiligo. This also would have the advantage of sparing uninvolved skin and having a lower cumulative dos-age and shorter treatment times, all of which may impact the side effects of long-term phototherapy.

B. H. Thiers, MD

Reference

1. Casacci M, Thomas P, Pacifico A, Bonnevalle A, Paro Vidolin A, Leone G. Comparison between 308-nm monochromatic excimer light and narrowband UVB phototherapy (311–313 nm) in the treatment of vitiligo—a multicentre controlled study. *J Eur Acad Dermatol Venereol.* 2007;21:956-963.

Comparison between 308-nm monochromatic excimer light and narrowband UVB phototherapy (311–313 nm) in the treatment of vitiligo—a multicentre controlled study
Casacci M, Thomas P, Pacifico A, et al (Univ of Lille, France; San Gallicano Dermatological Inst, Rome)
J Eur Acad Dermatol Venereol 21:956-963, 2007

Background.—Vitiligo is an acquired pigmentary disorder characterized by areas of depigmented skin resulting from loss of epidermal melanocytes. Recently, it has been shown that narrowband ultraviolet B (NB-UVB) phototherapy may be more effective than psoralen and ultraviolet A (PUVA) photochemotherapy in treating vitiligo, and that 308-nm monochromatic excimer light (MEL) may present some advantages as compared to NB-UVB for the treatment of vitiligo.

Aim.—The aim of this study was to compare the effectiveness of NB-UVB phototherapy and 308-nm MEL in vitiligo patients.

Methods.—The study was done in a randomized, investigator-blinded and half-side comparison design. Twenty-one subjects with symmetrical vitiligo lesions were enrolled in this study. Vitiligo lesions on one body side were treated twice weekly for 6 months with 308-nm MEL, while NB-UVB phototherapy was used to treat lesions on the opposite side.

Results.—At the end of the study six lesions (37.5%) treated with 308-nm MEL and only one lesion (6%) treated with NB-UVB achieved an excellent repigmentation (score 4) while four lesions (25%) treated with 308-nm MEL and five lesions (31%) treated with NB-UVB showed a good repigmentation (score 3).

Conclusions.—It appears that 308-nm MEL is more effective than NB-UVB in treating vitiligo lesions and it induces repigmentation more rapidly.

▶ Casacci et al suggest that 308-nm monochromatic excimer light might be more effective than conventional NBUVB phototherapy in the treatment of vitiligo. This also would have the advantage of sparing uninvolved skin and having lower cumulative dosage and shorter treatment times, all of which may impact the side effects of long-term phototherapy. In another article, Sitek et al[1] found the repigmentation after NBUVB to be quite durable, although their data were compromised by the small number of patients who reported for follow-up examination.

B. H. Thiers, MD

Reference

1. Sitek JC, Loeb M, Ronnevig JR. Narrowband UVB therapy for vitiligo: does the repigmentation last? *J Eur Acad Dermatol Venereol.* 2007;21:891-896.

Psoralen and ultraviolet A and narrow-band ultraviolet B in inducing stability in vitiligo, assessed by vitiligo disease activity score: an open prospective comparative study

Bhatnagar A, Kanwar AJ, Parsad D, et al (Postgraduate Inst of Med Education and Research, Chandigarh, India)
J Eur Acad Dermatol Venereol 21:1381-1385, 2007

Background.—Vitiligo is a common pigmentary disorder with significant cosmetic and psychological morbidity. The course of vitiligo is unpredictable; although usually one of slow progression, it may exacerbate rapidly or stabilize. Vitiligo may also spontaneously repigment, although only partially. No treatment is available as a definitive cure. Systemic psoralen and ultraviolet A (PUVA) has been the treatment of choice for many decades. Narrow-band UVB (NBUVB) was introduced in 1997 for the treatment of vitiligo, and many subsequent trials have found it effective in vitiligo. The purpose of the present study was to compare the effectiveness of PUVA and NBUVB in inducing stability in vitiligo, as assessed by using the vitiligo disease activity (VIDA) score.

Methods.—An open, prospective study of 50 patients was conducted from January 2004 to June 2005. The patients were divided equally into PUVA and NBUVB groups. This study was undertaken as part of a larger project to compare the efficacy of these two methods in the degree of repigmentation.

Results.—In the NBUVB group, disease activity was present in 40% of patients before the start of therapy, which was reduced to 16% at the end of therapy. The figures for the PUVA group were 20% and 16%, respectively. In the NBUVB group, 50% of patients whose disease was active before commencement of therapy had less than 50% repigmentation, whereas an equal number of patients had repigmentation of more than 50%. Almost an equal number of stable patients had less than 50% and more than 50% repigmentation. In the PUVA group, 80% of patients who had active disease had less than 50% repigmentation, whereas only 20% with active disease had more than 50% repigmentation. The time to attain stability was 3.6 ± 2.1 months in the NBUVB group and 3.22 ± 3.1 months in the PUVA group. Stability was obtained in 80% of patients with unstable disease in the NBUVB group, compared with 40% of similar patients in the PUVA group.

Conclusions.—NBUVB was more effective than PUVA for treatment of vitiligo in terms of stability and efficacy in both active and stable disease in a comparable time period.

▶ Bhatnagar et al compared NBUVB to TMP PUVA in the treatment of vitiligo and found the former to be superior. Fortunately, NBUVB and PUVA phototherapy each are associated with a quite low incidence of acute adverse effects, although the carcinogenic potential of PUVA must be kept in mind if such therapy is considered for long-term application.

B. H. Thiers, MD

Rate of acute adverse events for narrow-band UVB and Psoralen-UVA phototherapy
Martin JA, Laube S, Edwards C, et al (Univ Hosp of Wales, Cardiff; Aberdeen Royal Infirmary, England; Royal Gwent Hosp, Newport, Wales)
Photodermatol Photoimmunol Photomed 23:68-72, 2007

Background.—Ultraviolet (UV) radiation therapies are commonly used to treat a wide range of dermatological conditions. However, no published data exist regarding the rate of acute adverse events occurring within the different UV therapy modalities.

Aim.—The aim of this study was to determine the rate of acute adverse events experienced by patients receiving narrow-band UVB or photochemotherapy in 3 neighboring dermatology units.

Method.—Standardized adverse event forms from all 3 units were retrospectively analysed over a 12-month period between October 2003 and September 2004. The treatments included were narrow-band UVB and systemic, bath and hand/foot PUVA.

Results.—A total of 8784 treatments were given over the study period. The total number of acute adverse events recorded for all phototherapy treatments was 70 (0.8%). The rates of acute adverse events for each treatment modality were 0.6% for narrow-band UVB, 1.3% for systemic PUVA, 1.3% for bath PUVA and 0.8% for hand/foot PUVA. Adverse events were due to patient non-compliance with standard operating procedures in 15 cases (21%) and operator error in 2 (3%). Only 4 of the acute adverse events were considered to be severe, accounting for 0.05% of all treatments.

Conclusions.—The rates of acute adverse events with phototherapy in this analysis were low, in particular the rate of severe adverse events. The highest rate was seen with both systemic and bath PUVA. The number of adverse events resulting from operator error was low. These published rates for adverse events associated with narrow-band UVB and PUVA may help other units when analyzing their own rate of adverse events.

▶ Any studies that review the efficacy of phototherapy in the treatment of vitiligo are subject to a number of variables that can affect treatment outcome. Clearly, the quality of the reported data depends on how well the authors adjust for duration of disease and location of the depigmented skin. Fortunately, NBUVB and PUVA phototherapy each are associated with a quite low incidence of acute adverse effects, although the carcinogenic potential of PUVA must be kept in mind if such therapy is considered for long-term application.

B. H. Thiers, MD

9 Collagen Vascular and Related Disorders

A Serology-Based Approach Combined With Clinical Examination of 125 Ro/SSA-Positive Patients to Define Incidence and Prevalence of Subacute Cutaneous Lupus Erythematosus
Popovic K, Nyberg F, Wahren-Herlenius M, et al (Karolinska Institutet, Stockholm; AstraZeneca Pharmaceuticals, Mölndal, Sweden)
Arthritis Rheum 56:255-264, 2007

Objective.—To estimate the incidence and prevalence of Ro/SSA-positive subacute cutaneous lupus erythematosus (SCLE) in Stockholm County, Sweden (1.8 million inhabitants) and to investigate the frequency of photosensitivity and other clinical manifestations associated with Ro/SSA autoantibodies.

Methods.—Ro/SSA-positive patients in Stockholm were identified via registry-based searches. All patients who tested positive for the presence of Ro/SSA autoantibodies during 1996–2002 (n = 1,323; 85% women) were identified. A questionnaire was sent to all patients still living in Stockholm in 2003 (n = 1,048). Patients who reported having skin symptoms and photosensitivity (n = 125) underwent a clinical examination.

Results.—Of the 741 (71%) of 1,048 Ro/SSA-positive patients who responded to the questionnaire, 400 (54%) reported having photosensitivity, and of these patients, 125 agreed to be clinically examined. A diagnosis of LE was confirmed in 59 of the 125 patients (SCLE in 20, systemic LE [SLE] in 33, and chronic CLE in 6). Eighty-six patients reported experiencing symptoms consistent with polymorphous light eruption (PLE). Comorbidities such as cardiovascular disease, autoimmune disease, and other skin diseases were common. The incidence of Ro/SSA-positive SCLE during the study period was estimated to be 0.7 cases per 100,000 persons per year and the prevalence was ~6.2–14 in 100,000 persons.

Conclusion.—The incidence of Ro/SSA-positive SCLE in Stockholm County, Sweden is estimated to be 0.7 per 100,000 persons per year as compared with an incidence of SLE in Sweden of 4.8 per 100,000 persons per year. The prevalence is estimated to be 6.2–14 in 100,000 persons. Self-reported photosensitivity commonly corresponds to a history of PLE in Ro/SSA-positive patients, even when the clinical profile of SCLE is absent.

Photoprotection should therefore be included in the treatment recommendations for these patients.

▶ The incidence of photosensitivity was quite high (54%) in the Ro/SSA-positive patients reported in this study. Of the 125 patients actually examined, 86 (69%) reported a history consistent with polymorphous light eruption. The prevalence of polymorphous light eruption was particularly high in patients with Sjögren's syndrome, an association not previously reported. The results emphasize the importance of photoprotection in counseling patients with Ro/SSA-positive SCLE.

B. H. Thiers, MD

Mycophenolate sodium for subacute cutaneous lupus erythematosus resistant to standard therapy

Kreuter A, Tomi NS, Weiner SM, et al (Ruhr-Univ Bochum, Germany)
Br J Dermatol 156:1321-1327, 2007

Background.—Approximately 75–95% of patients with cutaneous lupus erythematosus respond to antimalarial therapy and/or topical glucocorticosteroids. Immunosuppressive agents are usually considered a second-line approach in patients with resistant disease.

Objectives.—This was a prospective, nonrandomized, open pilot study to evaluate the efficacy of mycophenolate sodium monotherapy in patients with recalcitrant subacute cutaneous lupus erythematosus (SCLE).

Methods.—Monotherapy with oral enteric-coated mycophenolate sodium 1440 mg daily was given for a total of 3 months. Treatment outcome was evaluated by means of a validated clinical score for cutaneous lupus erythematosus, the Cutaneous Lupus Erythematosus Disease Area and Severity Index (CLASI), as well as 20-MHz ultrasound measurements and colorimetry. Safety assessment included the monitoring of adverse effects and clinical laboratory parameters.

Results.—Ten patients with active SCLE resistant to at least one standard therapy were included in the trial. Mycophenolate sodium led to a remarkable improvement of skin lesions, resulting in a significant decrease of the mean ± SD CLASI from 10.8 ± 6.0 at the beginning to 2.9 ± 2.6 at the end of therapy. Clinical improvement was confirmed by ultrasonographic assessments and colorimetry. No serious side-effects were noted.

Conclusions.—Mycophenolate sodium is beneficial and safe in the treatment of patients with SCLE that failed standard therapy. However, these preliminary data must be confirmed by randomized controlled trials including a larger sample size.

▶ Whereas most patients with SCLE respond well to photoprotection, topical corticosteroids, and antimalarial drugs, some require second-line drugs of variable efficacy and side effects. Kreuter et al treated 10 patients with SCLE resistant to at least 1 standard of therapy with an enteric-coated preparation of mycophenolate sodium 1440 mg daily for 3 months. This dose corresponds to 2000 mg of the mycophenolate mofetil preparation available in the United States. All patients experienced "remarkable improvement" according to the authors. Certainly, the results need to be confirmed in a larger double-blind study. It would also be interesting to learn whether other forms of cutaneous LE respond equally well to this drug.

B. H. Thiers, MD

Libman-Sacks Endocarditis in Systemic Lupus Erythematosus: Prevalence, Associations, and Evolution

Moyssakis I, Tektonidou MG, Vasilliou VA, et al (Laiko Gen Hosp, Athens, Greece; Natl Univ of Athens, Greece)
Am J Med 120:636-642, 2007

Purpose.—We evaluated the prevalence and progression of Libman-Sacks endocarditis in patients with systemic lupus erythematosus and any association between this valvulopathy and their clinical and laboratory characteristics.

Methods.—Doppler echocardiography was performed in 342 consecutive patients with systemic lupus erythematosus (297 females and 45 males). The clinical and laboratory data were recorded. Patients were reevaluated after a follow-up period of 4 years.

Results.—Libman-Sacks endocarditis was found in 38 patients (11%). In 24 of 38 patients, mitral valve involvement was found, resulting in regurgitation in all (mild in 18, moderate in 4, and severe in 2), whereas stenosis co-occurred with regurgitation in 9 patients (mild in 6 and moderate in 3). Thirteen (34%) of 38 patients had aortic valve involvement; 11 had regurgitation (mild) and 8 had stenosis (mild), coexistent with regurgitation in 6 of them. One patient had mild tricuspid regurgitation. A significant association was found between Libman-Sacks endocarditis and disease duration and activity, thromboses, stroke, thrombocytopenia, anticardiolipin antibodies, and antiphospholipid syndrome. During the follow-up period, 252 of 342 patients were reevaluated echocardiographically. Among the 38 patients with Libman-Sacks vegetations, 5 with mild mitral regurgitation at the beginning developed moderate (n = 4) and severe mitral regurgitation (n = 1), 2 patients with mitral stenosis (mild in 1 and moderate in 1) developed severe mitral regurgitation, and 2 patients with mild aortic regurgitation developed moderate and severe mitral regurgitation, whereas a significant deterioration of aortic stenosis was found. Two patients who were candidates for surgery died. Among the 213 patients without vegetations at the beginning, 8 developed new Libman-Sacks lesions.

Conclusions.—Libman-Sacks vegetations can be found in approximately 1 of 10 patients with systemic lupus erythematosus, and they are associated with lupus duration, disease activity, anticardiolipin antibodies, and antiphospholipid syndrome manifestations. A progression of valve lesions may occur during long-term follow-up.

▶ Valvular disease is an important manifestation of cardiac involvement in patients with systemic lupus erythematosus. The valvular vegetations noted in this disease have been referred to as Libman-Sacks endocarditis. These vegetations are noninfective verrucous lesions that develop most often on the mitral valve. Moyssakis and colleagues found such vegetations in approximately 1 in 10 patients with systemic lupus erythematosus. Patients with Libman-Sacks vegetations tended to have a longer disease duration, higher disease activity, and positive antiphospholipid antibodies. They also appeared to be at an increased risk for thrombotic events, including stroke and transient ischemic attacks. After the mitral valve, the second most common site of involvement was the aortic valve. The progression of valvular lesions—especially of aortic valve stenosis—was noted during long-term follow-up.

B. H. Thiers, MD

Smoking, Alcohol Consumption, and Raynaud's Phenomenon in Middle Age
Suter LG, Murabito JM, Felson DT, et al (VA Connecticut Healthcare System, West Haven; Yale Univ, New Haven, Conn; Natl Heart, Lung, and Blood Inst's Framingham Heart Study, Mass; et al)
Am J Med 120:264-271, 2007

Background.—Data suggest Raynaud's phenomenon shares risk factors with cardiovascular disease. Studies of smoking, alcohol consumption, and Raynaud's have produced conflicting results and were limited by small sample size and failure to adjust for confounders. Our objective was to determine whether smoking and alcohol are independently associated with Raynaud's in a large, community-based cohort.

Methods.—By using a validated survey to classify Raynaud's in the Framingham Heart Study Offspring Cohort, we performed sex-specific analyses of Raynaud's status by smoking and alcohol consumption in 1840 women and 1602 men. Multivariable logistic regression analyses were used to examine the relationship of Raynaud's to smoking and alcohol consumption.

Results.—Current smoking was not associated with Raynaud's in women but was associated with increased risk in men (adjusted odds ratio [OR] 2.59, 95% confidence interval [CI], 1.11-6.04). Heavy alcohol consumption in women was associated with increased risk of Raynaud's (adjusted OR 1.69, 95% CI, 1.02-2.82), whereas moderate alcohol consumption in men was associated with reduced risk (adjusted OR 0.51, 95% CI, 0.29-0.89). In both genders, red wine consumption was associated with a reduced risk of Raynaud's (adjusted OR 0.59, 95% CI, 0.36-0.96 in women and adjusted OR 0.30, 95% CI, 0.15-0.62 in men).

Conclusions.—Our data suggest that middle-aged women and men may have distinct physiologic mechanisms underlying their Raynaud's, and thus sex-specific therapeutic approaches may be appropriate. Our data also support the possibility that moderate red wine consumption may protect against Raynaud's.

▶ Suter et al found that smoking was associated with increased risk of Raynaud's phenomenon in men but not women. This association was particularly strong in men with underlying cardiovascular disease. Although heavy alcohol consumption appeared to be associated with increased risk of Raynaud's phenomenon in women, red wine seemed to be protective against this problem in both men and women. Although the authors suggest the possibility of sex-specific therapy for managing Raynaud's phenomenon, a more generalizable recommendation may be to suggest smoking cessation and a glass of red wine with dinner for possible symptomatic relief.

B. H. Thiers, MD

Assessment of nailfold capillaroscopy by × 30 digital epiluminescence (dermoscopy) in patients with Raynaud phenomenon
Beltrán E, Toll A, Pros A, et al (Hosp del Mar, Barcelona)
Br J Dermatol 156:892-898, 2007

Background.—Dermoscopy is a useful tool for dermatologists to study melanocytic lesions. Its possible usefulness in the assessment of capillary nailfold morphological changes (capillaroscopy) has recently been advocated.

Objectives.—To assess the practical utility of digital epiluminescence microscopy as a capillaroscopic instrument in patients with Raynaud phenomenon (RP). To compare the sensitivity and specificity rates obtained by epiluminescence microscopy with those previously reported with conventional capillaroscopic devices.

Methods.—Fifty-six consecutive patients with primary RP (PRP; $n = 5$) or secondary RP (SRP; $n = 51$) (11 men and 45 women in total) were included in the study. A control group of 10 healthy subjects was also evaluated. Twenty-six patients (46%) had systemic sclerosis (SS), 12 (21%) presystemic sclerosis (pre-SS), one (2%) dermatopolymyositis–SS, one (2%) mixed connective tissue disease, two (4%) Sjögren syndrome, two (4%) an overlap syndrome, one (2%) rheumatoid arthritis and six (11%) other connective tissue diseases. Capillary nailfold changes were studied using a nonportable digital epiluminescence device (magnification × 30). Following a systematized protocol, capillary nailfold morphology, density and distribution were evaluated. Several capillaroscopic patterns were identified (normal, sclerodermic, nonspecific, nondiagnostic) as previously defined. A possible relationship between capillary nailfold changes and the intensity of RP or the presence of associated autoimmune diseases was assessed.

Results.—The sclerodermic pattern showed a sensitivity of 76.9% and a specificity of 90.9% in SS. A typical capillaroscopic SS pattern was observed in 73% of cases of limited SS and in 82% of cases of diffuse SS. Patients with Sjögren syndrome and dermatopolymyositis–SS showed a nonspecific capillaroscopic pattern. All patients with PRP presented a normal capillaroscopic pattern. A normal capillaroscopic pattern was also observed in 11 of 12 patients with pre-SS. In one of two patients presenting severe sclerodactyly and in all patients showing hand oedema (three of 56), capillaroscopic changes could not be evaluated. Avascular areas correlated significantly with severe RP ($P < 0.002$), bone resorption ($P < 0.007$) and diffuse SS ($P < 0.008$).

Conclusions.—Digital epiluminescence seems to be a useful and reliable technique in the evaluation of capillary nailfold morphological changes. This technical variation allows the identification of specific capillaroscopic patterns associated with connective tissue diseases. It also permits us to differentiate PRP from SRP. The results obtained with this technique are similar to those previously reported using standard capillaroscopy devices.

▶ Beltrán et al found dermoscopy to be useful in evaluating the morphology of periungual capillaries, allowing the detection of capillaroscopic changes in different autoimmune diseases. The technique could differentiate primary RP from SRP. An association was observed between severe RP and avascular areas on capillaroscopy. This avascular pattern appeared to correlate with distal digital bone resorption and was occasionally associated with diffuse SS. Thus, the dermoscopic appearance of the periungual capillaries seemed to have prognostic value as well.

B. H. Thiers, MD

A Polymorphism in the *CTGF* Promoter Region Associated with Systemic Sclerosis

Fonseca C, Lindahl GE, Ponticos M, et al (Royal Free and Univ College Med School, London; Univ of Siena, Italy; Imperial College London; et al)
N Engl J Med 357:1210-1220, 2007

Background.—Systemic sclerosis (scleroderma) is a life-threatening autoimmune disease that is characterized by the presence of specific autoantibodies and fibrosis of the skin and major internal organs.

Methods.—We genotyped a polymorphism (G–945C) in the promoter of the connective-tissue growth factor (*CTGF*) gene in 1000 subjects in two groups: group 1, consisting of 200 patients with systemic sclerosis and 188 control subjects; and group 2, consisting of 300 patients with systemic sclerosis and 312 control subjects. The combined groups represented an estimated 10% of patients with systemic sclerosis in the United Kingdom. We tested the effect of the polymorphism on the transcription of *CTGF*.

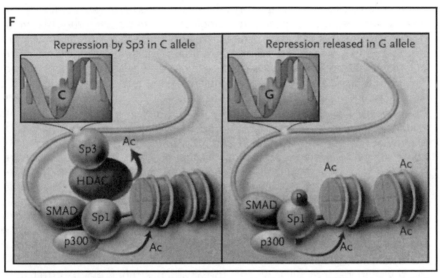

FIGURE 2F.—Panel F shows a proposed model of interaction of the polymorphic site with the proximal promoter in the *CTGF* gene. The balance of complex components and transcriptional activity—for example, through acetylation (Ac) and phosphorylation (P)—is probably affected by the loss of Sp3 binding at position -945. Histone deacetylase (HDAC) and p300, a histone acetylase, may form parts of this complex together with Sp1, Sp3, SMAD protein, and other factors. (Reprinted by permission of Fonseca C, Lindahl GE, Ponticos M, et al. A polymorphism in the *CTGF* promoter region associated with systemic sclerosis. *N Engl J Med*. 2007;357:1210-1220. Copyright 2007, Massachusetts Medical Society. All rights reserved.)

Results.—The GG genotype was significantly more common in patients with systemic sclerosis than in control subjects in both groups, with an odds ratio for the combined group of 2.2 (95% confidence interval [CI], 1.5 to 3.2; P<0.001 for trend). Analysis of the combined group of patients with systemic sclerosis showed a significant association between homozygosity for the G allele and the presence of anti–topoisomerase I antibodies (odds ratio, 3.3; 95% CI, 2.0 to 5.6; P<0.001) and fibrosing alveolitis (odds ratio, 3.1; 95% CI, 1.9 to 5.0; P<0.001). We observed that the substitution of cytosine for guanine created a binding site of the transcriptional regulators Sp1 and Sp3. The C allele has high affinity for Sp3 and is associated with severely reduced transcriptional activity. A chromatin immunoprecipitation assay showed a marked shift in the ratio of Sp1 to Sp3 binding at this region, demonstrating functional relevance in vivo.

Conclusions.—The G–945C substitution represses *CTGF* transcription, and the −945G allele is significantly associated with susceptibility to systemic sclerosis (Fig 2F).

▶ This is an important study that not only detected a genetic risk factor for systemic sclerosis but also revealed a mechanistic basis for the susceptibility. The investigators elected to search for candidate genetic polymorphisms within the promoter region of the *CTGF* gene, which appears to be upregulated in systemic sclerosis. They identified a common single nucleotide polymorphism located within a putative nuclear factor binding site; subsequent genotyping of their study population revealed significant differences in distribution of the polymorphic variants between patients and control subjects. Specifically, there was an increased frequency of the homozygous GG genotype in patients with systemic sclerosis, and this difference reached even greater significance in patients who possessed autoantibodies to topoisomerase I. Although the G allele of this polymorphism is the less common variant, it is by no means rare; from the data presented in this article, the allele frequencies can be calculated as 0.542 for the more common C allele and 0.458 for the G variant. The investigators subsequently examined the effect of this polymorphism on gene transcription, using human lung fibroblasts transfected with promoter constructs containing either the C or the G allele. The data obtained clearly showed that the transcriptional activity in thrombin-activated cells was 3 times greater in cells containing the G allele than those with the C allele construct. Further studies revealed that the C allele, but not the G variant, strongly binds the transcription factor Sp3, resulting in suppression of *CTGF* gene transcription. The authors hypothesize that without Sp3 binding, the G allele favors the increased transcription of the *CTGF* gene observed in systemic sclerosis (Fig 2F).

G. M. P. Galbraith, MD

TRAF1-C5 as a Risk Locus for Rheumatoid Arthritis—A Genomewide Study

Plenge RM, Seielstad M, Padyukov L, et al (Broad Inst of Harvard and Massachusetts Inst of Technology, Cambridge, Mass; Brigham and Women's Hosp, Boston; Genome Inst of Singapore; et al)
N Engl J Med 357:1199-1209, 2007

Background.—Rheumatoid arthritis has a complex mode of inheritance. Although *HLA-DRB1* and *PTPN22* are well-established susceptibility loci, other genes that confer a modest level of risk have been identified recently. We carried out a genomewide association analysis to identify additional genetic loci associated with an increased risk of rheumatoid arthritis.

Methods.—We genotyped 317,503 single-nucleotide polymorphisms (SNPs) in a combined case–control study of 1522 case subjects with rheumatoid arthritis and 1850 matched control subjects. The patients were seropositive for autoantibodies against cyclic citrullinated peptide (CCP). We obtained samples from two data sets, the North American Rheumatoid Arthritis Consortium (NARAC) and the Swedish Epidemiological Investigation of Rheumatoid Arthritis (EIRA). Results from NARAC and EIRA for 297,086 SNPs that passed quality-control filters were combined with the use of Cochran–Mantel–Haenszel stratified analysis. SNPs showing a significant association with disease ($P<1\times10^{-8}$) were genotyped in an independent set of case subjects with anti–CCP-positive rheumatoid arthritis (485 from NARAC and 512 from EIRA) and in control subjects (1282 from NARAC and 495 from EIRA).

Results.—We observed associations between disease and variants in the major-histocompatibility-complex locus, in *PTPN22*, and in a SNP (rs3761847) on chromosome 9 for all samples tested, the latter with an odds ratio of 1.32 (95% confidence interval, 1.23 to 1.42; $P=4\times10^{-14}$). The SNP is in linkage disequilibrium with two genes relevant to chronic inflammation: *TRAF1* (encoding tumor necrosis factor receptor–associated factor 1) and *C5* (encoding complement component 5).

Conclusions.—A common genetic variant at the *TRAF1-C5* locus on chromosome 9 is associated with an increased risk of anti–CCP-positive rheumatoid arthritis.

▶ Current technology permits the increasingly fine dissection of the human genome to tease out associations between a selected disease and a genetic locus. Not surprisingly, several recent studies have focused on diseases with a known familial predisposition. Two articles by essentially the same group of investigators, Plenge et al and Remmers et al,[1] describe the genotyping of literally thousands of SNPs in patients with rheumatoid arthritis and, in the study by Remmers et al, in patients with systemic lupus erythematosus also. Samples were obtained from patients and controls of self-reported white ancestry who belong to large cohorts of well-characterized patients in the United States and in Sweden. The results of the 2 studies are quite similar in that modest disease associations were found with the less common alleles of a polymorphism linked to *TRAF1* and *C5* on chromosome 9 and of another within the *STAT4* gene on chromosome 2. Replication studies of different individuals within the same cohorts confirmed the findings. In each case, the statistical significance of the association was strong but the odds ratio low (<1.5), and the significance values and odds ratios were even lower in the Swedish population of patients with rheumatoid arthritis.

In this article, Plenge et al calculated that the rarer allele of the *TRAF1–C5*-linked allele conferred approximately 7% risk of disease. This contrasts markedly with the known susceptibility variants at the HLA-DRB1 locus, which may contribute up to 50% of risk in rheumatoid arthritis. However, it is possible that as additional minor risk factors are detected in different populations, recognizable constellations of markers may prove useful in clarifying the molecular basis of these and other autoimmune diseases.

G. M. P. Galbraith, MD

Reference

1. Remmers EF, Plenge RM, Lee AT, et al. *STAT4* and the risk of rheumatoid arthritis and systemic lupus erythematosus. *N Engl J Med*. 2007;357:977-986.

STAT4 and the Risk of Rheumatoid Arthritis and Systemic Lupus Erythematosus

Remmers EF, Plenge RM, Lee AT, et al (Natl Inst of Arthritis and Musculoskeletal and Skin Diseases, Bethesda, Md; Broad Inst, Cambridge, Mass; Brigham and Women's Hosp; et al)
N Engl J Med 357:977-986, 2007

Background.—Rheumatoid arthritis is a chronic inflammatory disease with a substantial genetic component. Susceptibility to disease has been linked with a region on chromosome 2q.

Methods.—We tested single-nucleotide polymorphisms (SNPs) in and around 13 candidate genes within the previously linked chromosome 2q region for association with rheumatoid arthritis. We then performed fine mapping of the *STAT1–STAT4* region in a total of 1620 case patients with established rheumatoid arthritis and 2635 controls, all from North America. Implicated SNPs were further tested in an independent case–control series of 1529 patients with early rheumatoid arthritis and 881 controls, all from Sweden, and in a total of 1039 case patients and 1248 controls from three series of patients with systemic lupus erythematosus.

Results.—A SNP haplotype in the third intron of *STAT4* was associated with susceptibility to both rheumatoid arthritis and systemic lupus erythematosus. The minor alleles of the haplotype-defining SNPs were present in 27% of chromosomes of patients with established rheumatoid arthritis, as compared with 22% of those of controls (for the SNP rs7574865, $P=2.81\times10^{-7}$; odds ratio for having the risk allele in chromosomes of patients vs. those of controls, 1.32). The association was replicated in Swedish patients with recent-onset rheumatoid arthritis ($P=0.02$) and matched controls. The haplotype marked by rs7574865 was strongly associated with lupus, being present on 31% of chromosomes of case patients and 22% of those of controls ($P=1.87\times10^{-9}$; odds ratio for having the risk allele in chromosomes of patients vs. those of controls, 1.55). Homozygosity of the risk allele, as compared with absence of the allele, was associated with a more than doubled risk for lupus and a 60% increased risk for rheumatoid arthritis.

Conclusions.—A haplotype of *STAT4* is associated with increased risk for both rheumatoid arthritis and systemic lupus erythematosus, suggesting a shared pathway for these illnesses.

▶ Current technology permits the increasingly fine dissection of the human genome to tease out associations between a selected disease and a genetic locus. Not surprisingly, several recent studies have focused on diseases with a known familial predisposition. Two articles by essentially the same group of investigators, Plenge et al[1] and Remmers et al, describe the genotyping of literally thousands of SNPs in patients with rheumatoid arthritis and, in this study by Remmers et al, in patients with systemic lupus erythematosus also. Samples were obtained from patients and controls of self-reported white ancestry who belong to large cohorts of well-characterized patients in the United States and in Sweden. The results of the 2 studies are quite similar in that modest disease associations were found with the less common alleles of a polymorphism linked to *TRAF1* and *C5* on chromosome 9 and of another within the *STAT4* gene on chromosome 2. Replication studies of different individuals within the same cohorts confirmed the findings. In each case, the statistical significance of the association was strong but the odds ratio low (<1.5), and the significance values and odds ratios were even lower in the Swedish population of patients with rheumatoid arthritis.

In the study by Plenge et al,[1] the authors calculated that the rarer allele of the *TRAF1–C5*-linked allele conferred approximately 7% risk of disease. This contrasts markedly with the known susceptibility variants at the HLA-DRB1 locus, which may contribute up to 50% of risk in rheumatoid arthritis. However, it is possible that as additional minor risk factors are detected in different populations, recognizable constellations of markers may prove useful in clarifying the molecular basis of these and other autoimmune diseases.

G. M. P. Galbraith, MD

Reference

1. Plenge RM, Seielstad M, Padyukov L, et al. *TRAF1-C5* as a risk locus for rheumatoid arthritis—a genomewide study. *N Engl J Med.* 2007;357:1199-1209.

Interstitial lung disease associated with amyopathic dermatomyositis: Review of 18 cases
Ideura G, Hanaoka M, Koizumi T, et al (Shinshu Univ, Matsumoto, Japan)
Respir Med 101:1406-1411, 2007

Interstitial lung disease (ILD) associated with amyopathic dermatomyositis (ADM) is a rare and sometimes fatal condition whose clinical features are not well understood. The goal of this study was to clarify the characteristics of ILD based on its development.

Eighteen patients diagnosed with ILD associated with ADM were assigned to 1 of 2 groups: (1) a rapidly progressing group, which included patients who developed abnormal lung findings within 1 month of being diagnosed with ADM ($n = 9$); or (2) a slowly progressing group, which included patients who developed lung findings greater than 1 month after diagnosis of ADM ($n = 9$).

Serum creatine phosphokinase and C-reactive protein levels were higher in the rapidly progressing group than in the slowly progressing group. Further, arterial pH was higher and PaO_2/F_iO_2 was lower in the rapidly progressing group than in the slowly progressing group. On thoracic high-resolution CT, traction bronchiectasis was present in 4 of the 9 rapidly progressing patients but not in any patients of the slowly progressing group. All 9 slowly progressing patients survived with proper treatment, but only 4 of the 9 rapidly progressing patients survived.

In ADM, appropriate investigations are likely required for the early diagnosis of ILD. Our data suggest that ILD associated with ADM can be classified into 2 clinical subtypes based on the time course of pulmonary involvement. Patients with rapid progression in respiratory symptoms should undergo intensive treatment as soon as possible to promote favorable outcomes.

▶ This article is interesting in several respects. First, it demonstrates that systemic disease, in this case ILD, can occur in patients with dermatomyositis, even in the absence of muscle symptoms. Second, it shows that the clinical course of ILD associated with ADM correlates with the time interval to the development of pulmonary symptoms and that patients with rapid onset of pulmonary involvement (ie, <1 month) are likely to experience rapid progression of their lung disease and an associated poor prognosis. This suggests that such patients may benefit from early, intensive immunosuppressive therapy. Prospective studies with larger patient populations need to be done to confirm these results.

B. H. Thiers, MD

Cutaneous manifestations of Wegener's granulomatosis: a clinicopathologic study of 17 patients and correlation to antineutrophil cytoplasmic antibody status

Comfere NI, Macaron NC, Gibson LE (Mayo Clinic, Rochester, Minn)
J Cutan Pathol 34:739-747, 2007

Background.—Wegener's granulomatosis (WG), a systemic vasculitis, can be associated with cutaneous signs and symptoms before, during or after the diagnosis of systemic disease.

Methods.—We reviewed clinical and histologic features of cutaneous lesions from 17 patients with WG. The temporal relationship between development of cutaneous symptoms and onset of systemic disease was determined, and antineutrophil cytoplasmic antibody (ANCA) status of the patients was also established.

Results.—In six patients, systemic and cutaneous disease developed concurrently. In eight patients, cutaneous disease developed after patients received the diagnosis of systemic disease. In three patients, cutaneous disease preceded systemic disease. Cytoplasmic ANCA or proteinase-3-ANCA [c-ANCA/proteinase 3 (PR3)-ANCA] serologic test results were negative for one patient when cutaneous disease developed, and one patient had c-ANCA/PR3-ANCA seroconversion a year before systemic disease developed. Histopathologic features of cutaneous WG were not limited to leukocytoclastic vasculitis; they also included acneiform perifollicular and dermal granulomatous inflammation and palisaded neutrophilic and granulomatous inflammation.

Conclusions.—Patients with WG can present initially with cutaneous symptoms. Histopathologic patterns vary, but leukocytoclastic vasculitis is most commonly noted. Patients with WG and skin lesions are likely to have positive c-ANCA/PR3-ANCA serologic test results.

▶ Although one-half of patients with WG have cutaneous signs and symptoms, Comfere et al found that fewer, approximately 15%, have specific cutaneous lesions that are directly related to the disorder and are not the result of infection, drug hypersensitivity, or other definable causes. Cutaneous findings are more frequent in patients with multiple organ involvement, including the lungs, upper respiratory tract, the orbit, and joints. The most common clinical presentation noted in their patients was palpable purpura, although nodules, including deep erythema nodosum-like lesions, papules, and ulcers completed the clinical spectrum. The most common histopathologic finding was a leukocytoclastic vasculitis; this was especially frequent in those with palpable purpura, but was also observed in patients with nodules and ulceration. Pyoderma gangrenosum-like lesions were also seen; these showed a palisaded neutrophilic and granulomatous dermatitis with a prominent granulomatous and neutrophilic vasculitis and basophilic collagen degeneration. This contrasts with classic pyoderma gangrenosum, which more often shows striking neutrophilic epidermal and dermal necrosis with mononuclear cell-dominant vascular inflammation.

B. H. Thiers, MD

ANCA Are Detectable in Nearly All Patients with Active Severe Wegener's Granulomatosis

Finkielman JD, for the WGET Research Group (Mayo Clinic and Foundation, Rochester, Minn; et al)
Am J Med 120:643.e9-e14, 2007

Background.—The pathogenic significance of antineutrophilic cytoplasmic antibodies (ANCA) in Wegener's granulomatosis is controversial. Their presence is influenced by the extent, severity, and activity of the disease at the time of sampling. The objective of this study was to determine the frequency of ANCA in patients with active Wegener's granulomatosis and to assess the influence of disease severity on test results.

Methods.—Baseline serum samples from the 180 participants in a multicentric prospective trial were tested for ANCA by indirect immunofluorescence, direct enzyme-linked immunosorbent assay (ELISA), and capture ELISA. Disease activity was measured using the Birmingham Vasculitis Activity Score for Wegener's granulomatosis. All patients had active disease at enrollment. Patients were categorized as having severe (n = 128) or limited (n = 52) Wegener's granulomatosis.

Results.—When all ANCA detection methods were combined, 166 patients (92%) were ANCA positive, including 96% with severe disease and 83% with limited disease.

Conclusion.—ANCA are detectable in nearly all patients with active severe Wegener's granulomatosis, but approximately 1 of 5 patients with active limited disease are ANCA negative. Immunofluorescence and both direct and capture ELISAs are required for optimal detection, suggesting that ANCA are not recognized equally well by all testing methods.

▶ Finkielman and colleagues found that almost all patients with active severe Wegener's granulomatosis had ANCA. A combination of different studies, including immunofluorescence and both direct and capture ELISA, were required to ensure the optimal detection of these antibodies. This suggests that ANCA are a heterogeneous group of antibodies that are not recognized equally by the different testing methods.

B. H. Thiers, MD

Treatment of Antineutrophil Cytoplasmic Antibody–Associated Vasculitis: A Systematic Review
Bosch X, Guilabert A, Espinosa G, et al (Univ of Barcelona)
JAMA 298:655-669, 2007

Context.—Immunosuppressive therapies for antineutrophil cytoplasmic antibody (ANCA)–associated vasculitis have greatly advanced patient survival but have turned ANCA-associated vasculitis (AAV) into chronic, relapsing disorders. Long-term treatment and disease-related morbidity are major threats. The last decade has seen a collaborative international effort to determine effective treatment.

Objective.—To analyze the reported evidence on AAV therapy in order to provide physicians with a rational approach for dealing with various clinical scenarios.

Data Sources.—We searched English-language articles on the medical treatment of AAV published between 1966 and March 2007 using MEDLINE. Articles from the reference lists of the most relevant articles retrieved were also analyzed.

Study Selection.—Studies of current available drug treatments or medical interventions for patients with AAV were included. Duplicate publications, case reports, and uncontrolled trials and series including fewer than 10 patients were excluded.

Data Synthesis.—We included 2 meta-analyses, 20 randomized controlled prospective trials, and 62 uncontrolled trials with more than 10 patients or observational studies. Outcome measures and treatment protocols were heterogeneous across trials. Cotrimoxazole can be used alone or in

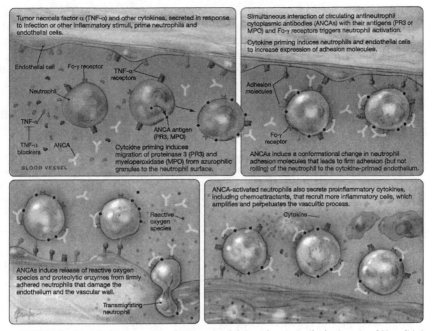

FIGURE 2.—Model of Pathogenesis of Antineutrophil Cytoplasmic Antibody–Associated Vasculitis in Wegener Granulomatosis, Microscopic Polyangiitis, and Churg-Strauss Syndrome and Therapeutic Immune Response Targets. Immune response therapies and targets are indicated in blue boldface text. (Courtesy of Bosch X, Guilabert A, Espinosa G, et al. Treatment of antineutrophil cytoplasmic antibody–associated vasculitis: a systematic review. *JAMA.* 2007;298:655-669. Copyright 2007, American Medical Association.)

combination with corticosteroids to induce and maintain remission in cases of isolated upper respiratory tract involvement. To induce remission, methotrexate plus corticosteroids can be used instead of cyclophosphamide for patients with generalized, non–organ-threatening disease. When methotrexate is used as maintenance therapy, the likelihood of relapse is high and rigorous monitoring is mandatory. Pulse cyclophosphamide with corticosteroids can be used to induce remission in patients with generalized organ-threatening disease. The combination of azathioprine and daily prednisone is effective in maintaining remission. Plasma exchange is at present the best complement to immunosuppressants in advanced renal disease. In Churg-Strauss syndrome, treatment can be started with high doses of corticosteroids, tapering them when the clinical situation improves. In patients with a high risk of death, cyclophosphamide should be introduced.

Conclusions.—Although AAV therapies should be tailored to the patient's specific clinical situation, evidence for treatment of several disease states is lacking. There is a need for safer and more effective drugs (Fig 2).

▶ Antineutrophil cytoplasmic antibody–associated vasculitis describes a spectrum of disorders that affect small- to medium-sized blood vessels. The diverse clinical manifestations of these life-threatening conditions include signs and symptoms recognized as Wegener's granulomatosis, Churg-

Strauss syndrome, and microscopic polyangiitis. The authors propose a model for the pathogenesis of these disorders (Fig 2) and review the literature on their treatment. They found a surprising lack of evidence-based data to support the effectiveness of traditional immunosuppressive treatment and suggest that future research efforts explore new immunosuppressive drugs and biologic agents such as rituximab and infliximab that have shown promise in limited early trials.

B. H. Thiers, MD

Randomized Trial of Pulsed Corticosteroid Therapy for Primary Treatment of Kawasaki Disease

Newburger JW, for the Pediatric Heart Network Investigators (Harvard Med School; et al)

N Engl J Med 356:663-675, 2007

Background.—Treatment of acute Kawasaki disease with intravenous immune globulin and aspirin reduces the risk of coronary-artery abnormalities and systemic inflammation, but despite intravenous immune globulin therapy, coronary-artery abnormalities develop in some children. Studies have suggested that primary corticosteroid therapy might be beneficial and that adverse events are infrequent with short-term use.

Methods.—We conducted a multicenter, randomized, double-blind, placebo-controlled trial to determine whether the addition of intravenous methylprednisolone to conventional primary therapy for Kawasaki disease reduces the risk of coronary-artery abnormalities. Patients with 10 or fewer days of fever were randomly assigned to receive intravenous methylprednisolone, 30 mg per kilogram of body weight (101 patients), or placebo (98 patients). All patients then received conventional therapy with intravenous immune globulin, 2 g per kilogram, as well as aspirin, 80 to 100 mg per kilogram per day until they were afebrile for 48 hours and 3 to 5 mg per kilogram per day thereafter.

Results.—At week 1 and week 5 after randomization, patients in the two study groups had similar coronary dimensions, expressed as z scores adjusted for body-surface area, absolute dimensions, and changes in dimensions. As compared with patients receiving placebo, patients receiving intravenous methylprednisolone had a somewhat shorter initial period of hospitalization (P=0.05) and, at week 1, a lower erythrocyte sedimentation rate (P=0.02) and a tendency toward a lower C-reactive protein level (P=0.07). However, the two groups had similar numbers of days spent in the hospital, numbers of days of fever, rates of retreatment with intravenous immune globulin, and numbers of adverse events.

Conclusions.—Our data do not provide support for the addition of a single pulsed dose of intravenous methylprednisolone to conventional intravenous immune globulin therapy for the routine primary treatment of children with Kawasaki disease.

▶ Kawasaki disease can be difficult to diagnose, especially in young children who may present with only 2 or 3 of the clinical signs and in whom the disease may mimic other acute infectious diseases. Fortunately, the disease generally responds well to treatment with high-dose intravenous immune globulin (IVIG) and aspirin. Aspirin is initially given at a high dosage for its anti-inflammatory effects and subsequently at a low dosage to mitigate the hypercoagulable state and platelet activation that contribute to the risk of thrombosis in the in-flamed coronary arteries. This combination therapy has reduced the incidence of coronary artery aneurysms from as high as 25% in untreated children to 3% to 5%. Because acute vasculitis appears to be a part of the pathology of Ka-wasaki disease and because aneurysms develop in a small percentage of pa-tients despite IVIG and aspirin, the addition of corticosteroids to the treatment regimen would seem to be of potential benefit. A multicenter, randomized, double-blind, placebo-controlled trial using a single pulsed dose of intravenous methylprednisolone given immediately before IVIG therapy was conducted between December 2002 and December 2004. No therapeutic benefit was seen with a single pulsed dose of methylprednisolone.

S. Raimer, MD

Clinical features and natural course of Behçet's disease in 661 cases: a multicentre study
Alpsoy E, Donmez L, Onder M, et al (Akdeniz Univ School of Medicine, Antalya, Turkey; Gazi Univ School of Medicine, Ankara, Turkey; Cukurova Univ School of Medicine, Adana, Turkey; et al)
Br J Dermatol 157:901-906, 2007

Background.—Behçet's disease (BD) is a systemic inflammatory disease with unpredictable exacerbations and remissions. The natural course of BD is not fully known.

Objectives.—We aimed retrospectively to determine the occurrence of the symptoms in chronological order. We also evaluated the influence of the treatment and follow-up on the clinical severity and tried to identify the fac-tors determining severe organ involvement.

Methods.—Six hundred and sixty-one patients were involved in this mul-ticentre study. The symptoms of the disease were recorded retrospectively in the time order of the manifestations in each patient.

Results.—Oral ulcers were the most common manifestation (100%), fol-lowed by genital ulcers (85.3%), papulopustular lesions (55.4%), erythema nodosum (44.2%), skin pathergy reaction (37.8%), and articular (33.4%) and ocular involvement (29.2%). Oral ulcers were the most common onset manifestation (88.7%). The mean ± SD duration between the onset symp-tom and the fulfilment of diagnostic criteria was calculated to be 4.3 ± 5.7 years. The clinical severity score was significantly increased in the noncom-pliant treatment group compared with the compliant group with the passage of time ($P < 0.001$). The frequency of ocular involvement and genital ulcers was significantly higher in patients whose disease onset was at < 40 years.

Genital ulcers, ocular involvement, papulopustular lesions, thrombophlebitis and skin pathergy reaction were found to be significantly more frequent in males.

Conclusions.—Mucocutaneous lesions are the hallmarks of the disease, and especially oral ulcers precede other manifestations. The increase in clinical severity score is more pronounced in patients without regular treatment and follow-up. Male sex and a younger age at onset are associated with more severe disease.

▶ Alpsoy et al reviewed 661 cases of Behçet's disease and confirmed that mucocutaneous lesions are the hallmark of the condition, with oral ulcers tending to precede other manifestations. Ocular manifestations were also common. More severe disease occurred most often in men and in patients with disease onset at a younger age. The authors suggested that patients who present with oral or genital ulcers, erythema nodosum, ocular symptoms such as uveitis, or any combination of these should be evaluated and followed for the possible development of Behçet's disease.

B. H. Thiers, MD

Sweet's syndrome: a spectrum of unusual clinical presentations and associations
Neoh CY, Tan AWH, Ng SK (Natl Skin Centre, Singapore)
Br J Dermatol 156:480-485, 2007

Background.—Sweet's syndrome (SS) is the prototypic neutrophilic dermatosis. First described in 1964, the characterization of new clinical associations, unique histopathological findings and clinical variants have stimulated much interest and discussion recently. However, the prevalence of these unusual variants and clinical associations within a single cohort of patients, has not been described.

Objectives.—To describe and evaluate the prevalence of unusual clinical and histopathological features, as well as the clinical associations of SS seen in patients from the National Skin Centre, Singapore.

Methods.—This is a retrospective study of all consecutive cases of SS seen at our centre over a 5.5-year period (June 1999–December 2004). Data on associated systemic diseases was obtained from the medical records and matched with information from the National Cancer Registry, Singapore. Patients not actively followed up for more than 3 months were contacted for their updated health status.

Results.—Thirty-seven patients were identified. Ten (27%) had non-idiopathic SS. These were associated with haematological disorders, connective tissue disorders, infections or a drug. Twenty-nine patients (78%) had at least one atypical clinical or histopathological feature. Atypical clinical features included bullous lesions, SS with hand involvement or neutrophilic dermatoses of the hands and the concomitant existence of subcutaneous SS with pyoderma gangrenosum. SS was the presenting feature in three patients with infections caused by atypical organisms, including *Mycobacterium chelonae*, *Penicillium* species and *Salmonella* type D. Unique histopathological variants included subcutaneous SS and lesions containing an admixture of mature and immature neutrophils. Subcutaneous neutrophilic inflammation seemed to be more common in patients with an underlying haematological disorder. This group of patients also had a lower mean haemoglobin level.

Conclusions.—Unusual clinical and histopathological variants of SS described in the literature are similarly encountered in our cohort of patients, with some features being more common than others. We highlight and discuss some unique clinical and histopathological observations seen in our patients with SS.

▶ Neoh et al present a comprehensive review of the presentation and clinical associations of SS. They confirm the association of anemia with an underlying hematologic disorder and describe bullous and drug-induced variants of the disease. They suggest that the various neutrophilic dermatoses, including pyoderma gangrenosum and SS may form a spectrum of entities rather than distinct diseases, a logical concept in this reviewer's opinion.

B. H. Thiers, MD

10 Blistering Disorders

Rituximab in the adjuvant treatment of pemphigus vulgaris: a prospective open-label pilot study in five patients
Goh MSY, McCormack C, Dinh HV, et al (Peter MacCallum Cancer Centre, Melbourne, Australia; Univ of Melbourne, Australia)
Br J Dermatol 156:990-996, 2007

Background.—Rituximab is a monoclonal antibody directed against the CD20 antigen expressed on B lymphocytes. There are reports of its efficacy in the treatment of autoimmune diseases, including pemphigus.

Objectives.—Prospectively to evaluate the efficacy of rituximab as adjuvant treatment for pemphigus vulgaris (PV).

Methods.—Patients with PV were treated with intravenous rituximab (375 mg m^{-2}) weekly for 4 weeks in this prospective open-label pilot study. Other concurrent immunosuppression was continued.

Results.—Of five patients, one achieved complete remission and was able to cease all medication, while two achieved clearance of clinical lesions but continued on systemic therapy. Two patients had progressive disease. Time to response was 2–8 months, with a 13- to 18-month response duration. Response was associated with reduction in serum antiepithelial antibodies. Two patients had significant infectious complications (one developed community-acquired pneumonia associated with delayed-onset neutropenia and the other developed cytomegalovirus infection).

Conclusions.—Rituximab has shown efficacy in the treatment of PV. Patients on multiple immunosuppressives should be closely monitored for infectious complications.

▶ A number of recent studies have evaluated the efficacy of IV rituximab with or without other immunosuppressive agents or IV immunoglobulin G in the treatment of autoimmune blistering diseases. Although most reports have suggested a positive therapeutic effect, it is clear that B-cell depletion by rituximab, especially when administered with concurrent immunosuppressive therapy, may be associated with substantial adverse effects that are often infectious in nature and may be fatal. Clearly, the use of this agent should be restricted to those individuals with severe disease who do not respond to more conventional therapy.

B. H. Thiers, MD

Rituximab in autoimmune bullous diseases: mixed responses and adverse effects

Schmidt E, Seitz CS, Benoit S, et al (Univ of Würzburg, Germany; Univ of Heidelberg, Mannheim, Germany)

Br J Dermatol 156:352-356, 2007

Background.—Intolerably high doses of systemic corticosteroids and additional immunosuppressants may be required to control disease activity in autoimmune bullous skin diseases. New therapeutic options are needed for such patients.

Objectives.—To determine the efficacy and adverse effects of adjuvant rituximab.

Methods.—Seven patients with refractory autoimmune blistering diseases (pemphigus vulgaris, PV, $n = 4$; bullous pemphigoid, BP, $n = 2$; mucous membrane pemphigoid, MMP, $n = 1$) were treated four times with rituximab at an individual dose of 375 mg m^{-2} at weekly intervals.

Results.—All lesions cleared in three patients (two PV, one BP), while they were reduced by more than 50% in three others (two PV, one BP). The concomitant immunosuppressive medication was reduced in five patients (four PV, one BP). The patient with MMP developed bilateral blindness while nasopharyngeal lesions resolved. Three patients (two BP, one PV) experienced severe adverse events including fatal pneumonia.

Conclusions.—Adjuvant B-cell depletion by rituximab is effective in otherwise therapy-resistant bullous autoimmune disorders but may be associated with substantial adverse effects including fatal outcomes.

▶ A number of recent studies have evaluated the efficacy of IV rituximab with or without other immunosuppressive agents or IV immunoglobulin G in the treatment of autoimmune blistering diseases. Although most reports have suggested a positive therapeutic effect, it is clear that B-cell depletion by rituximab, especially when administered with concurrent immunosuppressive therapy, may be associated with substantial adverse effects that are often infectious in nature and may be fatal. Clearly, the use of this agent should be restricted to those individuals with severe disease who do not respond to more conventional therapy.

B. H. Thiers, MD

A Single Cycle of Rituximab for the Treatment of Severe Pemphigus

Joly P, Mouquet H, Roujeau J-C, et al (Rouen Univ Hosp, France; Henri Mondor Univ Hosp, Créteil, France; Clermont-Fernand Univ Hosp, France; et al)

N Engl J Med 357:545-552, 2007

Background.—The combination of multiple cycles of rituximab and intravenous immune globulins has been reported to be effective in patients with severe pemphigus. The aim of this study was to assess the efficacy of a single cycle of rituximab in severe types of pemphigus.

Methods.—We studied 21 patients with pemphigus whose disease had not responded to an 8-week course of 1.5 mg of prednisone per kilogram of body weight per day (corticosteroid-refractory disease), who had had at least two relapses despite doses of prednisone higher than 20 mg per day (corticosteroid-dependent disease), or who had severe contraindications to corticosteroids. The patients were treated with four weekly infusions of 375 mg of rituximab per square meter of body-surface area. The primary end point was complete remission 3 months after the end of rituximab treatment; complete remission was defined as epithelialization of all skin and mucosal lesions.

Results.—Eighteen of 21 patients (86%; 95% confidence interval, 64 to 97%) had a complete remission at 3 months. The disease relapsed in nine patients after a mean of 18.9 ± 7.9 months. After a median follow-up of 34 months, 18 patients (86%) were free of disease, including 8 who were not receiving corticosteroids; the mean prednisone dose decreased from 94.0 ± 10.2 to 12.0 ± 7.5 mg per day (P=0.04) in patients with corticosteroid-refractory disease and from 29.1 ± 12.4 to 10.9 ± 16.5 mg per day (P=0.007) in patients with corticosteroid-dependent disease. Pyelonephritis developed in one patient 12 months after rituximab treatment, and one patient died of septicemia 18 months after rituximab treatment. These patients had a profound decrease in the number of circulating B lymphocytes but normal serum levels of IgG.

Conclusions.—A single cycle of rituximab is an effective treatment for pemphigus. Because of its potentially severe side effects, its use should be limited to the most severe types of the disease.

▶ A number of earlier case reports and small case series have demonstrated the efficacy of rituximab for the treatment of pemphigus vulgaris and pemphigus foliaceus. This is perhaps the first large series to confirm these beneficial effects, even after a single 4-week cycle of the drug. Because of the increased risk of infection with rituximab, this clearly is not an innocuous approach, and long-term efficacy as well as long-term risks are still unknown. Thus, for now, its use should be restricted to those patients with severe disease that does not respond to conventional therapy.[1]

B. H. Thiers, MD

Reference

1. Diaz LA. Rituximab and pemphigus—a therapeutic advance. *N Engl J Med.* 2007;357:605-607.

Treatment of Severe Pemphigus With Rituximab: Report of 12 Cases and a Review of the Literature

Cianchini G, Corona R, Frezzolini A, et al (Istituto di Ricovero e Cura a Carrattere Scientifico, Rome)
Arch Dermatol 143:1033-1038, 2007

Background.—Treatment of pemphigus vulgaris can be challenging. Systemic steroids associated with other immunosuppressant agents are the mainstay of therapy and have dramatically reduced morbidity and mortality from pemphigus vulgaris. In some patients, however, these agents are not able to control the disease or have severe adverse effects. Rituximab (MabThera; Roche, Basel, Switzerland), a chimeric monoclonal anti-CD20 antibody, induces depletion of B cells in vivo and has shown efficacy in patients with refractory antibody-mediated autoimmune disorders. We report 10 cases of pemphigus vulgaris and 2 cases of pemphigus foliaceous treated with rituximab—to our knowledge the largest series of patients so far—and review the existing literature on the topic.

Observation.—The 12 patients were selected for treatment with the anti-CD20 antibody. Rituximab was administered intravenously at a dosage of 375 mg/m^2 once weekly for 4 weeks. The treatment was well tolerated, and all 12 patients showed a good clinical response during an 18-month follow-up period, along with a consensual decline of the serum antidesmoglein titers. No infectious complications were observed.

Conclusions.—Rituximab is able to induce a prolonged clinical remission in patients with both pemphigus vulgaris and pemphigus foliaceous after a single course of 4 treatments. The preliminary experiences worldwide make rituximab a promising therapeutic option for patients with autoimmune diseases. The high costs and the limited knowledge of long-term adverse effects, however, limit its use to selected patients with treatment-resistant or life-threatening disease.

▶ The efficacy of the monoclonal anti-CD20 antibody, rituximab, in the amelioration of treatment-resistant pemphigus vulgaris and pemphigus foliaceus has been reported previously. The authors suggest that the increased rate of opportunistic infections in patients so treated may be relevant primarily for patients receiving coincident immunosuppressive therapy rather than for those treated with rituximab alone. The long-term side effect profile of rituximab is unknown, and controlled clinical trials involving larger numbers of patients will be necessary to determine its true place in the treatment of autoimmune blistering diseases.

B. H. Thiers, MD

Development of Psoriasis After B Cell Depletion With Rituximab
Dass S, Vital EM, Emery P (Univ of Leeds, England)
Arthritis Rheum 56:2715-2718, 2007

The B cell–depleting monoclonal antibody rituximab is a novel therapy for the rheumatic diseases, with an increasing body of evidence regarding its safety and efficacy in an expanding range of indications. However, there is uncertainty over its potential use in, and impact on, autoantibody-negative diseases. We describe 3 patients, with no known risk factor for psoriasis, who developed psoriasis (and 1 who also developed features of psoriatic arthritis) after receiving rituximab for a variety of indications, namely, seropositive and seronegative rheumatoid arthritis and systemic lupus erythematosus. In all cases, the underlying disease responded well to rituximab. The interpretation of this possible side effect of rituximab remains unclear, but a B cell–depleted environment may induce abnormal T cell responses, possibly provoked either by subclinical infection or by the removal of mechanisms whereby B cells regulate T cells. These cases suggest that the pathogenesis of psoriasis may not require normal numbers of B cells and that proposed treatment of psoriasis and psoriatic arthritis with rituximab may result in unpredictable responses.

▶ The occurrence of psoriasis in patients treated with the B cell–depleting anti-CD20 monoclonal antibody, rituximab, suggests that normal numbers of B cells are not necessary for the initiation of the disease. The authors speculate that B cells may have a role in the regulation of T cell–mediated immune responses and suggest further studies into the interactions between B and T cells in the pathogenesis of psoriasis.

B. H. Thiers, MD

Role of different pathways of the complement cascade in experimental bullous pemphigoid
Nelson KC, Zhao M, Schroeder PR, et al (Univ of North Carolina at Chapel Hill; Univ of Texas Health Science Ctr)
J Clin Invest 116:2892-2900, 2006

Bullous pemphigoid (BP) is an autoimmune subepidermal blistering disease associated with autoantibodies directed against the hemidesmosomal proteins BP180 and BP230 and inflammation. Passive transfer of antibodies to the murine BP180 (mBP180) induces a skin disease that closely resembles human BP. In the present study, we defined the roles of the different complement activation pathways in this model system. Mice deficient in the alternative pathway component factor B (Fb) and injected with pathogenic anti-mBP180 IgG developed delayed and less intense subepidermal blisters. Mice deficient in the classical pathway component complement component 4 (C4) and WT mice pretreated with neutralizing antibody against the first component of the classical pathway, C1q, were resistant to experimental BP.

These mice exhibited a significantly reduced level of mast cell degranulation and polymorphonuclear neutrophil (PMN) infiltration in the skin. Intradermal administration of compound 48/80, a mast cell degranulating agent, restored BP disease in C4$^{-/-}$ mice. Furthermore, C4$^{-/-}$ mice became susceptible to experimental BP after local injection of PMN chemoattractant IL-8 or local reconstitution with PMNs. These findings provide the first direct evidence to our knowledge that complement activation via the classical and alternative pathways is crucial in subepidermal blister formation in experimental BP.

▶ More than 10 years ago, Liu et al[1] demonstrated that complement activation was essential for lesion formation in murine experimental bullous pemphigoid, using mice with partial deletion of the *C5* gene, and cobra venom to deplete C3. Dr Liu is also the senior author of this article, which describes the examination of the relative contributions of the classical and alternative complement activation pathways; this could not be determined in the earlier study since components C3 and C5 participate in both. The results clearly show that the classical pathway plays the major role in triggering of mast cell degranulation and recruitment of neutrophils, culminating in disease induction. This is very nicely illustrated in Figure 1 of the original article. It is likely that in this model, administration of antibodies analogous to the autoantibodies found in the human disease results in binding to the hemidesmosome antigens in the basement membrane zone of the skin; complement component C1q then binds to the immune complexes formed and activates the classic pathway. The products of the pathway include component fragments C3a and C5a, which as anaphylatoxins, activate mast cells. In addition, C5a is a potent chemoattractant for neutrophils. The authors suggest that the key involvement of the complement cascade in this model is, in fact, the generation of C5a.

G. M. P. Galbraith, MD

Reference

1. Liu Z, Giudice GJ, Swartz SJ, et al. The role of complement in experimental bullous pemphigoid. *J Clin Invest.* 1995;95:1539-1544.

The Cartilage Matrix Protein Subdomain of Type VII Collagen Is Pathogenic for Epidermolysis Bullosa Acquisita
Chen M, Doostan A, Bandyopadhyay P, et al (Univ of Southern California, Los Angeles; Univ of North Carolina, Chapel Hill)
Am J Pathol 170:2009-2018, 2007

Epidermolysis bullosa acquisita (EBA) is an acquired bullous disease of the skin characterized by IgG autoantibodies against type VII (anchoring fibril) collagen. We previously defined four immunodominant antigenic epitopes within the noncollagenous 1 (NC1) domain of type VII collagen. In this study, we produced an additional recombinant fusion protein from the NC1 domain corresponding to the N-terminal 227 amino acids (residues

1 to 227), which contains homology with cartilage matrix protein (CMP). Using enzyme-linked immunosorbent assay and immunoblot analysis, we tested sera from EBA patients ($n = 32$), bullous systemic lupus erythematosus patients ($n = 3$), bullous pemphigoid patients ($n = 15$), and normal humans ($n = 12$). Twenty-six of 32 EBA sera and two of three bullous systemic lupus erythematosus sera reacted with the CMP domain, whereas none of the control sera did. Affinity-purified anti-CMP EBA antibodies injected into hairless mice produced the clinical, histological, immunological, and ultrastructural features of EBA. $F(ab')_2$ fragments generated from anti-CMP EBA autoantibodies did not induce disease. Our studies provide the first evidence that EBA autoantibodies to the CMP subdomain of NC1 are pathogenic and induce blister formation. This is the first antigenic epitope on type VII collagen demonstrated to be a pathogenic target for EBA autoantibodies.

▶ Chen et al characterize a previously unrecognized new antigenic epitope, cartilage matrix protein (CMP), that is recognized by the sera of most patients with epidermolysis bullosa acquisita (EBA). Autoantibodies against CMP were pathogenic when passively transferred to hairless immunocompetent mice. The data presented here further elucidate the pathogenetic mechanisms underlying EBA, and will also help investigators develop effective therapies for this notoriously treatment-resistant condition.

B. H. Thiers, MD

Dermatitis Herpetiformis: No Evidence of Bone Disease Despite Evidence of Enteropathy
Abuzakouk M, Barnes L, O'Gorman N, et al (St James's Hosp, Dublin; St Vincent's Univ, Dublin)
Dig Dis Sci 52:659-664, 2007

The majority of patients with dermatitis herpetiformis (DH) have small intestinal enteropathy that may result in bone loss. The objective of this study was to evaluate bone mineral density (BMD) in DH and to examine whether dietary treatment or degree of the small intestinal lesion correlate with BMD. Twenty-five patients with DH (18 men) were investigated. Detailed dietary assessment and duodenal biopsies were performed on all patients before entry into the study. BMD at lumbar spine and femur was determined by DXA scan. Bone biomarkers, vitamin D, and parathyroid status were assessed. Twenty patients had enteropathy. None of the patients had hypovitaminosis D or secondary hyperparathyroidism. Resorption and formation markers were within normal limits. BMD Z-scores were not significantly different from expected (-0.38; CI, -0.84 to 0.07) and femur (0.46; CI, -0.06 to 0.97). There was no relationship between BMD Z-scores and the severity of the degree of enteropathy. We conclude that enteropathy of differing severity is present in 80% of patients with DH, but this is not associated with bone disease.

▶ The gluten-sensitive enteropathy associated with DH is similar to, but less severe than, that found in patients with celiac disease (CD). Complications of untreated CD include an increased prevalence of gastrointestinal malignancy as well as reduced bone mineral density (BMD). The latter can be associated with bone pain, pathologic fractures, and osteoporosis. Abuzakouk et al studied vitamin D and parathyroid status, bone turnover, and BMD in patients with DH, and investigated the relationship between BMD and the extent of enteropathy. They found that enteropathy of varying degrees commonly occurs in patients with DH but is not associated with bony abnormalities. They do nevertheless recommend a strict gluten-free diet to offset the risk of malignancy and to reduce reliance on dapsone therapy.

B. H. Thiers, MD

Antiphospholipid antibodies in patients with autoimmune blistering disease
Echigo T, Hasegawa M, Inaoki M, et al (Kanazawa Univ, Japan; Kawasaki Med School, Kurashiki, Japan; Nagasaki Univ, Japan)
J Am Acad Dermatol 57:397-400, 2007

Objective.—Our purpose was to determine the serum levels and frequency of antiphospholipid antibodies (aPLs) and confirm the clinical importance of these antibodies in patients with autoimmune blistering disease (ABD).

Methods.—IgG and IgM anticardiolipin antibodies (aCL), IgG anticardiolipin-β_2 glycoprotein I complex antibody (aCL/β_2GPI), and IgG antiphosphatidylserine-prothrombin complex antibody (aPS/PT) were examined with an enzyme-linked immunosorbent assay in 71 patients with ABD, including pemphigus vulgaris, pemphigus foliaceus, and bullous pemphigoid.

Results.—The prevalence of IgG aCL, IgM aCL, aCL/β_2GPI, and IgG aPS/PT was positive for 22.4%, 9.1%, 9.9%, and 25.4% of the ABD patients, respectively, whereas these antibodies were not detected in any of the normal control subjects. Ten of 20 patients with ABD who were attending our hospital in 2004 tested positive for aPLs, and thromboembolism was detected in 7 of 10 patients with aPLs.

Limitations.—Follow-up studies, especially with a large patient group, will be needed to clarify the clinical relevance of aPLs in ABD.

Conclusion.—aPLs are frequently detected in patients with ABD. Careful examination and follow-up for thromboembolism may be necessary in ABD patients with aPLs.

▶ The authors demonstrate the presence of aPLs in a group of patients with ABD. Although thromboembolism was not uncommon, most cases were asymptomatic, which suggests that the tendency for coagulation in these patients may be modest compared with that in patients with primary antiphospholipid syndrome or lupus erythematosus. It should be remembered that systemic corticosteroid treatment, which often is used for the treatment of ABD, may enhance the tendency for coagulation.

B. H. Thiers, MD

11 Genodermatoses

Hereditary Leiomyomatosis and Renal Cell Cancer: A Syndrome Associated With an Aggressive Form of Inherited Renal Cancer
Grubb RL III, Franks ME, Toro J, et al (NIH, Bethesda, Md)
J Urol 177:2074-2080, 2007

Purpose.—Hereditary leiomyomatosis and renal cell cancer is a recently described hereditary cancer syndrome in which affected individuals are at risk for cutaneous and uterine leiomyomas, and kidney cancer. Our initial experience revealed the aggressive behavior of these renal tumors, often with early metastasis, despite small primary tumor size. We report the clinical characteristics and urological treatment of patients with hereditary leiomyomatosis and renal cell cancer associated renal tumors.

Materials and Methods.—A total of 19 patients with hereditary leiomyomatosis and renal cell cancer associated renal tumors were evaluated. The 11 women and 8 men had a median age at diagnosis of 39 years (range 22 to 67), and a median clinical and radiological followup of 34 months (range 6 to 141). Hereditary leiomyomatosis and renal cell cancer manifestations in pa-

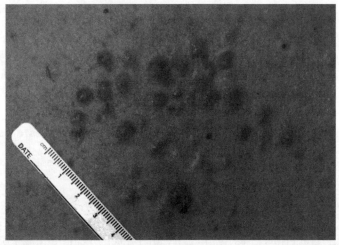

FIGURE 1.—Leiomyoma is characteristic cutaneous lesion of HLRCC. (Reprinted from Grubb RL III, Franks ME, Toro J, et al. Hereditary leiomyomatosis and renal cell cancer: a syndrome associated with an aggressive form of inherited renal cancer. *J Urol.* 2007;177:2074-2080. Copyright 2007, with permission from the American Urological Association.)

tients with renal tumors included cutaneous leiomyomas in 11 of 17 evaluable patients (65%) and uterine leiomyomas in 7 of 7 evaluable females (100%).

Results.—Median pathological tumor size was 7.8 cm (range 1.5 to 20). Histological subtypes were consistent with hereditary leiomyomatosis and renal cell cancer renal carcinoma. Four of 7 patients with 2.0 to 6.7 cm T1 tumors had spread to regional lymph nodes or metastases at nephrectomy. Overall 9 of 19 patients (47%) presented with nodal or distant metastases.

Conclusions.—Renal tumors in patients with hereditary leiomyomatosis and renal cell cancer syndrome are significantly more aggressive than those in patients with other hereditary renal tumor syndromes. In contrast to other familial renal cancer syndromes, the observation of 3 cm or less renal tumors associated with hereditary leiomyomatosis and renal cell cancer is not recommended. Careful followup of affected and at risk individuals in families is necessary (Fig 1).

▶ Kiuru and colleagues first reported in 2001 the link between cutaneous and uterine leiomyomas and renal cell carcinoma (Fig 1).[1] Different studies have shown that affected kindreds carry germ line mutations of the FH gene that encodes the Krebs cycle enzyme located at 1q43.2-42.3. This gene is inherited in an autosomal-dominant manner. Grubb and colleagues found that the renal cancers in these patients are particularly aggressive as compared with those found in patients with other hereditary renal tumor syndromes. Grubb et al advised that a family history of renal cancer (especially of those tumors that cause death at a young age), small tumors with early metastatic spread that is out of proportion with tumor size, early hysterectomy as a result of symptomatic fibroids, and the presence of cutaneous leiomyomas should alert clinicians to the possibility of this syndrome.

B. H. Thiers, MD

References

1. Kiuru M, Launonen V, Hietala M, et al. Familial cutaneous leiomyomatosis is a two-hit condition associated with renal cancer of characteristic histopathology. *Am J Pathol.* 2001;159:825-829.

Reprogramming of keratin biosynthesis by sulforaphane restores skin integrity in epidermolysis bullosa simplex
Kerns ML, DePianto D, Dinkova-Kostova AT, et al (Johns Hopkins Univ, Baltimore, Md)
Proc Natl Acad Sci U S A 104:14460-14465, 2007

Epidermolysis bullosa simplex (EBS) is a rare inherited condition in which the epidermis loses its integrity after mechanical trauma. EBS is typified by the dysfunction of intermediate filaments in basal keratinocytes of epidermis. Most cases of EBS are due to mutations in the keratin 5 or 14 gene (*K5* and *K14*), whose products copolymerize to form intermediate filaments in basal keratinocytes. Available treatments for this disorder are only palliative. Here we exploit functional redundancy within the keratin gene family as the basis for therapy. We show that genetic activation of Gli2 or treatment with a pharmacological activator of Nrf2, two transcription factors eliciting distinct transcriptional programs, alleviates the blistering caused by a K14 deficiency in an EBS mouse model, correlating with K17 induction in basal epidermal keratinocytes. Nrf2 induction is brought about by treatment with sulforaphane, a natural product. Sulforaphane thus represents an attractive option for the prevention of skin blistering associated with K14 mutations in EBS.

▶ EBS is characterized by mutations in the genes controlling keratin synthesis, leading to defects in intermediate filament formation and a weakened, structurally deficient epidermis that tears after minor trauma. Kerns et al found that sulforaphane, a natural product derived from broccoli, could induce keratin 17 synthesis in basal keratinocytes and alleviate blistering in a mouse model of keratin 14-deficient EBS. The same group has observed a protective effect of sulforaphane against UV-induced erythema, inflammation, and edema.[1]

B. H. Thiers, MD

Reference

1. Talalay P, Fahey JW, Healy ZR, et al. Sulforaphane mobilizes cellular defenses that protect skin against damage by UV radiation. *Proc Natl Acad Sci U S A.* 2007;104: 17500-17505.

Missense Mutations in the *BCS1L* Gene as a Cause of the Björnstad Syndrome
Hinson JT, Fantin VR, Schönberger J, et al (Harvard Med School; Howard Hughes Med Inst, Boston; Univ Hosp Würzburg, Germany; et al)
N Engl J Med 356:809-819, 2007

Background.—The Björnstad syndrome, an autosomal recessive disorder associated with sensorineural hearing loss and pili torti, is caused by mutation of a previously unidentified gene on chromosome 2q34–36.

Methods.—Refined genetic mapping and DNA sequencing of 44 genes between *D2S2210* and *D2S2244* revealed *BCS1L* mutations. Functional analyses elucidated how *BCS1L* mutations cause the Björnstad syndrome.

Results.—*BCS1L* encodes a member of the AAA family of ATPases that is necessary for the assembly of complex III in the mitochondria. In addition to the Björnstad syndrome, *BCS1L* mutations cause complex III deficiency and the GRACILE syndrome, which in neonates are lethal conditions that have multisystem and neurologic manifestations typifying severe mitochondrial disorders. Patients with the Björnstad syndrome have mutations that alter residues involved in protein–protein interactions, whereas mutations in patients with complex III deficiency alter ATP-binding residues, as deduced from the crystal structure of a related AAA-family ATPase. Biochemical studies provided evidence to support this model: complex III deficiency mutations prevented ATP-dependent assembly of BCS1L-associated complexes. All mutant BCS1L proteins disrupted the assembly of complex III, reduced the activity of the mitochondrial electron-transport chain, and increased the production of reactive oxygen species. However, only mutations associated with complex III deficiency increased mitochondrial content, which further increased the production of reactive oxygen species.

Conclusions.—*BCS1L* mutations cause disease phenotypes ranging from highly restricted pili torti and sensorineural hearing loss (the Björnstad syndrome) to profound multisystem organ failure (complex III deficiency and the GRACILE syndrome). All *BCS1L* mutations disrupted the assembly of mitochondrial respirasomes (the basic unit for respiration in human mitochondria), but the clinical expression of the mutations was correlated with the production of reactive oxygen species. Mutations that cause the Björnstad syndrome illustrate the exquisite sensitivity of ear and hair tissues to mitochondrial function, particularly to the production of reactive oxygen species.

▶ Hinson et al show that recessive *BCS1L* mutations cause sensorineural hearing loss and pili torti in patients with the Björnstad syndrome. The mutations disrupt mitochondrial respiration with specific mutations correlating with the production of reactive oxygen species and the observed pathologic features. Presumably, although all *BCS1L* mutations increase the production of reactive oxygen species, the amount of the increase is mutation-specific and correlates with the ultimate clinical manifestations.

B. H. Thiers, MD

12 Drug Actions, Reactions, and Interactions

A Randomized, Double-blind, Placebo-Controlled Trial of Pentoxifylline for the Treatment of Recurrent Aphthous Stomatitis
Thornhill MH, Baccaglini L, Theaker E, et al (Univ of Sheffield School of Clinical Dentistry, England; Univ Dental Hosp of Manchester, England; Univ of Florida College of Dentistry, Gainesville)
Arch Dermatol 143:463-470, 2007

Objective.—To evaluate pentoxifylline for the treatment of recurrent aphthous stomatitis.

Design.—A 60-day, randomized, double-blind, placebo-controlled trial with a 60-day no treatment follow-up.

Setting.—An oral medicine specialist referral center in Manchester.

Participants.—Forty-nine volunteers who passed the initial assessment for recurrent aphthous stomatitis entered a pretrial phase in which their eligibility for the trial phase of the study was assessed. Sixteen subjects were deemed ineligible, and 7 failed to attend or withdrew. The remaining 26 subjects were randomized to placebo or treatment. Six subjects withdrew because of adverse effects, and 1 was unavailable for follow-up.

Intervention.—Pentoxifylline (also called oxpentifylline), 400 mg 3 times daily, or matching placebo.

Main Outcome Measure.—A reduction in the median pain score, ulcer size, number of ulcers, or total number of ulcer episodes.

Results.—Patients taking pentoxifylline had less pain and reported smaller and fewer ulcers compared with baseline. Patients taking placebo reported no improvement in these variables. Patients taking pentoxifylline also reported more ulcer-free days than those taking placebo. However, the differences were small and, with the exception of median ulcer size ($P = .05$), did not reach statistical significance. Adverse effects were common with pentoxifylline, but not significantly different from those experienced by patients taking placebo.

Conclusions.—Although pentoxifylline may have some benefit in the treatment of recurrent aphthous stomatitis, the benefit is limited. It may have a role in the treatment of patients unresponsive to other treatments, but cannot yet be recommended as a first-line treatment.

▶ Pentoxifylline has been suggested as a treatment for aphthous stomatitis by virtue of its activity as a tumor necrosis factor α inhibitor and its ability to inhibit neutrophil chemotaxis and function. This study by Thornhill and colleagues shows that the drug has a rather modest clinical benefit. I have found it to be only marginally useful for the treatment of this condition.

B. H. Thiers, MD

Chronic Eczematous Eruptions of the Elderly Are Associated with Chronic Exposure to Calcium Channel Blockers: Results from a Case–Control Study
Joly P, Benoit-Corven C, Baricault S, et al (Rouen Univ Hosp, France; Nancy Univ Hosp, France; Lille Univ Hosp, France; et al)
J Invest Dermatol 127:2766-2771, 2007

It has been suggested that chronic eczematous eruptions of the elderly could be associated with chronic drug exposure. To determine the drugs associated with these eruptions, we conducted a case–control study on 102 cases and 204 controls. Cases were consecutive patients older than 60 years presenting with an eczematous eruption that had evolved continuously or recurrently for more than 3 months without a reliable cause. Two controls were matched to each case on age, sex, in/outpatient origin, and center. Information about drug exposure was obtained from patients and their pharmacists. Drug use for more than 3 months within the year preceding the eruption was compared between cases and controls. An association was found between calcium channel blockers (CCB) and eczema, with a matched OR (odds ratio) of 2.5 (95% CI (confidence interval): 1.3–4.6). To ascertain the course of patients after CCB withdrawal, two ancillary studies were performed on 74 patients with eczematous eruptions from our department before the case–control study period, and on 101 patients registered in the French "Pharmacovigilance" database. Healing of these eruptions after CCB withdrawal occurred in 83 and 68% of these cases, respectively. The long-term use of CCB is a risk factor for chronic eczematous eruptions of the elderly.

▶ The authors suggest that the administration of CCBs may underlie a significant number of unexplained eczematous eruptions occurring in older individuals. The overall incidence may be quite low, especially in community practices as opposed to tertiary care referral centers. The association between CCBs and acute cutaneous eruptions has previously been reported.[1]

B. H. Thiers, MD

Reference

1. Stern RS. Chronic medication use in inflammatory skin diseases: the power and limitations of the case-control study. *J Invest Dermatol.* 2007;127:2709-2710.

Appropriate prescribing in elderly people: how well can it be measured and optimised?
Spinewine A, Schmader KE, Barber N, et al (Université catholique de Louvain, Brussels, Belgium; Duke Univ Med Ctr, Durham, NC; Veterans Affairs Med Ctr, Durham, NC; et al)
Lancet 370:173-184, 2007

Background.—The prescription of medicines is a basic component of health care for elderly persons, and the optimization of drug prescription for this segment of the population has become an important public health issue throughout the world. One challenging aspect of prescribing for elderly persons is the increasing heterogeneity of the population. Although there are increasing numbers of fit, healthy elderly people, there are also increasing numbers of those who are vulnerable and frail and have limited physiologic reserve, reduced homeostasis, dysregulations in immune and inflammation mechanisms, have several comorbidities, and take several prescription drugs. This was the first report that demonstrated completion of 3 primary objectives: (1) appropriate prescribing in elderly persons was defined and categorized; (2) the instruments available for its measurement and their predictive validity were discussed; and (3) recent randomized controlled studies that assessed the effect of optimization strategies on the appropriateness of prescribing in elderly persons were critically reviewed, with suggestions made for the direction of future research and practice.

Overview.—There is evidence that elderly patients are often prescribed inappropriate drugs, partly, because of the complexities of prescribing in addition to other patient, provider, and health system factors. However, the evidence is mixed and often contradictory. Some studies have shown a positive relation between inappropriate prescribing and mortality, use of health care services, adverse drug events, and quality of life; however, other studies have reported mixed or negative results. These findings have called into question the validity of existing process measures of appropriateness in prescribing for elderly persons. Prescribing to this population could be optimized by the addition of trials complemented by evidence from well-designed, nonexperimental studies that estimate causal effects. Another promising approach is the involvement of patients or their caregivers in decision making relevant to prescribing. Information technology should also improve the use of drugs through 3 interacting databases—the patient's drug history, a scientific drug information reference and guideline database, and patient-specific clinical information.

Conclusions.—Drug prescription among geriatric populations is an important public health issue worldwide. The measurement and optimization of appropriate prescribing is a complex challenge. This article sought to define and categorize appropriate prescribing in elderly persons, to review the instruments currently in use for assessing such prescribing, and to suggest directions for future research and practice.

▶ Prescribing to the elderly patient is a challenging undertaking. Patients come in with long lists of medications; many of which appear to be redundant. Some patients are quite organized and understand their medications, whereas others are confused and uncertain as to what medications they are taking and why they are taking them. Polypharmacy is rampant, and most of our elderly patients are, in this reviewer's opinion, heavily overmedicated. The challenge for us as physicians is to identify, manage, and prevent drug interactions that can cause real harm. Software is helpful but not the total answer. A team-based approach where information is shared and communicated among providers will provide maximum benefit to the patient.

B. H. Thiers, MD

The challenge of managing drug interactions in elderly people
Mallet L, Spinewine A, Huang A (Univ of Montreal; Université catholique de Louvain, Brussels, Belgium; McGill Univ, Montreal)
Lancet 370:185-191, 2007

Drug therapy is essential when caring for elderly patients, but clearly it is a double-edged sword. Elderly patients are at high risk of having drug interactions, but the prevalence of these interactions is not well documented. Several types of interactions exist: drug–drug, drug–disease, drug–food, drug–alcohol, drug–herbal products, and drug–nutritional status. Factors such as age-related changes in pharmacokinetics and pharmacodynamics, frailty, interindividual variability, reduced homoeostatic mechanisms, and psychosocial issues need to be considered when drug interactions are assessed. Software can help clinicians to detect drug interactions, but many programmes have not been updated with the evolving knowledge of these interactions, and do not take into consideration important factors needed to optimise drug treatment in elderly patients. Any generated recommendations have to be tempered by a holistic, geriatric, multiprofessional approach that is team-based. This second paper in a series of two on prescribing in elderly people proposes an approach to categorise drug interactions, along with strategies to assist in their detection, management, and prevention.

▶ Prescribing to the elderly is a challenging undertaking. Patients come in with long lists of medications, many of which appear to be redundant. Some patients are quite organized and understand their medications, whereas others are confused and uncertain as to what medications they are taking and why they are taking them. Polypharmacy is rampant, and most of our elderly patients are in this reviewer's opinion heavily overmedicated. The challenge for us as physicians is to identify, manage, and prevent drug interactions that can cause real harm. Software is helpful but not the total answer. A team-based approach where information is shared and communicated among providers will provide maximum benefit to the patient.

B. H. Thiers, MD

Fixed-Dose Combinations Improve Medication Compliance: A Meta-Analysis
Bangalore S, Kamalakkannan G, Parkar S, et al (St Luke's-Roosevelt Hosp and Columbia Univ, New York)
Am J Med 120:713-719, 2007

Background.—Compliance with treatment is a sine qua non for successful treatment of chronic conditions like hypertension. Fixed-dose combinations are designed to simplify the medication regimen and potentially improve compliance. However the data on comparison of fixed-dose combination with free-drug regimen to improve patient's medication compliance is limited.

Methods.—We conducted a MEDLINE search of studies using the words fixed-dose combinations, compliance and/or adherence. The inclusion criteria were studies which involved fixed-dose combination versus free-drug components of the regimen given separately. Only studies which reported patient's compliance were included.

Results.—Of the 68 studies on fixed-dose combinations, only 9 studies fulfilled the inclusion criteria. Two studies were in patients with tuberculosis, 4 in the hypertensive population, 1 in patients with human immunodeficiency virus (HIV) disease and 2 in the diabetic population. A total of 11,925 patients on fixed-dose combination were compared against 8317 patients on free-drug component regimen. Fixed-dose combination resulted in a 26% decrease in the risk of non-compliance compared with free-drug component regimen (pooled relative risk [RR] 0.74; 95% confidence interval [CI], 0.69-0.80; P <.0001). There was no evidence of heterogeneity in this analysis ($\chi^2 = 14.49$, df = 8; P = .07). A subgroup analysis of the 4 studies on hypertension showed that fixed-dose combination (pooled RR 0.76; 95% CI, 0.71-0.81; P <.0001) decreased the risk of medication non-compliance by 24% compared with free-drug combination regimen.

Conclusions.—Fixed-dose combination decreases the risk of medication non-compliance and should be considered in patients with chronic conditions like hypertension for improving medication compliance which can translate into better clinical outcomes.

▶ Complex treatment regimens and polypharmacy are frequent causes of poor treatment compliance, which obviously leads to increased patient morbidity. Bangalore et al found that fixed-dose combinations reduce the risk of poor patient compliance. Although they limited their investigation to patients under treatment for a variety of systemic conditions, there is little doubt the results could be extrapolated to skin disorders as well. How many of our patients leave our offices with just a single prescription? The FDA has often frowned upon fixed-dose combination drugs, but that philosophy may be changing.

B. H. Thiers, MD

Mortality in Randomized Trials of Antioxidant Supplements for Primary and Secondary Prevention: Systematic Review and Meta-analysis
Bjelakovic G, Nikolova D, Gluud LL, et al (Copenhagen Univ; Univ of Nis, Serbia; Ospedale V Cervello, Palermo, Italy)
JAMA 297:842-857, 2007

Context.—Antioxidant supplements are used for prevention of several diseases.

Objective.—To assess the effect of antioxidant supplements on mortality in randomized primary and secondary prevention trials.

Data Sources and Trial Selection.—We searched electronic databases and bibliographies published by October 2005. All randomized trials involving adults comparing beta carotene, vitamin A, vitamin C (ascorbic acid), vitamin E, and selenium either singly or combined vs placebo or vs no intervention were included in our analysis. Randomization, blinding, and follow-up were considered markers of bias in the included trials. The effect of antioxidant supplements on all-cause mortality was analyzed with random-effects meta-analyses and reported as relative risk (RR) with 95% confidence intervals (CIs). Meta-regression was used to assess the effect of covariates across the trials.

Data Extraction.—We included 68 randomized trials with 232,606 participants (385 publications).

Data Synthesis.—When all low- and high-bias risk trials of antioxidant supplements were pooled together there was no significant effect on mortality (RR, 1.02; 95% CI, 0.98-1.06). Multivariate meta-regression analyses showed that low-bias risk trials (RR, 1.16; 95% CI, 1.05-1.29) and selenium (RR, 0.998; 95% CI, 0.997-0.9995) were significantly associated with mortality. In 47 low-bias trials with 180,938 participants, the antioxidant supplements significantly increased mortality (RR, 1.05; 95% CI, 1.02-1.08). In low-bias risk trials, after exclusion of selenium trials, beta carotene (RR, 1.07; 95% CI, 1.02-1.11), vitamin A (RR, 1.16; 95% CI, 1.10-1.24), and vitamin E (RR, 1.04; 95% CI, 1.01-1.07), singly or combined, significantly increased mortality. Vitamin C and selenium had no significant effect on mortality.

Conclusions.—Treatment with beta carotene, vitamin A, and vitamin E may increase mortality. The potential roles of vitamin C and selenium on mortality need further study.

▶ In previous studies, the authors found that with the potential exception of selenium, antioxidant supplements were without a significant effect on the incidence of gastrointestinal cancers and actually were associated with increased all-cause mortality.[1] In the current study, they analyzed the effects of antioxidant supplements (beta carotene, vitamins A and E, vitamin C, and selenium) on all-cause mortality of adults included in primary and secondary prevention trials, and again found an increase in mortality associated with some of them. The findings contradict those in some previously published observational studies claiming that antioxidants improve health. Intense marketing efforts are used to support this claim, and 10% to 20% of the adult population in North America and Europe consume these supplements. Thus, the public health consequences under discussion here are substantial. Why could antioxidants have a negative effect on mortality? The authors hypothesize that although oxidative stress may have a role in the pathogenesis of many chronic diseases, it may also be the consequence of certain pathologic conditions.[1] By eliminating free radicals, antioxidants may interfere with essential defense mechanisms including apoptosis, phagocytosis, and detoxification. Certainly, a better understanding of antioxidant metabolism in relation to disease pathogenesis and resolution is urgently needed.

B. H. Thiers, MD

Reference

1. Halliwell B. Free radicals, antioxidants, and human disease: curiosity, cause, or consequence? *Lancet.* 1994;344:721-724.

Corticosteroid-induced clinical adverse events: frequency, risk factors and patient's opinion
Fardet L, Flahault A, Kettaneh A, et al (Hôpital Saint-Antoine, Paris; Univ Pierre et Marie Curie, Paris; Nouvelles Cliniques Nantaises, Nantes, France; et al)
Br J Dermatol 157:142-148, 2007

Background.—More than 50 years after the introduction of corticosteroids, few studies have focused on corticosteroid-induced adverse events after long-term systemic therapy.

Objectives.—To assess the frequency, risk factors and patient's opinion regarding clinical adverse events occurring early during prednisone therapy.

Patients and Methods.—We conducted a cohort study in two French centres. All consecutive patients starting long-term ($\geq$ 3 months), high dosage ($\geq$ 20 mg day^{-1}) prednisone therapy were enrolled. The main clinical adverse events attributable to corticosteroids were assessed after 3 months of therapy, by comparison with baseline status. The patient's opinion regarding the disability induced by these adverse events was recorded. Risk factors of frequently observed adverse effects were identified by using logistic regression.

Results.—Eighty-eight patients were enrolled and 80 were monitored for at least 3 months (women 76%; mean age 59.1 ± 18.7 years; giant cell arteritis 39%; mean baseline prednisone dosage 54 ± 17 mg day^{-1}). Lipodystrophy was the most frequent adverse event [63.0% (51.0–73.1)], was considered the most distressing by the patients and was most frequent in women and young patients. Neuropsychiatric disorders occurred in 42 patients [52.5% (41.0–63.8)], necessitating hospitalization in five cases. Skin disorders were noted by 37 patients [46.2% (35.0–57.7)] and were more frequent in women. Muscle cramp and proximal muscle weakness were reported by 32.5% (22.5–43.9) and 15% (8.0–24.7) of patients, respectively. Newly developed hypertension occurred in 8.7% (2.9–20.3) of patients. Lastly, 39% (19.7–61.4) of the premenopausal women reported menstrual disorders.

Conclusions.—Lipodystrophy and neuropsychiatric disorders are common adverse events of long-term prednisone therapy and are particularly distressing for the patients concerned. The impact of these adverse events on adherence to corticosteroid therapy is not known.

▶ Although corticosteroid-induced clinical adverse advents can be frequent and debilitating, there is a surprising lack of reliable data on them. Fardet et al found a surprisingly high incidence of lipodystrophy and neuropsychiatric disorders in corticosteroid-treated patients. These were the most distressing adverse events from the patients' standpoint, and their long-term impact on patient health and treatment compliance is worthy of consideration.

B. H. Thiers, MD

Chronic hepatitis B reactivation: a word of caution regarding the use of systemic glucocorticosteroid therapy
Yang C-H, Wu T-S, Chiu CT (Chang Gung Univ, Taoyuan, Taiwan; Chang Gung Inst of Technology, Taoyuan, Taiwan)
Br J Dermatol 157:587-590, 2007

Background.—The potentially fatal complications associated with viral hepatitis B (HBV) reactivation have not been characterized in bullous/connective tissue disease patients receiving prolonged systemic glucocorticosteroids (GCs).

Objectives.—This study reports HBV reactivation following GC therapy for a case series of pemphigus vulgaris and dermatomyositis.

Methods.—The retrospective study cohort comprised 98 patients who received at least 6 months of systemic GC therapy.

Results.—Four cases of HBV carriers with viral hepatitis flare were identified. Two patients suffered fulminant hepatitis and died, while the remaining two patients experienced recurrent hepatitis flare following antiviral medication. The mean time from the start of GCs to the time of HBV reactivation was 10.5 months.

Conclusions.—HBV infection is an important global public health problem. Fatal HBV reactivation may occur following long-term systemic GC therapy. Given the risk of mortality, all bullous/connective tissue disease patients should be screened for serum hepatitis B markers before commencing systemic GC therapy.

▶ As noted by the authors, autoimmune bullous diseases and collagen vascular diseases are but 2 of the major dermatologic disorders that require long-term GC therapy, which may reactivate latent infections. They show that GC-induced HBV reactivation is a serious but preventable complication. Similarly, in areas where tuberculosis has been a major public health problem, PPD (purified protein derivative) screening should be considered in patients in whom long-term GC therapy may be necessary. Another not uncommon but preventable complication of long-term steroid therapy is osteoporosis, for which calcium and vitamin D supplementation and bisphosphonate administration may be recommended.

B. H. Thiers, MD

Anaphylaxis and toxic epidermal necrolysis or Stevens–Johnson syndrome after nonmucosal topical drug application: fact or fiction?
Sachs B, Fischer-Barth W, Erdmann S, et al (Fed Inst for Drugs and Med Devices, Bonn, Germany; Aachen Univ, Germany)
Allergy 62:877-883, 2007

Background.—Drug-induced anaphylaxis and toxic epidermal necrolysis (TEN) or Stevens-Johnson syndrome (SJS) represent severe immediate and delayed-type adverse drug reactions (ADRs), respectively. Occurrence of such reactions after topical drug application has only rarely been reported. Hence, we compiled a large number of such cases which we systematically analyzed.

Methods.—All such cases contained in the ADR database of the competent pharmacovigilance authority in Germany and cases reported in literature were identified, evaluated and analyzed with regard to potential risk factors. Since the application of drugs to mucous membranes facilitates their entry to the systemic circulation only cases occurring after non-mucosal topical drug application were considered.

Results.—After evaluation 28 anaphylaxis database cases and 48 anaphylaxis literature cases remained for analysis. Application to skin wounds or to skin with impaired barrier function was identified as a risk factor in 10/28 (36%) of the database cases and in 42/48 (88%) of the literature cases. In 9/28 database cases (32%), anaphylaxis was induced by drugs used for their hyperemizing effect and, in 8/28 cases (29%) by antibiotics or antiseptics. In the literature cases, anaphylaxis was induced by antibiotics or antiseptics in 35/48 cases (73%). Only one SJS database case and one TEN literature case remained after case evaluation.

Conclusion.—Anaphylaxis does occur after non-mucosal topical drug administration. Application of drugs to skin wounds or to skin with impaired barrier function may pose a risk factor for its occurrence. TEN or SJS following non-mucosal topical drug application seems to be extremely rare.

▶ Sachs et al searched the literature and several databases to confirm that anaphylaxis can indeed occur after nonmucosal topical drug application. Impaired barrier function appears to be a risk factor. They found that 7% to 8% of such cases may be prevented by taking an adequate history regarding preexisting drug sensitivities. TEN or SJS after nonmucosal drug application was reported only rarely.

B. H. Thiers, MD

Vancomycin-Induced Immune Thrombocytopenia

Von Drygalski A, Curtis BR, Bougie DW, et al (Med College of Wisconsin, Milwaukee; BloodCenter of Wisconsin, Milwaukee; Baylor College of Medicine, Houston)

N Engl J Med 356:904-910, 2007

Background.—Vancomycin has only rarely been implicated as a cause of thrombocytopenia, and there is only limited evidence that this complication is caused by immune mechanisms. We conducted a study to determine whether thrombocytopenia is caused by vancomycin-dependent antibodies in patients being treated with vancomycin.

Methods.—We identified and characterized vancomycin-dependent, platelet-reactive antibodies in patients who had been referred for testing during a 5-year period because of a clinical suspicion of vancomycin-induced thrombocytopenia. We obtained clinical information about the patients from their referring physicians.

Results.—Drug-dependent, platelet-reactive antibodies of the IgG class, the IgM class, or both were identified in 34 patients, and clinical follow-up information was obtained from 29 of these patients. The mean nadir platelet count in these patients was 13,600 per cubic millimeter, and severe bleeding occurred in 10 patients (34%). Platelet levels returned to baseline in all 26 surviving patients after vancomycin was stopped. In 15 patients, the drug was continued for 1 to 14 days while other possible causes of thrombocytopenia were investigated. Vancomycin-dependent antibodies were not found in 25 patients who had been given vancomycin and in whom thrombocytopenia did not develop.

Conclusions.—Severe bleeding can occur in patients with vancomycin-induced immune thrombocytopenia. The detection of vancomycin-dependent antiplatelet antibodies in patients receiving the antibiotic in whom thrombocytopenia develops, and the absence of antibodies in patients given the drug in whom platelet counts remain stable, indicate that these antibodies are the cause of the thrombocytopenia.

▶ This article probably is of special significance to dermatologists working in tertiary care settings, where patient exposure to vancomycin is quite common. Interestingly, all 29 patients in this study in whom vancomycin-dependent antibodies were detected had been exposed to the drug before thrombocytopenia developed. Von Drygalski et al present strong evidence that the vancomycin-induced antibodies were the cause of the thrombocytopenia in these patients. As life-threatening bleeding can occur from vancomycin-induced thrombocytopenia, awareness of its existence is critical, especially because patients given the drug often have life-threatening bacterial sepsis and are receiving heparin, which initially may be considered responsible for any associated bleeding.[1]

B. H. Thiers, MD

Reference

1. Warkentin TE. Drug-induced immune-mediated thrombocytopenia—from purpura to thrombosis. *N Engl J Med*. 2007;356:891-893.

Intertriginous Eruption Associated With Chemotherapy in Pediatric Patients
Webber KA, Kos L, Holland KE, et al (Med College of Wisconsin, Milwaukee)
Arch Dermatol 143:67-71, 2007

Background.—Cutaneous eruptions commonly occur in children receiving chemotherapy, and the clinical situation often demands immediate diagnosis and initiation of treatment. Several patterns of cutaneous eruptions to chemotherapy have been reported; however, the nomenclature used to describe these entities has been derived from the histologic findings. The morphologic characteristics, distribution, and natural history of these reactions have not been well established.

Observations.—We report the clinical features of 16 pediatric patients with a distinctive chemotherapy-induced eruption. The eruption is most prominent in or limited to intertriginous regions and areas of occlusion. We were not able to identify any single chemotherapeutic agent or even a group of agents in the same pharmacologic family that seemed to be associated with this reaction. The eruption did not appear to be related to sex, age, ethnicity, underlying malignancy, or genetic disease.

Conclusions.—Recognition of this distinct clinical pattern can help rule out more serious entities, avoid a biopsy, and reassure the physician and patient of the benign and self-resolving clinical course. This entity may be observed with many chemotherapeutic agents and underlying diseases, but most often with high-dose chemotherapy protocols.

▶ The authors describe a rather dramatic yet asymptomatic eruption in children undergoing high-dose chemotherapy. It is important to be aware of this phenomenon, as it seems to be a toxic reaction rather than a hypersensitivity eruption and will resolve despite continuation of chemotherapy. When an erythematous eruption occurs in intertriginous areas of severely immunocompromised children, staphylococcal scalded skin syndrome should be in the differential diagnosis. The eruption associated with chemotherapy is described as beginning as papules, which are dusky red in color and tend to coalesce in intertriginous areas. In contrast, staphylococcal scalded skin syndrome usually begins as bright red patches in intertriginous areas and periorally that later denude. Although the authors are confident that a skin biopsy is unnecessary in most cases, obtaining 1 in these critically ill children seems prudent when the diagnosis is uncertain. Initiation of antibiotics should be considered if a possible diagnosis of staphylococcal scalded skin syndrome is of serious concern.

S. Raimer, MD

13 Drug Development and Promotion

Institutional Academic–Industry Relationships
Campbell EG, Weissman JS, Ehringhaus S, et al (Massachusetts Gen Hosp, Boston; Univ of Michigan, Ann Arbor; Association of American Med Colleges, Boston)
JAMA 298:1779-1786, 2007

Context.—Institutional academic–industry relationships have the potential of creating institutional conflicts of interest. To date there are no empirical data to support the establishment and evaluation of institutional policies and practices related to managing these relationships.

Objective.—To conduct a national survey of department chairs about the nature, extent, and consequences of institutional–academic industry relationships for medical schools and teaching hospitals.

Design, Setting, and Participants.—National survey of department chairs in the 125 accredited allopathic medical schools and the 15 largest independent teaching hospitals in the United States, administered between February 2006 and October 2006.

Main Outcome Measure.—Types of relationships with industry.

Results.—A total of 459 of 688 eligible department chairs completed the survey, yielding an overall response rate of 67%. Almost two-thirds (60%) of department chairs had some form of personal relationship with industry, including serving as a consultant (27%), a member of a scientific advisory board (27%), a paid speaker (14%), an officer (7%), a founder (9%), or a member of the board of directors (11%). Two-thirds (67%) of departments as administrative units had relationships with industry. Clinical departments were more likely than nonclinical departments to receive research equipment (17% vs 10%, $P = .04$), unrestricted funds (19% vs 3%, $P < .001$), residency or fellowship training support (37% vs 2%, $P < .001$), and continuing medical education support (65% vs 3%, $P < .001$). However, nonclinical departments were more likely to receive funding from intellectual property licensing (27% vs 16%, $P = .01$). More than two-thirds of chairs perceived that having a relationship with industry had no effect on their professional activities, 72% viewed a chair's engaging in more than 1 industry-related activity (substantial role in a start-up company, consulting, or serving on a company's board) as having a negative impact on a department's ability to conduct independent unbiased research.

Conclusion.—Overall, institutional academic–industry relationships are highly prevalent and underscore the need for their active disclosure and management.

▶ Campbell et al present data to document that institutional academic–industry relationships are quite prevalent in medical schools and teaching hospitals. Future research is needed to better understand their impact on the performance of independent unbiased research and on the education and research missions of medical schools.

Thoughtful management and disclosure of these relationships is mandatory. As noted by the authors, failure to do so can endanger the trust of the public in United States medical schools and teaching hospitals.

B. H. Thiers, MD

A National Survey of Physician–Industry Relationships
Campbell EG, Gruen RL, Mountford J, et al (Harvard Med School, Boston; Univ of Melbourne, Australia; Mediphase, Newton, Mass; et al)
N Engl J Med 356:1742-1750, 2007

Background.—Relationships between physicians and pharmaceutical, medical device, and other medically related industries have received considerable attention in recent years. We surveyed physicians to collect information about their financial associations with industry and the factors that predict those associations.

Methods.—We conducted a national survey of 3167 physicians in six specialties (anesthesiology, cardiology, family practice, general surgery, internal medicine, and pediatrics) in late 2003 and early 2004. The raw response rate for this probability sample was 52%, and the weighted response rate was 58%.

Results.—Most physicians (94%) reported some type of relationship with the pharmaceutical industry, and most of these relationships involved receiving food in the workplace (83%) or receiving drug samples (78%). More than one third of the respondents (35%) received reimbursement for costs associated with professional meetings or continuing medical education, and more than one quarter (28%) received payments for consulting, giving lectures, or enrolling patients in trials. Cardiologists were more than twice as likely as family practitioners to receive payments. Family practitioners met more frequently with industry representatives than did physicians in other specialties, and physicians in solo, two-person, or group practices met more frequently with industry representatives than did physicians practicing in hospitals and clinics.

Conclusions.—The results of this national survey indicate that relationships between physicians and industry are common and underscore the variation among such relationships according to specialty, practice type, and professional activities.

▶ The public, and now the medical and scientific community, have turned the spotlight on relationships between the medical profession and the drug industry. As demonstrated by Campbell et al, such relationships are almost universal among American doctors. While such relationships usually involve free food, drink, or drug samples, some physicians have received expenses for attending meetings or payments for consulting, lecturing, or enrolling patients in clinical trials. Campbell et al noted that cardiologists were significantly more likely than other hospital specialists or primary care physicians to receive payments for professional services and postulated that drug companies might target specialists whose prescribing habits are likely to influence others. Primary care doctors reported 16 meetings per month with drug company representatives; internists had 10; cardiologists, 9; and anesthesiologists, 2. For comparison, 7 years earlier the average number of monthy meetings was about 4. The authors indicated a response rate of only 52% to their survey and suggested that those who did reply probably underreported the extent of their involvement with industry.

Our medical center has taken steps to implement a strict conflict-of-interest policy that includes a prohibition against the iconic drug company–sponsored "free lunch." To bring back a quote from the 1960s, "The whole world is watching!"

B. H. Thiers, MD

Direct-to-Consumer Advertising of Pharmaceuticals
Gellad ZF, Lyles KW (Duke Univ, Durham, NC; Durham VA Med Ctr, NC)
Am J Med 120:475-480, 2007

Since the US Food and Drug Administration (FDA) released new guidelines on broadcast direct-to-consumer advertising in 1997 (Table 1), the prevalence of direct-to-consumer advertising of prescription drugs has increased exponentially. The impact on providers, patients, and the health care system is varied and dynamic, and the rapid changes in the last several years have markedly altered the health care landscape. To continue providing optimal medical care, physicians and other health care providers must be able to manage this influence on their practice, and a more thorough understanding of this phenomenon is an integral step toward this goal. This review will summarize the history of direct-to-consumer drug advertisements and the current regulations governing them. It will summarize the evidence concerning the impact of direct-to-consumer advertising on the public, providers, and the health care system, and conclude with observations regarding the future of direct-to-consumer advertising.

TABLE 1.—FDA Guidelines on Direct-to-Consumer Drug Advertisements

Print Advertisements*	Broadcast Advertisements†
Brief Summary—Advertisements must disclose each side effect, warning, precaution and contraindication from the approved product professional labeling. FDA-approved patient labeling that focuses on the most serious risks and less serious, but most frequently occurring, adverse reactions is also acceptable. The latter must include:	Major Statement—Advertisements must disclose a product's major risks and most commonly occurring adverse effects in either the audio or audio and visual parts of the presentation
(1) All contraindications	and
(2) All warnings	Adequate Provision—In place of brief summary, advertisements may make "adequate provision" for dissemination of package labeling with four alternative souces of information:
(3) Major precautions, including any that describe serious adverse events	(1) Toll-free telephone number
(4) The 3-5 most common non-serious adverse reactions most likely to affect the patient's quality of life or compliance with drug therapy	(2) Referral to a print advertisement in a concurrently running print publication, or provision of enough brochures, with required product information, in convenient outlets
	(3) Referral to a health care provider
	(4) Internet web page address

*Amended in 2004 draft guidance from the FDA's Division of Drug Marketing, Advertising, and Communications in the Center for Drug Evaluation and Research, available at www.fda.gov/cder/Guidance/5669dft.pdf.

†Based on 1999 final FDA guidelines on consumer-directed broadcast advertisements, available at www.fda.gov/cder/guidance/1804fnl.pdf.
(Courtesy of Gellad ZF, Lyles KW. Direct-to-consumer advertising of pharmaceuticals. *Am J Med.* 2007;120:475-480. Copyright 2007, Association of Professors of Medicine.)

▶ Among industrialized countries, only the United States and New Zealand allow direct-to-consumer advertising of prescription drugs. Such advertising has increased dramatically since 1997, when the FDA released new guidelines regulating broadcast advertisements (Table 1). Although the rationale behind such advertising is to stimulate discussion between patients and providers, it unquestionably increases prescription drug use, much of which may be unnecessary. Although many physicians (myself included) would like to see direct-to-consumer advertising cease, this is highly unlikely and, in fact, pharmaceutical companies can be expected to continue to increase funding of it.

B. H. Thiers, MD

A Decade of Direct-to-Consumer Advertising of Prescription Drugs
Donohue JM, Cevasco M, Rosenthal MB (Univ of Pittsburgh Graduate School of Public Health, Pa; Harvard School of Public Health, Boston; Vanderbilt School of Medicine, Nashville, Tenn)
N Engl J Med 357:673-681, 2007

Background.—Evidence suggests that direct-to-consumer advertising of prescription drugs increases pharmaceutical sales and both helps to avert underuse of medicines and leads to potential overuse. Concern about such advertising has increased recently owing to the withdrawal from the market of heavily advertised drugs found to carry serious risks. Moreover, the Food and Drug Administration (FDA) has been criticized for its weak enforcement of laws regulating such advertising.

Methods.—We examined industry-wide trends in spending by pharmaceutical companies on direct-to-consumer advertising and promotion to physicians during the past decade. We characterized the drugs for which such advertising is used and assessed the timing of advertising after a drug is introduced. Finally, we examined trends in the FDA's regulation of drug advertising.

Results.—Total spending on pharmaceutical promotion grew from $11.4 billion in 1996 to $29.9 billion in 2005. Although during that time spending on direct-to-consumer advertising increased by 330%, it made up only 14% of total promotional expenditures in 2005. Direct-to-consumer campaigns generally begin within a year after the approval of a product by the FDA. In the context of regulatory changes requiring legal review before issuing letters, the number of letters sent by the FDA to pharmaceutical manufacturers regarding violations of drug-advertising regulations fell from 142 in 1997 to only 21 in 2006.

Conclusions.—Spending on direct-to-consumer advertising has continued to increase in recent years in spite of the criticisms leveled against it. Our findings suggest that calls for a moratorium on such advertising for new drugs would represent a dramatic departure from current practices.

▶ Many drugs promoted directly to the consumer are used regularly in dermatologic practice. Although promotion to physicians continues to be the dominant marketing strategy for pharmaceutical companies, spending on direct-to-consumer advertising continues to increase both in absolute terms and as a percentage of pharmaceutical sales. Total promotional expenses as percentage of sales, driven largely by increases in direct-to-consumer advertising, have increased substantially during the past 5 years. Consumers very likely will bear the increased costs of such promotional activity, although some would argue that marketing costs are unlikely to have a direct effect on pharmaceutical prices.[1] Donohue et al show that advertising campaigns generally begin within 1 year after the introduction of a pharmaceutical product, which raises the question of whether such advertising increases the use of drugs with still-unknown safety profiles. Although the Institute of Medicine recommended that the FDA restrict advertising for newer prescription drugs, such a mandatory waiting period appears unlikely.[2] Conversely, the sharp fall in regulatory actions taken by the FDA against companies marketing prescription drugs to consumers suggests that FDA oversight of such advertising is weakening.

B. H. Thiers, MD

References

1. Berndt ER. Pharmaceuticals in U.S. health care: determinants of quantity and price. *J Econ Perspect*. 2002;16:45-66.
2. Smith SW. Sidelining safety—the FDA's inadequate response to the IOM. *N Engl J Med*. 2007;357:960-963.

Factors Associated with Findings of Published Trials of Drug–Drug Comparisons: Why Some Statins Appear More Efficacious than Others
Bero L, Oostvogel F, Bacchetti P, et al (Univ of California, San Francisco; Univ of Leiden, The Netherlands)
PLoS Med 4:e184, 2007

Background.—Published pharmaceutical industry–sponsored trials are more likely than non-industry-sponsored trials to report results and conclusions that favor drug over placebo. Little is known about potential biases in drug–drug comparisons. This study examined associations between research funding source, study design characteristics aimed at reducing bias, and other factors that potentially influence results and conclusions in randomized controlled trials (RCTs) of statin–drug comparisons.

Methods and Findings.—This is a cross-sectional study of 192 published RCTs comparing a statin drug to another statin drug or non-statin drug. Data on concealment of allocation, selection bias, blinding, sample size, disclosed funding source, financial ties of authors, results for primary outcomes, and author conclusions were extracted by two coders (weighted kappa 0.80 to 0.97). Univariate and multivariate logistic regression identified associations between independent variables and favorable results and conclusions. Of the RCTs, 50% (95/192) were funded by industry, and 37% (70/192) did not disclose any funding source. Looking at the totality of available evidence, we found that almost all studies (98%, 189/192) used only surrogate outcome measures. Moreover, study design weaknesses common to published statin–drug comparisons included inadequate blinding, lack of concealment of allocation, poor follow-up, and lack of intention-to-treat analyses. In multivariate analysis of the full sample, trials with adequate blinding were less likely to report results favoring the test drug, and sample size was associated with favorable conclusions when controlling for other factors. In multivariate analysis of industry-funded RCTs, funding from the test drug company was associated with results (odds ratio = 20.16 [95% confidence interval 4.37–92.98], $p < 0.001$) and conclusions (odds ratio = 34.55 [95% confidence interval 7.09–168.4], $p < 0.001$) that favor the test drug when controlling for other factors. Studies with adequate blinding were less likely to report statistically significant results favoring the test drug.

Conclusions.—RCTs of head-to-head comparisons of statins with other drugs are more likely to report results and conclusions favoring the sponsor's product compared to the comparator drug. This bias in drug–drug comparison trials should be considered when making decisions regarding drug choice.

▶ The results, which are hardly surprising, demonstrate that the type of sponsorship used to fund RCTs may strongly influence the results and conclusions of these studies. This can be due to many reasons. For example, drug companies may deliberately choose low doses for the comparison drug when they carry out "head-to-head" trials; this would obviously increase the chance that the sponsor's product would perform in a superior manner. Several years ago when oral terbinafine was tested against what was in my opinion a subtherapeutic dose of griseofulvin in the treatment of tinea capitis,[1] the former drug showed the better result. Guess which drug came out better? Selective publication, in which trials that produce unfavorable results are not submitted for publication, may also mislead the medical community on the effectiveness of a drug or a class of drugs. Whatever the reasons, the findings here are undoubtedly relevant to dermatology, and suggest that so-called evidence-based medicine may not always be based on all the evidence.

B. H. Thiers, MD

Reference

1. Fuller LC, Smith CH, Cerio R, et al. A randomized comparison of 4 weeks of terbinafine vs. 8 weeks of griseofulvin for the treatment of tinea capitis. *Br J Dermatol.* 2001;144:321-327.

Medicine Residents' Understanding of the Biostatistics and Results in the Medical Literature

Windish DM, Huot SJ, Green ML (Yale Univ School of Medicine, New Haven, Conn)
JAMA 298:1010-1022, 2007

Context.—Physicians depend on the medical literature to keep current with clinical information. Little is known about residents' ability to understand statistical methods or how to appropriately interpret research outcomes.

Objective.—To evaluate residents' understanding of biostatistics and interpretation of research results.

Design, Setting, and Participants.—Multiprogram cross-sectional survey of internal medicine residents.

Main Outcome Measure.—Percentage of questions correct on a biostatistics/study design multiple-choice knowledge test.

Results.—The survey was completed by 277 of 367 residents (75.5%) in 11 residency programs. The overall mean percentage correct on statistical knowledge and interpretation of results was 41.4% (95% confidence interval [CI], 39.7%-43.3%) vs 71.5% (95% CI, 57.5%-85.5%) for fellows and general medicine faculty with research training ($P<.001$). Higher scores in residents were associated with additional advanced degrees (50.0% [95% CI, 44.5%-55.5%] vs 40.1% [95% CI, 38.3%-42.0%]; $P<.001$); prior biostatistics training (45.2% [95% CI, 42.7%-47.8%] vs 37.9% [95% CI, 35.4%-40.3%]; $P=.001$); enrollment in a university-based training program (43.0% [95% CI, 41.0%-45.1%] vs 36.3% [95% CI, 32.6%-40.0%]; $P=.002$); and male sex (44.0% [95% CI, 41.4%-46.7%] vs 38.8% [95% CI, 36.4%-41.1%]; $P=.004$). On individual knowledge questions, 81.6% correctly interpreted a relative risk. Residents were less likely to know how to interpret an adjusted odds ratio from a multivariate regression analysis (37.4%) or the results of a Kaplan-Meier analysis (10.5%). Seventy-five percent indicated they did not understand all of the statistics they encountered in journal articles, but 95% felt it was important to understand these concepts to be an intelligent reader of the literature.

Conclusions.—Most residents in this study lacked the knowledge in biostatistics needed to interpret many of the results in published clinical research. Residency programs should include more effective biostatistics training in their curricula to successfully prepare residents for this important lifelong learning skill.

▶ Physicians with busy practices find it difficult to keep up with the onslaught of information that awaits them regularly in the medical journals. This is unfortunate, given the current emphasis on evidence-based medicine. Many of us must resort to shortcuts, including dependence on abstracts, summaries, and updates. These often omit important parts of the original article and leave the reader unable to critically appraise the design and conduct of the study and analyze the data generated. Even when presented with this information, many physicians have little background in epidemiology and biostatistics and a poor understanding of commonly used statistical tests. Statistics are easy to manipulate, and statisticians have many methods to choose from to produce the "desired" result. Some journals will not consider an article for publication unless its authors consent to independent statistical analysis of their work. Recently, a manuscript was withdrawn from *JAMA* after its authors would not agree to this condition; their article was subsequently published elsewhere.

B. H. Thiers, MD

Comparison of treatment effects between animal experiments and clinical trials: systematic review

Perel P, Roberts I, Sena E, et al (London School of Hygiene and Tropical Medicine; Univ of Edinburgh, Scotland; WHO Collaborative Centre in Maternal and Child Health, Rosario, Argentina; et al)

BMJ 334:197, 2007

Objective.—To examine concordance between treatment effects in animal experiments and clinical trials.

Study Design.—Systematic review.

Data Sources.—Medline, Embase, SIGLE, NTIS, Science Citation Index, CAB, BIOSIS.

Study Selection.—Animal studies for interventions with unambiguous evidence of a treatment effect (benefit or harm) in clinical trials: head injury, antifibrinolytics in haemorrhage, thrombolysis in acute ischaemic stroke, tirilazad in acute ischaemic stroke, antenatal corticosteroids to prevent neonatal respiratory distress syndrome, and bisphosphonates to treat osteoporosis.

Review Methods.—Data were extracted on study design, allocation concealment, number of randomised animals, type of model, intervention, and outcome.

Results.—Corticosteroids did not show any benefit in clinical trials of treatment for head injury but did show a benefit in animal models (pooled odds ratio for adverse functional outcome 0.58, 95% confidence interval 0.41 to 0.83). Antifibrinolytics reduced bleeding in clinical trials but the data were inconclusive in animal models. Thrombolysis improved outcome in patients with ischaemic stroke. In animal models, tissue plasminogen activator reduced infarct volume by 24% (95% confidence interval 20% to 28%) and improved neurobehavioural scores by 23% (17% to 29%). Tirilazad was associated with a worse outcome in patients with ischaemic stroke. In animal models, tirilazad reduced infarct volume by 29% (21% to 37%) and improved neurobehavioural scores by 48% (29% to 67%). Antenatal corticosteroids reduced respiratory distress and mortality in neonates whereas in animal models respiratory distress was reduced but the effect on mortality was inconclusive (odds ratio 4.2, 95% confidence interval 0.85 to 20.9). Bisphosphonates increased bone mineral density in patients with osteoporosis. In animal models the bisphosphonate alendronate increased bone mineral density compared with placebo by 11.0% (95% confidence interval 9.2% to 12.9%) in the combined results for the hip region. The corresponding treatment effect in the lumbar spine was 8.5% (5.8% to 11.2%) and in the combined results for the forearms (baboons only) was 1.7% (−1.4% to 4.7%).

Conclusions.—Discordance between animal and human studies may be due to bias or to the failure of animal models to mimic clinical disease adequately.

▶ Differences between species have brought into question the relevance of animal models to human disease. Perel et al found that most studies in animal models suffer from methodological problems. They suggest that the lack of concordance between animal experiments and clinical trials may result from a number of factors including bias, random error, and the failure of animal models to adequately correlate with human disease. These findings are no less applicable to skin disease than to the conditions studied by the authors.

B. H. Thiers, MD

Eligibility Criteria of Randomized Controlled Trials Published in High-Impact General Medical Journals: A Systematic Sampling Review
Van Spall HGC, Toren A, Kiss A, et al (Univ of Toronto; Univ of Ottawa, Ont, Canada)
JAMA 297:1233-1240, 2007

Context.—Selective eligibility criteria of randomized controlled trials (RCTs) are vital to trial feasibility and internal validity. However, the exclusion of certain patient populations may lead to impaired generalizability of results.

Objective.—To determine the nature and extent of exclusion criteria among RCTs published in major medical journals and the contribution of exclusion criteria to the representation of certain patient populations.

Data Sources and Study Selection.—The MEDLINE database was searched for RCTs published between 1994 and 2006 in certain general medical journals with a high impact factor. Of 4827 articles, 283 were selected using a series technique.

Data Extraction.—Trial characteristics and the details regarding exclusions were extracted independently. All exclusion criteria were graded independently and in duplicate as either strongly justified, potentially justified, or poorly justified according to previously developed and pilot-tested guidelines.

Data Synthesis.—Common medical conditions formed the basis for exclusion in 81.3% of trials. Patients were excluded due to age in 72.1% of all trials (60.1% in pediatric populations and 38.5% in older adults). Individuals receiving commonly prescribed medications were excluded in 54.1% of trials. Conditions related to female sex were grounds for exclusion in 39.2% of trials. Of all exclusion criteria, only 47.2% were graded as strongly justified in the context of the specific RCT. Exclusion criteria were not reported in

12.0% of trials. Multivariable analyses revealed independent associations between the total number of exclusion criteria and drug intervention trials (risk ratio, 1.35; 95% confidence interval, 1.11-1.65; $P = .003$) and between the total number of exclusion criteria and multicenter trials (risk ratio, 1.26; 95% confidence interval, 1.06-1.52; $P = .009$). Industry-sponsored trials were more likely to exclude individuals due to concomitant medication use, medical comorbidities, and age. Drug intervention trials were more likely to exclude individuals due to concomitant medication use, medical comorbidities, female sex, and socioeconomic status. Among such trials, justification for exclusions related to concomitant medication use and comorbidities were more likely to be poorly justified.

Conclusions.—The RCTs published in major medical journals do not always clearly report exclusion criteria. Women, children, the elderly, and those with common medical conditions are frequently excluded from RCTs. Trials with multiple centers and those involving drug interventions are most likely to have extensive exclusions. Such exclusions may impair the generalizability of RCT results. These findings highlight a need for careful consideration and transparent reporting and justification of exclusion criteria in clinical trials.

▶ Van Spall et al sought to determine the nature and extent of exclusion criteria among the RCTs published in major medical journals and how these criteria contribute to the underrepresentation of certain patient populations. They found that RCTs published in major medical journals often exclude large segments of the general population and also specific patient populations. The most frequent exclusions were children, the elderly, pregnant women, patients taking common medications, and those with common medical comorbidities. This information is essential to adequately interpret the reported data, which might therefore not be generalizable to the overall patient population. As an example relevant to dermatology, it would be important to know whether studies of systemic treatments for toenail onychomycosis excluded diabetics or patients with peripheral vascular disease, as such individuals are disproportionally affected with fungal nail disease and would be less likely to respond to therapy than those without metabolic or circulatory abnormalities.

B. H. Thiers, MD

Reporting of study design in titles and abstracts of articles published in clinically oriented dermatology journals
Ubriani R, Smith N, Katz KA (Univ of Pennsylvania, Philadelphia; Christiana Hosp, Newark, Del)
Br J Dermatol 156:557-559, 2007

Background.—Dermatologists may have difficulty in identifying the types of study design used in published articles, hindering their ability to appraise the literature critically.

Objectives.—To assess the frequency with which titles or abstracts of articles published in clinically oriented dermatology journals reported the type of study design using standard key words, including 'randomized control trial', 'nonrandomized control trial', 'double-blind', 'placebo control', 'crossover trial', 'before–after trial', 'gold standard', 'blinded or masked comparison', 'cohort', 'inception cohort', 'validation cohort', 'validation sample', 'survey', 'case series', 'cost-effectiveness analysis', 'cost-benefit analysis', 'cost-utility analysis', 'cross-sectional study' and 'case-control'.

Methods.—A cross-sectional study analysed articles published between December 2004 and November 2005 in the 'Epidemiology and Health Services Research' and 'Therapeutics' sections of the *British Journal of Dermatology (BJD)*, in the 'Studies' section of the *Archives of Dermatology (Arch Dermatol)* and in the 'Reports' section of the *Journal of the American Academy of Dermatology (JAAD)*.

Results.—In the *BJD*, 15 of 37 articles (40.5%, 95% confidence interval, CI 24.8–57.9%) included at least one standard key word in the title or abstract, compared with 43 of 87 articles (49.4%, 95% CI 38.5–60.4%) in the *Arch Dermatol* and 19 of 93 articles (20.4%, 95% CI 12.8–30.1%) in the *JAAD* ($P < 0.001$).

Conclusions.—Most articles in the three journals did not report the study design used in the title or abstract. A consistent and clear indication of the design used in studies may better enable editors, reviewers and readers to assess critically articles published in clinically oriented dermatology journals.

▶ The first step in assessing the validity of an article published in a medical journal is to understand the "rules" under which the study was conducted. The authors observed that some journal abstracts fail to report the type of study design used or report a study design using nonstandard terminology. In the current article, Ubriani et al investigated the frequency with which articles published in 3 clinically oriented dermatology journals reported study design using standard terminology, and found that fewer than half included a standard study design key word in the title or abstract. Reporting study design types in a standardized manner would aid in the evaluation of the reported data and move dermatology further along on the road to evidence-based medicine.

B. H. Thiers, MD

Characteristics and completeness of clinical trial registrations in psoriasis and atopic dermatitis
Quain RD, Katz KA (Univ of Pennsylvania, Philadelphia)
Br J Dermatol 156:106-110, 2007

Background.—Controversy over the failure to publish results of clinical trials linking antidepressant treatment to suicidal behaviour in adolescents has increased interest in clinical trial registration.

Objective.—To assess numbers, characteristics and completeness of registrations of trials for psoriasis and atopic dermatitis registered at two web-based trial registries: ClinicalTrials.gov and isrctn.org.

Methods.—In this cross-sectional study we identified trials by searching ClinicalTrials.gov and isrctn.org on 18 January 2006 for trials registered up to 31 December 2005. We included only trials of therapeutic interventions for atopic dermatitis or psoriasis. We ascertained the date of submission of registration, the funding source of the trial, and whether a registration listed the specific name of the intervention studied, the specific outcome measure used (e.g. "Psoriasis Area and Severity Index"), the criterion used to gauge success on the outcome measure (e.g. ≥75% decrease), and the time at which the outcome would be assessed (e.g. at 12 weeks).

Results.—There were 156 registered trials, including 128 (82%) at ClinicalTrials.gov [36 (23%) in atopic dermatitis, 92 (59%) in psoriasis] and 28 (18%) at isrctn.org [23 (15%) in atopic dermatitis, 5 (3%) in psoriasis]. Pharmaceutical companies funded 87 trials (56%), federal or governmental agencies 28 (18%), universities or organizations 21 (13%), and a combination of funders 20 (13%). Of atopic dermatitis trials (13 of 36) and (24 of 92) of psoriasis trials at ClinicalTrials.gov were registered in September 2005. The specific name of the intervention studied was listed in 150 registrations (96%), 89 (57%) listed the specific measure used, 69 (44%) listed the criteria to gauge success and 62 (40%) listed the time of assessment.

Conclusions.—While trial registrations in atopic dermatitis and psoriasis are increasing, more complete information in these registrations may increase their value for dermatologists and their patients.

▶ Selective publication, in which only favorable trial data are published, is a problem in all medical specialties. This can occur at least in part because the public is often unaware of what clinical trials are underway. More recently, an effort to require prospective trial registration has gained momentum. Quain and Katz assessed the completeness of trial registration for 2 diseases of intense research interest in dermatology, psoriasis, and atopic dermatitis. Although the number of registered trials increased dramatically over time, the information contained in many trial registrations was incomplete. More comprehensive disclosure would benefit both physicians and patients.

B. H. Thiers, MD

Single application of a fluorescent test cream by healthy volunteers: assessment of treated and neglected body sites
Ulff E, Maroti M, Kettis-Lindblad Å, et al (Ryhov Hosp, Jönköping, Sweden; Uppsala Univ, Sweden; Göteborg Univ, Sweden; et al)
Br J Dermatol 156:974-978, 2007

Background.—Management of dermatological self-treatment is demanding. Imperfect application of creams and ointments and poor adherence to topical treatment are common, resulting in unsatisfactory treatment outcome.

Objectives.—To assess the technique and precision of test subjects' self-application of a test cream. Treated and neglected skin sites were measured after intended widespread single application of a fluorescent test cream.

Methods.—Twenty healthy volunteers (10 women, 10 men) were included. They were asked to treat their whole skin surface with the fluorescent test cream, except the head and neck and skin covered by underwear. Treated and untreated sites were subsequently measured under Wood's ultraviolet radiation.

Results.—Thirty-one per cent of the skin surface that was a target for application did not show any fluorescence and thus was assumed to have been untreated. Typical neglected sites included the central back, the upper breast, the axilla with surrounding skin, the legs and the feet, particularly the sole. The posterior aspect of both trunk and extremities, not easily inspected, was more often neglected. In the treated sites the fluorescence was typically uneven.

Conclusions.—Qualified and motivated persons with no obvious physical limitations practised imperfect self-application of a test cream mimicking a therapeutic cream product. As much as 31% of the skin surface was neglected. Sites especially prone to nonapplication were identified. This might imply that dermatological patients on long-term self-treatment may practise local application very poorly, a problem of major therapeutic and economic importance. A fluorescent test cream can be used for research, and as an educational tool in the training of dermatological patients on how to apply local treatment.

▶ As disappointing as these findings are, they are by no means surprising and likely even overstate the completeness of home-based topical therapies. This study was conducted under ideal conditions with volunteers who were asked to apply a cream as a single application. Long-term treatment at home, where patients could be easily distracted by other concerns and obligations, is much more problematic. Imperfect application is probably quite common when large surface areas or difficult-to-reach anatomic sites are concerned, and such incomplete application could easily lead to treatment failure. The fluorescent cream used here could be a valuable educational tool for patients requiring topical therapy of their skin diseases.

B. H. Thiers, MD

14 Practice Management and Managed Care

Willing to wait?: The influence of patient wait time on satisfaction with primary care
Anderson RT, Camacho FT, Balkrishnan R (Wake Forest Univ Health Sciences, Winston-Salem, NC; Ohio State Univ, Columbus)
BMC Health Serv Res 7:31, 2007

Background.—This study examined the relationship between patient waiting time and willingness to return for care and patient satisfaction ratings with primary care physicians.

Methods.—Cross-sectional survey data on a convenience sample of 5,030 patients who rated their physicians on a web-based survey developed to collect detailed information on patient experiences with health care. The survey included self-reported information on wait times, time spent with doctor, and patient satisfaction.

Results.—Longer waiting times were associated with lower patient satisfaction ($p < 0.05$), however, time spent with the physician was the strongest predictor of patient satisfaction. The decrement in satisfaction associated with long waiting times is substantially reduced with increased time spent with the physician (5 minutes or more). Importantly, the combination of long waiting time to see the doctor and having a short doctor visit is associated with very low overall patient satisfaction.

Conclusion.—The time spent with the physician is a stronger predictor of patient satisfaction than is the time spent in the waiting room. These results suggest that shortening patient waiting times at the expense of time spent with the patient to improve patient satisfaction scores would be counterproductive.

▶ This is an interesting study with findings that appear to be equally applicable outside the primary care realm. Anderson et al report that what patients really want is time with the doctor. Their data showed that time spent with the physician is the most powerful determinant of overall patient satisfaction, despite long waiting room times. Indeed, the combination of long wait times and short visit times was associated with the lowest levels of patient satisfaction.

Patients give physicians considerable leeway in terms of wait times as long as they get what they consider to be adequate time with their physician.

B. H. Thiers, MD

The Primary Care–Specialty Income Gap: Why It Matters

Bodenheimer T, Berenson RA, Rudolf P (Univ of California, San Francisco; Urban Inst and Arent Fox, PLLC, Washington, DC)

Ann Intern Med 146:301-306, 2007

A large, widening gap exists between the incomes of primary care physicians and those of many specialists. This disparity is important because noncompetitive primary care incomes discourage medical school graduates from choosing primary care careers.

The Resource-Based Relative Value Scale, designed to reduce the inequality between fees for office visits and payment for procedures, failed to prevent the widening primary care–specialty income gap for 4 reasons: 1) The volume of diagnostic and imaging procedures has increased far more rapidly than the volume of office visits, which benefits specialists who perform those procedures; 2) the process of updating fees every 5 years is heavily influenced by the Relative Value Scale Update Committee, which is composed mainly of specialists; 3) Medicare's formula for controlling physician payments penalizes primary care physicians; and 4) private insurers tend to pay for procedures, but not for office visits, at higher levels than those paid by Medicare. Payment reform is essential to guarantee a healthy primary care base to the U.S. health care system.

▶ In an article by Maxwell et al,[1] the investigators examined how the distribution of payments under Medicare's resource-based relative value scale fee schedule changed over the decade since it was introduced in 1992. In fact, the relative values or fees for evaluation and management services increased, whereas those for imaging, major procedures, and other procedures decreased during that period. Nevertheless, despite the large increase in relative fees, in 2002, the share of Medicare spending on physicians for evaluation and management services was exactly the same as it was in 1992 (ie, 49.5%). Although the quantity of evaluation and management services grew by 18% over the following decade, the quantity of imaging services increased by 70%, and the quantity of nonmajor procedures increased by 21%. Moreover, these figures reflect only service codes that existed in 1992. Almost a quarter of the growth in the total quantity of physician services was attributable to the introduction of new codes, few of which were for evaluation and management services, and most of which were for imaging, procedures, or tests. So, why do so many primary care physicians feel short changed? One reason is the formula that Congress adopted in 1998 to limit the growth in spending on physician services per Medicare beneficiary to approximate the rate of growth in the gross domestic product. This limit reduces spending for evaluation and management services to accommodate the increase in spending for imaging services and new codes. Although Congress has ignored the formula in recent years, it has either given increases that were below the inflation rate or simply frozen fees. The net result? Medicare payments to physicians for evaluation and management services have not increased.[2] My prediction for dermatology: sharp cuts in services for procedures such as Mohs surgery. As one of my colleagues suggested to me, we are now in the eye of the "perfect storm," much as ophthalmologists were before the reduction in their fees for cataract surgery.

B. H. Thiers, MD

References

1. Maxwell S, Zuckerman S, Berenson RA. Use of physicians' services under Medicare's resource-based payments. *N Engl J Med.* 2007;356:1853-1861.
2. Newhouse JP. Medicare spending on physicians—no easy fix in sight. *N Engl J Med.* 2007;356:1883-1884.

Use of Physicians' Services under Medicare's Resource-Based Payments
Maxwell S, Zuckerman S, Berenson RA (Urban Inst, Washington, DC)
N Engl J Med 356:1853-1861, 2007

Background.—In 1992, Medicare implemented the resource-based relative-value scale, which established payments for physicians' services based on relative costs. We conducted a study to determine how the use of physicians' services changed during the first decade after the implementation of this scale.

Methods.—With the resource-based relative-value scale, Medicare payments are based on the number of relative-value units (RVUs) assigned to physicians' services. The total number of RVUs reflects the volume of physicians' work (the time, skill, and training required for a physician to provide the service), practice expenses, and professional-liability insurance. Using national data from Medicare on physicians' services and American Medical Association files on RVUs, we analyzed the growth in RVUs per Medicare beneficiary from 1992 to 2002 according to the type of service and specialty. We also examined this growth with respect to the quantity and mix of services, revisions in the valuation of RVUs, and new service codes.

Results.—Between 1992 and 2002, the volume of physicians' work per Medicare beneficiary grew by 50%, and the total RVUs per Medicare beneficiary grew by 45%. The quantity and mix of services were the largest sources of growth, increasing by 19% for RVUs for physicians' work and by 22% for total RVUs. Our findings varied among services and specialties. Revised valuation of RVUs was a key source of the growth in RVUs for physicians' work and total RVUs for evaluation and management and for tests. New service codes were the largest drivers of growth for major procedures (accounting for 36% of the growth in RVUs for physicians' work and 35% of the growth in total RVUs), and the quantity and mix of existing services were the largest drivers of growth for imaging. The growth in RVUs for phy-

TABLE 2.—Distribution and Sources of Growth of RVUs From 1992 to 2002, According to Specialty*

RVU Component and Specialty	Distribution of RVUs		10-Year Change in RVUs per Medicare Beneficiary			
				Due to Quantity and Mix of	Due to Revised Values for Existing	Due to
	1992	2002	Overall	Services	Codes	New Codes
			percent			
Physician's work						
Internal medicine	17.6	15.8	31.7	5.1	20.1	4.3
Cardiology	6.6	9.7	113.6	52.0	21.5	15.6
Ophthalmology	10.2	7.5	7.8	2.9	0.9	3.8
Diagnostic radiology	7.7	7.3	37.9	17.3	6.3	10.6
Family practice	8.4	7.6	32.4	9.4	16.4	3.9
Orthopedic surgery	4.6	4.9	56.7	30.0	9.0	10.5
General surgery	6.5	5.0	11.8	−19.5	23.8	12.2
Dermatology	2.6	2.9	62.0	41.4	−3.2	18.4
Urology	3.9	2.6	−1.0	−12.2	2.5	10.1
Gastroenterology	2.9	3.4	71.8	49.4	7.6	6.9
Physicians' work, practice expenses, and liability insurance						
Internal medicine	16.0	14.6	28.8	3.7	18.7	4.6
Cardiology	7.6	10.8	99.4	87.4	−4.3	11.2
Ophthalmology	12.1	8.6	−0.4	2.3	−7.4	5.2
Diagnostic radiology	8.5	8.1	33.6	26.8	−7.2	13.5
Family practice	7.5	7.5	40.8	8.9	24.1	4.2
Orthopedic surgery	5.4	5.6	44.4	29.0	2.0	9.7
General surgery	6.4	4.4	−3.7	−20.3	7.8	12.1
Dermatology	2.4	3.5	104.8	41.1	21.9	19.1
Urology	3.8	3.0	10.5	−14.1	14.3	12.6
Gastroenterology	3.1	2.9	33.2	52.3	−18.0	6.6

*Data are from physicians' Medicare claims and files on RVUs from 1992 to 2002. There were 33,956,000 Medicare beneficiaries in 1992 and 38,088,000 Medicare beneficiaries in 2002. (Health Care Financing Review statistical supplement. Baltimore: Centers for Medicare and Medicaid Services, 2005:29.)

(Reprinted by permission of Maxwell S, Zuckerman S, Berenson RA. Use of physicians' services under Medicare's resource-based payments. N Engl J Med. 356:1853-1861. Copyright 2007, Massachusetts Medical Society. All rights reserved.)

sicians' work was greatest in cardiology (114%) and gastroenterology (72%). The total growth in RVUs was greatest in cardiology (99%) and dermatology (105%) (Table 2).

Conclusions.—In the first 10 years after the implementation of the resource-based relative-value scale, RVUs per Medicare beneficiary grew substantially. The leading sources of growth varied among service types and specialties. An understanding of these sources of growth can inform policies to control Medicare spending.

▶ Maxwell et al examined how the distribution of payments under Medicare's resource-based relative-value scale fee schedule changed over the decade since it was introduced in 1992. In fact, the relative values or fees for evaluation and management services increased, whereas those for imaging, major procedures, and other procedures decreased during that period. Nevertheless, despite the large increase in relative fees, in 2002, the share of Medicare spending on physicians for evaluation and management services was exactly the same as it was in 1992 (ie, 49.5%). Although the quantity of evaluation and management services grew by 18% over the following decade, the quantity of imaging services increased by 70%, and the quantity of nonmajor procedures increased by 21%. Moreover, these figures reflect only service codes that existed in 1992. Almost a quarter of the growth in the total quantity of physician services was attributable to the introduction of new codes, few of which were for evaluation and management services, and most of which were for imaging, procedures, or tests. In this regard, note the prominent inclusion of dermatology in Table 2. So, why do so many primary care physicians feel short changed? One reason is the formula that Congress adopted in 1998 to limit the growth in spending on physician services per Medicare beneficiary to approximate the rate of growth in the gross domestic product. This limit reduces spending for evaluation and management services to accommodate the increase in spending for imaging services and new codes. Although Congress has ignored the formula in recent years, it has either given increases that were below the inflation rate or simply frozen fees. The net result? Medicare payments to physicians for evaluation and management services have not increased.[1] My prediction for dermatology: sharp cuts in services for procedures such as Mohs surgery. As one of my colleagues suggested to me, we are now in the eye of the "perfect storm," much as ophthalmologists were before the reduction in their fees for cataract surgery.

B. H. Thiers, MD

Reference

1. Newhouse JP. Medicare spending on physicians—no easy fix in sight. *N Engl J Med.* 2007;356:1883-1884.

Public Reporting and Pay for Performance in Hospital Quality Improvement
Lindenauer PK, Remus D, Roman S, et al (Baystate Med Ctr, Springfield, Mass; Tufts Univ, Boston; Premier Healthcare Informatics, Charlotte, NC; et al)
N Engl J Med 356:486-496, 2007

Background.—Public reporting and pay for performance are intended to accelerate improvements in hospital care, yet little is known about the benefits of these methods of providing incentives for improving care.

Methods.—We measured changes in adherence to 10 individual and 4 composite measures of quality over a period of 2 years at 613 hospitals that voluntarily reported information about the quality of care through a national public-reporting initiative, including 207 facilities that simultaneously participated in a pay-for-performance demonstration project funded by the Centers for Medicare and Medicaid Services; we then compared the pay-for-performance hospitals with the 406 hospitals with public reporting only (control hospitals). We used multivariable modeling to estimate the improvement attributable to financial incentives after adjusting for baseline performance and other hospital characteristics.

Results.—As compared with the control group, pay-for-performance hospitals showed greater improvement in all composite measures of quality, including measures of care for heart failure, acute myocardial infarction, and pneumonia and a composite of 10 measures. Baseline performance was inversely associated with improvement; in pay-for-performance hospitals, the improvement in the composite of all 10 measures was 16.1% for hospitals in the lowest quintile of baseline performance and 1.9% for those in the highest quintile (P<0.001). After adjustments were made for differences in baseline performance and other hospital characteristics, pay for performance was associated with improvements ranging from 2.6 to 4.1% over the 2-year period.

Conclusions.—Hospitals engaged in both public reporting and pay for performance achieved modestly greater improvements in quality than did hospitals engaged only in public reporting. Additional research is required to determine whether different incentives would stimulate more improvement and whether the benefits of these programs outweigh their costs.

▶ Many experts in health care delivery regard the fee-for-service system of provider payment an obstacle to achieving effective, coordinated, and efficient patient care. They claim it rewards the overuse of services, the duplication of services, the use of costly specialized services, and the involvement of multiple physicians in the treatment of individual patients. Conversely, it does not reward the prevention of hospitalization or rehospitalization, the effective control of chronic conditions, or the coordination of care. One strategy for moving from payment based solely on the quantity of services to payment based on the quality or efficiency of care is pay for performance, and Medicare is experimenting with different designs for its implementation.[1] A report by Pham et al[2] describes some of the difficulties in implementing a pay-for-performance system under the existing medical care structure in this country, where there exists a dispersion of care across physicians and practices, fragmentation of the health system, and lack of continuity in physician-patient relationships.[3] Pay for performance will be unsuccessful unless it incorporates strategies that address this dispersion.

B. H. Thiers, MD

References

1. Epstein AM. Pay for performance at the tipping point. N Engl J Med. 2007; 356:515-517.
2. Pham HH, Schrag D, O'Malley AS, Wu B, Bach PB. Care patterns in Medicare and their implications for pay for performance. N Engl J Med. 2007;356:1130-1139.
3. Davis K. Paying for care episodes and care coordination. N Engl J Med. 2007; 356:1166-1168.

Care Patterns in Medicare and Their Implications for Pay for Performance
Pham HH, Schrag D, O'Malley AS, et al (Ctr for Studying Health System Change, Washington, DC; Mem Sloan-Kettering Cancer Ctr, New York; Social and Scientific Systems, Silver Spring, Md)
N Engl J Med 356:1130-1139, 2007

Background.—Two assumptions underpin the implementation of pay for performance in Medicare: that with the use of claims data, patients can be assigned to a physician or to a practice that will have primary responsibility for their care, and that a meaningful fraction of the care physicians deliver is for patients for whom they have primary responsibility.

Methods.—We analyzed Medicare claims from 2000 through 2002 for 1.79 million fee-for-service beneficiaries treated by 8604 respondents to the Community Tracking Study Physician Survey in 2000 and 2001. In separate analyses, we assigned each patient to the physician or primary care physician with whom the patient had had the most visits. We determined the number of physicians and practices seen annually, the percentage of care received from the assigned physician or practice, the stability of assignments over time, and the percentage of physicians' Medicare patients who were their assigned patients.

Results.—Beneficiaries saw a median of two primary care physicians and five specialists working in four different practices. A median of 35% of beneficiaries' visits each year were with their assigned physicians; for 33% of beneficiaries, the assigned physician changed from one year to another. On the basis of all visits to any physician, a primary care physician's assigned patients accounted for a median of 39% of the physician's Medicare patients and 62% of Medicare visits. For medical specialists, the respective percentages were 6% and 10%. On the basis of visits to primary care physicians only, 79% of beneficiaries could be assigned to a physician, and a median of 31% of beneficiaries' visits were with that assigned primary care physician.

Conclusions.—In fee-for-service Medicare, the dispersion of patients' care among multiple physicians will limit the effectiveness of pay-for-performance initiatives that rely on a single retrospective method of assigning responsibility for patient care.

▶ Many experts in health care delivery regard the fee-for-service system of provider payment an obstacle to achieving effective, coordinated, and efficient patient care. They claim it rewards the overuse of services, the duplication of services, the use of costly specialized services, and the involvement of multiple physicians in the treatment of individual patients. Conversely, it does not reward the prevention of hospitalization or rehospitalization, the effective control of chronic conditions, or the coordination of care. One strategy for moving from payment based solely on the quantity of services to payment based on the quality or efficiency of care is pay for performance, and Medicare is experimenting with different designs for its implementation.[1] The report by Pham et al describes some of the difficulties in implementing a pay-for-performance system under the existing medical care structure in this country, where there exists a dispersion of care across physicians and practices, fragmentation of the health system, and lack of continuity in physician-patient relationships.[2] Pay for performance will be unsuccessful unless it incorporates strategies that address this dispersion.

B. H. Thiers, MD

References

1. Epstein AM. Pay-for-performance at the tipping point. N Engl J Med. 2007; 356:515-517.
2. Davis K. Paying for care episodes and care coordination. N Engl J Med. 2007; 356:1166-1168, 2007.

The Response of Physician Groups to P4P Incentives
Mehrotra A, Pearson SD, Coltin KL, et al (Univ of Pittsburgh Med School, Pa; Harvard Med School; Harvard Pilgrim Health Care, Boston; et al)
Am J Managed Care 13:249-255, 2007

Objectives.—Despite substantial enthusiasm among insurers and federal policy makers for pay-for-performance incentives, little is known about the current scope of these incentives or their influence on the delivery of care. To assess the scope and magnitude of pay-for-performance (P4P) incentives among physician groups and to examine whether such incentives are associated with quality improvement initiatives.

Study Design.—Structured telephone survey of leaders of physician groups delivering primary care in Massachusetts.

Assessed Methods.—Prevalence of P4P incentives among physician groups tied to specific measures of quality or utilization and prevalence of physician group quality improvement initiatives.

Results.—Most group leaders (89%) reported P4P incentives in at least 1 commercial health plan contract. Incentives were tied to performance on Health Employer Data and Information Set (HEDIS) quality measures (89% of all groups), utilization measures (66%), use of information technology (52%), and patient satisfaction (37%). Among the groups with P4P and knowledge of all revenue streams, the incentives accounted for 2.2% (range, 0.3%-8.8%) of revenue. P4P incentives tied to HEDIS quality measures were positively associated with groups' quality improvement initiatives (odds ratio, 1.6; $P = .02$). Thirty-six percent of group leaders with P4P incentives reported that they were very important or moderately important to the group's financial success.

Conclusions.—P4P incentives are now common among physician groups in Massachusetts, and these incentives most commonly reward higher clinical quality or lower utilization of care. Although the scope and magnitude of incentives are still modest for many groups, we found an association between P4P incentives and the use of quality improvement initiatives.

▶ "Pay for performance" has only recently become part of the American medical lexicon; however, it has been a reality for family practitioners in the United Kingdom since 2004. Performance measures involve measuring and monitoring the quality of care using standardized indicators. Recognition of substandard and uneven quality of care has led to calls for physicians to be more publicly accountable and for health care systems to change. Whether the "cure" will be worse than the disease remains to be seen.

B. H. Thiers, MD

Physician-level P4P—DOA? Can Quality-based Payment Be Resuscitated?
McMahon LF Jr, Hofer TP, Hayward RA (Univ of Michigan, Ann Arbor; Ann Arbor Veterans Affairs Health Research & Development Service, Mich)
Am J Managed Care 13:233-236, 2007

Unlike many areas of the economy where value is relatively easy to measure and reward, healthcare is "messy." Patients bring both clinical heterogeneity and illness-severity complexities to the interchange with their physician. The measurable outcomes or process measures are as likely to be due to patient characteristics as they are to be due to the actions (or inactions) of the patient's provider. Moreover, data suggest that the simplest fix for providers with bad metrics is to "dump" their sickest patients. Perhaps the most pernicious consequence of physician-level pay-for-performance (P4P) systems is how these systems can affect the neediest patients and their providers. As patient characteristics (eg, illness severity, preferences, resources) are more likely to be an issue in our poorer and minority communities, these patients' physicians will be at a financial disadvantage in a P4P system. It is likely that the widespread adoption of P4P systems will further limit these necessary resources.

▶ "Pay for performance" has only recently become part of the American medical lexicon; however, it has been a reality for family practitioners in the United Kingdom since 2004. Performance measures involve measuring and monitoring the quality of care using standardized indicators. Recognition of substandard and uneven quality of care has led to calls for physicians to be more publicly accountable and for health care systems to change. Whether the "cure" will be worse than the disease remains to be seen.

B. H. Thiers, MD

Impact of financial incentives on clinical autonomy and internal motivation in primary care: ethnographic study

McDonald R, Harrison S, Checkland K, et al (Univ of Manchester, England)
BMJ 334:1357, 2007

Objective.—To explore the impact of financial incentives for quality of care on practice organisation, clinical autonomy, and internal motivation of doctors and nurses working in primary care.

Design.—Ethnographic case study.

Setting.—Two English general practices.

Participants.—12 general practitioners, nine nurses, four healthcare assistants, and four administrative staff.

Main Outcome Measure.—Observation of practices over a five month period after the introduction of financial incentives for quality of care introduced in the 2004 general practitioner contract.

Results.—After the introduction of the quality and outcomes framework there was an increase in the use of templates to collect data on quality of care. New regimens of surveillance were adopted, with clinicians seen as "chasers" or the "chased," depending on their individual responsibility for delivering quality targets. Attitudes towards the contract were largely positive, although discontent was higher in the practice with a more intensive surveillance regimen. Nurses expressed more concern than doctors about changes to their clinical practice but also appreciated being given responsibility for delivering on targets in particular disease areas. Most doctors did not question the quality targets that existed at the time or the implications of the targets for their own clinical autonomy.

Conclusions.—Implementation of financial incentives for quality of care did not seem to have damaged the internal motivation of the general practitioners studied, although more concern was expressed by nurses.

▶ The British experience is critiqued and detailed in this article by McDonald et al and also in reports published in other journals.[1,2] McDonald et al describe a way 2 general practices changed to achieve high performance scores under the quality and outcomes framework. Similar measurement and reporting efforts have been adopted by the US Veterans Health Administration. Unfortunately, practices that serve socioeconomically disadvantaged patients tend to show poorer performance using many standard quality indicators than do practices serving more advantaged patients. Thus, when pay is linked to performance under these circumstances, providers who care for those most in need have been inadvertently penalized, creating adverse incentives to exclude such patients. In the United Kingdom, the government appears to have overpaid for gains in health improvement and performance, a situation that is not likely to persist. Overall, pay for performance is a work in progress and, in the end, may turn out to be much ado about nothing.

B. H. Thiers, MD

References

1. Bierman AS, Clark JT. Performance measure and equity. *BMJ*. 2007;334:1333-1334.
2. Campbell S, Reeves D, Kontopantelis E. Quality of primary care in England with the introduction of pay for performance. *N Engl J Med*. 2007;357:181-190.

15 Miscellaneous Topics in Clinical Dermatology

Gadolinium deposition in nephrogenic fibrosing dermopathy
Boyd AS, Zic JA, Abraham JL (Vanderbilt Univ, Nashville, Tenn; SUNY Upstate Med Univ, Syracuse, NY)
J Am Acad Dermatol 56:27-30, 2007

Background.—There is increasing recognition of an association between the use of gadolinium-containing radiocontrast agents for MRI and nephrogenic fibrosing dermopathy/nephrogenic systemic fibrosis (NFD/NSF), a serious dermal and systemic disease. However, in previous studies of this association, none of the patients demonstrated a monoclonal gammopathy. This case presented the first report of the presence of gadolinium (Gd) in cutaneous biopsies from patients with NFD.

Case Report.—Woman, 68, white was seen at a university-affiliated dermatology clinic in June 2006 with a 3-week history of thickened skin on her extremities, which began as painful soft-tissue swelling and rapidly became indurated. The patient's past history was significant for chronic hepatitis C infection–induced hepatic failure for which she received a liver transplant in 1995. Cyclosporine therapy–induced renal failure necessitated hemodialysis in January 2006. Three weeks later, the patient underwent an in-patient MRI heart scan using Gd-containing contrast material. Throughout this hospitalization the patient was consistently hypocalcemic, hyperphosphatemic, and acidotic. Medications included cyclosporine, metoprolol, coumadin, and amiodarone. The patient was not exposed to additional radiocontrast materials. Physical examination showed woody induration without appreciable color changes on her bilateral arms and forearms, calves, and shins. A punch biopsy from the left posterior arm demonstrated diffuse dermal fibroplasia with spindle cells extending into the subcutaneous tissues, mild interstitial mucin deposition, and minimal inflammation. These features were consistent with NFD. Scanning electron microscopy and energy dispersive x-ray spectroscopy (SEM/EDS) demonstrated Gd detected only in areas of calcium phosphate deposition in blood vessels. The patient is undergoing extracorporeal photophoresis and has experienced modest improvement.

Conclusions.—Cutaneous Gd deposition may serve as a nidus for the development of NFD. Gd deposition at sites other than those associated with discernible calcium phosphate deposition cannot be excluded because only retained, insoluble Gd is detectable in tissue samples with SEM/EDS methodology. It is unclear whether the presence of elevated circulating and/or tissue calcium and phosphate induce release of the toxic-free Gd from the contrast agent.

▶ Since Cowper et al reported in 2000 a series of 14 hemodialysis patients with scleromyxedema-like skin changes, many similar patients have been reported and investigators have moved rapidly to determine the underlying cause of this condition. As time has passed the name of the condition has evolved from nephrogenic fibrosing dermopathy to nephrogenic systemic fibrosis (NSF) to reflect the systemic nature of the manifestations. In 2006 an Austrian group reported an association between NSF and exposure to gadolinium-based contrast agents used in MRI. They observed that the disease appeared to selectively affect patients with renal disease who are acidotic at the time of imaging, although other investigators have reported patients with NSF who were not acidotic at the time of exposure. In this article by Boyd et al and an article by High et al,[1] the investigators provide evidence for tissue deposition of gadolinium in NSF-affected patients.

B. H. Thiers, MD

Reference

1. High WA, Ayers RA, Chandler J, Zito G, Cowper SE. Gadolinium is detectable within the tissue of patients with nephrogenic systemic fibrosis. *J Am Acad Dermatol.* 2007;56:24-26.

Gadolinium is detectable within the tissue of patients with nephrogenic systemic fibrosis
High WA, Ayers RA, Chandler J, et al (Univ of Colorado, Denver; Colorado School of Mines, Golden; Yale Univ, New Haven, Conn)
J Am Acad Dermatol 56:24-26, 2007

Background.—Nephrogenic systemic fibrosis (NSF) is a disease of unknown etiology that affects a subset of patients with renal insufficiency. Recent publications suggested an association between exposure to gadolinium-containing contrast agents and subsequent development of NSF. We sought to detect gadolinium within the skin and soft tissue of patients with NSF who were exposed to gadolinium-based contrast.

Methods.—Paraffin-embedded skin and soft tissue from NSF patients exposed to gadolinium, and from negative controls, was provided by the NSF Registry (New Haven, Conn). The tissue was searched for metals using a field emission scanning electron microscope that was equipped with energy dispersive spectroscopy. The presence of gadolinium and other metals was verified through identification of unique and requisite X-ray emission spectra.

Results.—Gadolinium was detected in 4 of 13 tissue specimens from 7 patients with documented NSF who were exposed to gadolinium-based radiographic contrast. No gadolinium was detected in a paraffin-embedded specimen from a negative control. Based upon the known exposure history of patients with detectable gadolinium, a tissue residence time of 4 to 11 months was observed.

Limitations.—As this was a pilot investigation, only a single control specimen and a single histological section from each block of tissue were utilized.

Conclusion.—In this pilot investigation, gadolinium was detected in the tissue of a number of patients with NSF. Although neither dispositive of a pathophysiologic mechanism, nor proof of causation, the detection of gadolinium within tissue of NSF patients is supportive of an epidemiologic association between exposure to gadolinium-containing contrast material and development of disease.

▶ Since Cowper et al reported in 2000 a series of 14 hemodialysis patients with scleromyxedema-like skin changes, many similar patients have been reported and investigators have moved rapidly to determine the underlying cause of this condition. As time has passed the name of the condition has evolved from nephrogenic fibrosing dermopathy to nephrogenic systemic fibrosis (NSF) to reflect the systemic nature of the manifestations. In 2006 an Austrian group reported an association between NSF and exposure to gadolinium-based contrast agents used in MRI. They observed that the disease appeared to selectively affect patients with renal disease who are acidotic at the time of imaging, although other investigators have reported patients with NSF who were not acidotic at the time of exposure. In this article by High et al and an article by Boyd et al,[1] the investigators provide evidence for tissue deposition of gadolinium in NSF-affected patients.

B. H. Thiers, MD

Reference

1. Boyd AS, Zic JA, Abraham JL. Gadolinium deposition in nephrogenic fibrosing dermopathy. *J Am Acad Dermatol.* 2007;56:27-30.

Gadodiamide-Associated Nephrogenic Systemic Fibrosis: Why Radiologists Should Be Concerned

Broome DR, Girguis MS, Baron PW, et al (Loma Linda Univ, Calif)
Am J Roentgenol 188:586-592, 2007

Objective.—Nephrogenic systemic fibrosis (NSF) is a rare multisystemic fibrosing disorder that principally affects the skin but may affect other organs of patients with renal insufficiency. The purpose of our study was to identify any common risk factors and determine whether IV gadodiamide is associated with the development of NSF.

Materials and Methods.—A retrospective chart review was performed for all 12 patients diagnosed with NSF at our institution between 2000 and 2006 to identify the clinical manifestations, timing, and dose of gadodiamide administration; dialysis records; concurrent medications; comorbid conditions and surgeries; laboratory findings; imaging findings; and clinical outcome. A review of the dialysis and MR records between 2000 and 2006 showed 559 MRI examinations on 168 dialysis patients (including 301 contrast-enhanced examinations).

Results.—NSF was diagnosed by clinical findings and tissue diagnosis. All 12 patients had renal insufficiency—eight with dialysis-dependent chronic renal insufficiency and four with acute hepatorenal syndrome. All 12 patients developed skin fibrosis within 2–11 weeks after gadodiamide administration. The odds ratio for development of NSF after gadodiamide exposure was 22.3. No other common event or exposure could be found. Four patients had abnormal scintigraphic bone scans with skin and muscle uptake and lower-extremity MRI finding of edema in the muscles, intermuscular fascia, and skin. Despite the fact that 10 patients were dialyzed within 2 days of gadodiamide administration, this did not prevent the development of NSF.

Conclusion.—Development of NSF was strongly associated with gadodiamide administration in the setting of either acute hepatorenal syndrome or dialysis-dependent chronic renal insufficiency.

▶ Broome et al reviewed the association of NSF with gadolinium exposure. All investigators, including Boyd et al[1] and High et al,[2] appear to agree that gadolinium-containing contrast material should be used with great caution in patients with advanced renal disease, particularly those who are acidotic.

B. H. Thiers, MD

References

1. Boyd AS, Zic JA, Abraham JL. Gadolinium deposition in nephrogenic fibrosing dermopathy. *J Am Acad Dermatol.* 2007;56:27-30.
2. High WA, Ayers RA, Chandler J, Zito G, Cowper SE. Gadolinium is detectable within the tissue of patients with nephrogenic systemic fibrosis. *J Am Acad Dermatol.* 2007;56:24-26.

Gadolinium-enhanced MR Imaging and Nephrogenic Systemic Fibrosis: Retrospective Study of a Renal Replacement Therapy Cohort
Collidge TA, Thomson PC, Mark PB, et al (Glasgow Royal Infirmary, Scotland; Western Infirmary, Glasgow, Scotland)
Radiology 245:168-175, 2007

Purpose.—To retrospectively compare the frequency of administration and cumulative dose of gadolinium-based contrast agent in dialysis-dependent patients who did and those who did not develop nephrogenic systemic fibrosis.

Materials and Methods.—The ethics committees granted exempt status for this study and also waived the need for informed consent. A retrospective analysis was performed of all adult patients undergoing dialysis in the west of Scotland between January 1, 2000, and July 1, 2006. Diagnoses of nephrogenic systemic fibrosis, episodes of gadolinium-enhanced magnetic resonance (MR) imaging, and cumulative doses of gadolinium-based contrast agent were recorded. Outcomes were analyzed by means of parametric and nonparametric testing.

Results.—Fourteen of 1826 patients had a diagnosis of nephrogenic systemic fibrosis. Mortality was similar for affected and nonaffected patients. Thirteen (93%) of 14 patients with nephrogenic systemic fibrosis had undergone gadolinium-enhanced MR imaging compared with 408 (22.5%) of 1812 nonaffected patients ($P<.001$). Patients with nephrogenic systemic fibrosis received a higher median cumulative dose of gadodiamide (0.39 vs 0.23 mmol per kilogram of body weight, $P=.008$) and underwent more gadolinium-enhanced MR imaging than their nonaffected gadolinium-exposed counterparts.

Conclusion.—The data support a positive association between gadolinium-based contrast agent administration and development of nephrogenic systemic fibrosis in the established renal failure population; in addition, there is a positive association between cumulative dose of gadodiamide used and dosing events.

▶ The association between gadolinium-enhanced MR imaging and the development of nephrogenic systemic fibrosis (NSF) in patients with renal failure is well established. The challenge now is to identify the risk factors for NSF in this subset of patients.

Collidge et al found a possible association between the total cumulative dose of gadodiamide and the development of NSF and recommended that the dose of gadolinium-based contrast material be minimized when contrast-enhanced MR imaging is necessary. When gadolinium-enhanced MR imaging must be performed in a hemodialysis patient, the patient should be dialyzed immediately after the conclusion of the study.

In an article by Todd et al,[1] the investigators present data to suggest that in patients receiving hemodialysis, NSF may, in fact, be more common than previously recognized. Unfortunately, no successful treatment exists for the condition, although I have seen 2 patients who have had a remarkable remission when their renal function was restored by renal transplantation.

B. H. Thiers, MD

Reference

1. Todd DJ, Kagan A, Chibnik LB, Kay J. Cutaneous changes of nephrogenic systemic fibrosis: predictor of early mortality and association with gadolinium exposure. *Arthritis Rheum.* 2007;56:3433-3441.

Cutaneous Changes of Nephrogenic Systemic Fibrosis: Predictor of Early Mortality and Association With Gadolinium Exposure
Todd DJ, Kagan A, Chibnik LB, et al (Harvard Med School)
Arthritis Rheum 56:3433-3441, 2007

Objective.—Nephrogenic systemic fibrosis (NSF) is a rapidly progressive, debilitating condition that causes cutaneous and visceral fibrosis in patients with renal failure. Little is known about its prevalence or etiology. The aim of this study was to establish the prevalence of NSF and associated risk factors.

Methods.—Two cohorts of patients were recruited from 6 outpatient hemodialysis centers and examined for cutaneous changes of NSF, which were defined using a scoring system based on hyperpigmentation, hardening, and tethering of skin on the extremities. Demographic data were gathered, mortality was followed up prospectively for 24 months, and gadolinium exposure was ascertained for a subgroup of patients in the second cohort.

Results.—Examination reproducibility was 97% in cohort 1. In cohort 2, 25 (13%) of 186 patients demonstrated cutaneous changes of NSF. Twenty-four–month mortality following examination was 48% and 20% in patients with and those without cutaneous changes of NSF, respectively (adjusted hazard ratio 2.9, 95% confidence interval [95% CI] 1.4–5.9). Cutaneous changes of NSF were observed in 16 (30%) of 54 patients with prior exposure to gadopentetate dimeglumine contrast during imaging studies. Exposure to gadolinium-containing contrast was associated with an increased risk of developing cutaneous changes of NSF (odds ratio 14.7, 95% CI 1.9–117.0) compared with nonexposed patients.

Conclusion.—In patients receiving hemodialysis, NSF is an underrecognized disorder that is associated with increased mortality. Exposure to gadolinium-containing contrast material appears to be a significant risk factor for the development of NSF.

▶ The association between gadolinium-enhanced MR imaging and the development of nephrogenic systemic fibrosis (NSF) in patients with renal failure is well established. The challenge now is to identify the risk factors for NSF in this subset of patients.

In an article by Collidge et al,[1] the investigators found a possible association between the total cumulative dose of gadodiamide and the development of

NSF, and recommended that the dose of gadolinium-based contrast material be minimized when contrast-enhanced MR imaging is necessary. When gadolinium-enhanced MR imaging must be performed in a hemodialysis patient, the patient should be dialyzed immediately after the conclusion of the study. In this report, Todd et al present data to suggest that in patients receiving hemodialysis, NSF may, in fact, be more common than previously recognized. Unfortunately, no successful treatment exists for the condition, although I have seen 2 patients who have had a remarkable remission when their renal function was restored by renal transplantation.

B. H. Thiers, MD

Reference

1. Collidge TA, Thomson PC, Mark PB, et al. Gadolinium-enhanced MR imaging and nephrogenic systemic fibrosis: retrospective study of a renal replacement therapy cohort. *Radiology.* 2007;245:168-175.

Clinicopathologic Correlation of Cutaneous Metastases: Experience From a Cancer Center

Sariya D, Ruth K, Adams-McDonnell R, et al (Fox Chase Cancer Ctr, Philadelphia; Hosp of the Univ of Pennsylvania, Philadelphia; Baldassano Dermatology PC, Blue Bell, Pa)
Arch Dermatol 143:613-620, 2007

Objective.—To analyze the clinical, histopathologic, and immunohistochemical characteristics of skin metastases.

Design.—Retrospective analysis (January 1, 1990, to December 31, 2005).

Setting.—Comprehensive cancer center.

Patients.—Fifty-one patients (21 men and 30 women) with biopsy-proven skin metastases and correlative clinical data.

Interventions.—Four dermatopathologists reviewed a random mixture of metastases and primary skin tumors. Immunohistochemical studies for 12 markers were performed on the metastases, with skin adnexal tumors as controls.

Main Outcome Measures.—Clinical characteristics of cutaneous lesions, clinical outcomes, histologic features, and immunohistochemical markers.

Results.—Eighty-six percent (43 of 50) of the patients had known stage IV cancer, and skin metastasis was the presenting sign in 12% (6 of 50). In 45% (21 of 47) of the biopsies, the lesions were not suspected of being metastases owing to unusual clinical presentations. Seventy-six percent of the patients died of disease (median survival, 5 months). On pathologic review, many metastases from adenocarcinomas were either recognized or suspected, but the primary site was not easily identified based on histologic findings alone. Metastases from small cell carcinomas and sarcomas were histologically misinterpreted as primary skin tumors. Immunohistochemical analysis using a panel including p63, B72.3, calretinin, and CK5/6 differentiated metastatic carcinoma from primary skin adnexal tumors.

Conclusions.—Cutaneous metastases can have variable clinical appearances and can mimic benign skin lesions. They are usually seen in patients with advanced disease, but they can be the presenting lesion. Although many metastatic adenocarcinomas can be recognized based on histologic findings alone, immunohistochemical analysis is an important diagnostic adjunct in some cases.

▶ Sariya and colleagues present a detailed study of 51 patients with biopsy-proven cutaneous metastases. Metastatic lesions must be differentiated clinically and histologically from primary cutaneous tumors that may have a similar clinical appearance. Clinicopathologic correlation is essential, and immunohistochemical studies are often necessary.

B. H. Thiers, MD

Risk of cancer after blood transfusion from donors with subclinical cancer: a retrospective cohort study

Edgren G, Hjalgrim H, Reilly M, et al (Karolinska Institutet, Stockholm; Statens Serum Institut, Copenhagen; Odense Univ, Denmark; et al)
Lancet 369:1724-1730, 2007

Background.—Although mechanisms for detection of short-term complications after blood transfusions are well developed, complications with delayed onset, notably transmission of chronic diseases such as cancer, have been difficult to assess. Our aim was to investigate the possible risk of cancer transmission from blood donors to recipients through blood transfusion.

Methods.—We did a register-based retrospective cohort study of cancer incidence among patients who received blood from donors deemed to have a subclinical cancer at the time of donation. These precancerous donors were diagnosed with a cancer within 5 years of the donation. Data from all computerised blood bank registers in Sweden and Denmark gathered between 1968 and 2002 were merged into a common database. Demographic and medical data, including mortality and cancer incidence, were ascertained through linkages with nationwide, and essentially complete, population and health-care registers. The risk of cancer in exposed recipients relative to that in recipients who received blood from non-cancerous donors was estimated with multivariate Poisson regression, adjusting for potential confounding factors.

Findings.—Of the 354,094 transfusion recipients eligible for this analysis, 12,012 (3%) were exposed to blood products from precancerous donors. There was no excess risk of cancer overall (adjusted relative risk 1.00, 95% CI 0.94–1.07) or in crude anatomical subsites among recipients of blood from precancerous donors compared with recipients of blood from non-cancerous donors.

Interpretation.—Our data provide no evidence that blood transfusions from precancerous blood donors are associated with increased risk of cancer among recipients compared with transfusions from non-cancerous donors.

▶ With the knowledge that certain cancers may be associated with infectious agents, for example, oncogenic viruses, such as the Kaposi's sarcoma (KS)-associated herpesvirus, possible transmission via blood transfusion has been a cause for concern. Indeed, transmission of both solid and nonsolid malignancies as well as oncogenic viruses such as KS-associated herpesvirus and Epstein-Barr virus (EBV) from organ donors to transplant recipients has been reported repeatedly, and transmission of KS-associated herpesvirus via blood transfusions has also been documented.[1] Edgren et al performed an epidemiologic investigation that was based on details in transfusion histories and health outcomes to investigate the possible risk of cancer transmission from blood donors to recipients. They could find no evidence of an increased risk of cancer among recipients of transfusions from precancerous blood donors compared with the risk of transfusion from noncancerous donors. This is an important step forward in evaluating concerns regarding potential long-term risks from blood transfusions.[2]

B. H. Thiers, MD

References

1. Hladik W, Dollard SC, Mermin J, et al. Transmission of human herpesvirus 8 by blood transfusion. *N Engl J Med*. 2006;355:1331-1338.
2. Utter GH. The risk of transmitting cancer with transfusion. *Lancet*. 2007;369: 1670-1671.

Subcutaneous fat necrosis of the newborn: a systematic evaluation of risk factors, clinical manifestations, complications and outcome of 16 children

Mahé E, Girszyn N, Hadj-Rabia S, et al (Assistance Publique-Hôpitaux de Paris)
Br J Dermatol 156:709-715, 2007

Background.—Subcutaneous fat necrosis (SFN) of the newborn is a rare acute transient hypodermatitis that develops within the first weeks of life in term infants. It often follows a difficult delivery. Prognosis is generally good except for the development of hypercalcaemia in severe cases. Only several case reports or small patients series have been published.

Objectives.—To evaluate risk factors, complications and outcomes of SFN in 16 consecutive patients seen from 1996 to 2002 in our Department of Paediatric Dermatology.

Methods.—On a case-report form created for the study, we recorded putative risk factors concerning the mother, pregnancy and delivery, clinical aspects of SFN, and early and late outcomes. The study was conducted in two stages: the first was a retrospective analysis of the observations and the second analysed data collected on children and their parents during a new consultation ($n = 10$).

Results.—All the children were born at term. Lesions appeared a mean of 4 days after delivery. Three-quarters of the children had diffuse SFN. Risk factors identified were newborn failure to thrive (12/16), forceps delivery (7/16), maternal high blood pressure (3/10) and/or diabetes (2/10), and newborn cardiac surgery (1/16). Putative novel risk factors were macrosomia (7/16), exposure to active (4/10) or passive (3/10) smoking during pregnancy, putative or known maternal, paternal or newborn risk factors for thrombosis (5/10), and dyslipidaemia (2/10). Complications were hypercalcaemia (9/16), pain (4/16), dyslipidaemia (1/16), renal insufficiency (1/16) and late subcutaneous atrophy (6/6).

Conclusions.—This study on 16 newborns with SFN provides new information. Familial or newborn risk factors for thrombosis are frequent. Macrosomia, familial dyslipidaemia and smoking should be evaluated. The main complications identified were severe pain, hypercalcaemia and subcutaneous atrophy.

▶ In this case series of 16 patients with subcutaneous fat necrosis (SFN), hypercalcemia appeared to be the most significant complication, affecting 9 of 13 children tested. However, in only 3 children was the calcium level high enough to require treatment. As noted in a previous case series reported by Burden and Krafchik,[1] infants with hypercalcemia tend to have extensive skin involvement. High blood calcium levels were detected up to 86 days after the diagnosis of SFN; therefore, monitoring of blood calcium levels is recommended for 2 to 3 months in infants with severe disease. The authors also observed subcutaneous atrophy in all 6 children examined between 9 months and 6 years of age. Long-term follow-up is generally not reported in children with subcutaneous fat necrosis, and this high incidence of residual atrophy previously has been unrecognized.

S. Raimer, MD

Reference

1. Burden AD, Krafchik BR. Subcutaneous fat necrosis of the newborn: a review of 11 cases. *Pediatr Dermatol.* 1999;16:384-387.

Treatment of Periodontitis and Endothelial Function
Tonetti MS, D'Aiuto F, Nibali L, et al (Univ of Connecticut, Farmington; Univ College London)
N Engl J Med 356:911-920, 2007

Background.—Systemic inflammation may impair vascular function, and epidemiologic data suggest a possible link between periodontitis and cardiovascular disease.

Methods.—We randomly assigned 120 patients with severe periodontitis to community-based periodontal care (59 patients) or intensive periodontal treatment (61). Endothelial function, as assessed by measurement of the diameter of the brachial artery during flow (flow-mediated dilatation), and inflammatory biomarkers and markers of coagulation and endothelial activation were evaluated before treatment and 1, 7, 30, 60, and 180 days after treatment.

Results.—Twenty-four hours after treatment, flow-mediated dilatation was significantly lower in the intensive-treatment group than in the control-treatment group (absolute difference, 1.4%; 95% confidence interval [CI], 0.5 to 2.3; P=0.002), and levels of C-reactive protein, interleukin-6, and the endothelial-activation markers soluble E-selectin and von Willebrand factor were significantly higher (P<0.05 for all comparisons). However, flow-mediated dilatation was greater and the plasma levels of soluble E-selectin were lower in the intensive-treatment group than in the control-treatment group 60 days after therapy (absolute difference in flow-mediated dilatation, 0.9%; 95% CI, 0.1 to 1.7; P=0.02) and 180 days after therapy (difference, 2.0%; 95% CI, 1.2 to 2.8; P<0.001). The degree of improvement was associated with improvement in measures of periodontal disease (r=0.29 by Spearman rank correlation, P=0.003). There were no serious adverse effects in either of the two groups, and no cardiovascular events occurred.

Conclusions.—Intensive periodontal treatment resulted in acute, short-term systemic inflammation and endothelial dysfunction. However, 6 months after therapy, the benefits in oral health were associated with improvement in endothelial function.

▶ A link between periodontitis and vascular disease has been suggested by clinical and epidemiologic studies, but these studies may be confounded by factors such as social status, smoking, and other classic risk factors for atherosclerosis. Tonetti et al addressed the possibility that low-grade chronic systemic inflammation may be linked to adverse cardiovascular outcomes, a concept similar to that proposed for psoriasis. They had previously shown that intensive periodontal therapy results in a reduction in both oral and systemic inflammation.[1-3] They here report the results of a randomized, controlled study to determine the effect on endothelial function of treatment of severe periodontitis. Endothelial dysfunction may represent a common pathway by which a multitude of risk factors, including inflammation, influence the development of atherosclerosis and cardiovascular disease. They found that intensive treatment of periodontitis leads to improvement in endothelial function after a transient acute inflammatory response characterized by endothelial function impairment.

B. H. Thiers, MD

References

1. D'Aiuto F, Parkar M, Andreou G, et al. Periodontitis and systemic inflammation: control of the local infection is associated with a reduction in serum inflammatory markers. *J Dent Res.* 2004;83:156-160.
2. D'Aiuto F, Nibali L, Parkar M, Suvan J, Tonetti MS. Short-term effects of intensive periodontal therapy on serum inflammatory markers and cholesterol. *J Dent Res.* 2005;84:269-273.

3. D'Aiuto F, Parkar M, Nibali L, Suvan J, Lessem J, Tonetti MS. Periodontal infections cause changes in traditional and novel cardiovascular risk factors: results from a randomized controlled clinical trial. *Am Heart J*. 2006;151:977-984.

Retinaldehyde represses adipogenesis and diet-induced obesity

Ziouzenkova O, Orasanu G, Sharlach M, et al (Harvard Med School; Merck Research Labs, Rahway, NJ; Boston Univ; et al)
Nature Med 13:695-702, 2007

The metabolism of vitamin A and the diverse effects of its metabolites are tightly controlled by distinct retinoid-generating enzymes, retinoid-binding proteins and retinoid-activated nuclear receptors. Retinoic acid regulates differentiation and metabolism by activating the retinoic acid receptor and retinoid X receptor (RXR), indirectly influencing RXR heterodimeric partners. Retinoic acid is formed solely from retinaldehyde (Rald), which in turn is derived from vitamin A. Rald currently has no defined biologic role outside the eye. Here we show that Rald is present in rodent fat, binds retinol-binding proteins (CRBP1, RBP4), inhibits adipogenesis and suppresses peroxisome proliferator-activated receptor-γ and RXR responses. *In vivo*, mice lacking the Rald-catabolizing enzyme retinaldehyde dehydrogenase 1 (Raldh1) resisted diet-induced obesity and insulin resistance and showed increased energy dissipation. In *ob/ob* mice, administrating Rald or a Raldh inhibitor reduced fat and increased insulin sensitivity. These results identify Rald as a distinct transcriptional regulator of the metabolic responses to a high-fat diet.

▶ Rald is an intermediate metabolite between vitamin A and retinoic acid that was previously thought to be active only in the visual system.[1] Ziouzenkova and colleagues show that active Rald concentrations exist in fat tissue, where the substance regulates adipogenesis and may improve insulin sensitivity. The authors' observations open new avenues of investigation into the metabolism of retinoic acid and its derivatives. Whether future studies will lead to a better understanding of obesity and improve its treatment (and thus make liposuction a thing of the past) remains doubtful.

B. H. Thiers, MD

Reference

1. Desvergne B. Retinaldehyde: more than meets the eye. *Nat Med*. 2007;13:671-673.

Effect of Smoking on Aging of Photoprotected Skin: Evidence Gathered Using a New Photonumeric Scale

Helfrich YR, Yu L, Ofori A, et al (Univ of Michigan, Ann Arbor)
Arch Dermatol 143:397-402, 2007

Objectives.—To develop a reproducible photonumeric scale to assess photoprotected skin aging and to determine whether health and lifestyle factors, such as smoking, affect skin aging in photoprotected sites.

Design.—Using standard photographs of participants' upper inner arms, we created a 9-point photonumeric scale. Three blinded reviewers used the scale to grade the photographs. Participants answered multiple lifestyle questions.

Setting.—Academic outpatient dermatology clinic.

Participants.—Eighty-two healthy men and women aged 22 to 91 years.

Interventions.—A professional medical photographer took standardized photographs of each participant's upper inner arm. Participants answered standardized health and lifestyle questions.

Main Outcome Measures.—(1) Interobserver agreement and reproducibility using the photonumeric scale and (2) health and lifestyle factors most predictive of the degree of aging in photoprotected skin.

Results.—There was good blinded interobserver agreement as measured by the maximum range of disagreement scores for each participant (mean, 0.91; 95% confidence interval, 0.76-1.06). Results were reproducible. We developed a multiple regression model showing that the best model for predicting the degree of aging in photoprotected skin includes 2 variables: age and packs of cigarettes smoked per day.

Conclusions.—This photonumeric scale demonstrates good interobserver agreement and good reproducibility. Using this scale, the degree of aging in photoprotected skin was significantly correlated with patient age and a history of cigarette smoking. Additional studies are needed to continue garnering information regarding independent risk factors for aging of photoprotected skin.

▶ Helfrich et al developed a 9-point scale to test the degree of aging in photoprotected skin. They found that 2 variables, age and packs of cigarettes smoked per day, correlated best with the degree of skin aging. The value of this scale appears to lie mainly in its reproducibility and its usefulness in evaluating future treatments for photoaging.

B. H. Thiers, MD

A single type of progenitor cell maintains normal epidermis

Clayton E, Doupé DP, Klein AM, et al (MRC Research Centre, Cambridge, England; Univ of Cambridge, England; Cancer Research UK Cambridge Research Inst, England)
Nature 446:185-189, 2007

According to the current model of adult epidermal homeostasis, skin tissue is maintained by two discrete populations of progenitor cells: self-renewing stem cells; and their progeny, known as transit amplifying cells, which differentiate after several rounds of cell division. By making use of inducible genetic labelling, we have tracked the fate of a representative sample of progenitor cells in mouse tail epidermis at single-cell resolution *in vivo* at time intervals up to one year. Here we show that clone-size distributions are consistent with a new model of homeostasis involving only one type of progenitor cell. These cells are found to undergo both symmetric and asymmetric division at rates that ensure epidermal homeostasis. The results raise important questions about the potential role of stem cells on tissue maintenance *in vivo*.

▶ Using mouse tail skin, Clayton at al present data compatible with a model involving a single proliferating cell compartment that may undergo an unlimited number of cell divisions. Whether such a single progenitor cell model is viable in other areas, such as back skin, could not be determined. It also is uncertain whether a small quiescent stem cell population may also be present that is active only under special circumstances (eg, wound healing).

B. H. Thiers, MD

Wnt-dependent *de novo* hair follicle regeneration in adult mouse skin after wounding

Ito M, Yang Z, Andl T, et al (Univ of Pennsylvania, Philadelphia)
Nature 447:316-320, 2007

The mammalian hair follicle is a complex 'mini-organ' thought to form only during development; loss of an adult follicle is considered permanent. However, the possibility that hair follicles develop *de novo* following wounding was raised in studies on rabbits, mice and even humans fifty years ago. Subsequently, these observations were generally discounted because definitive evidence for follicular neogenesis was not presented. Here we show that, after wounding, hair follicles form *de novo* in genetically normal adult mice. The regenerated hair follicles establish a stem cell population, express known molecular markers of follicle differentiation, produce a hair shaft and progress through all stages of the hair follicle cycle. Lineage analysis demonstrated that the nascent follicles arise from epithelial cells outside of the hair follicle stem cell niche, suggesting that epidermal cells in the wound assume a hair follicle stem cell phenotype. Inhibition of Wnt signalling after re-epithelialization completely abrogates this wounding-induced folliculogenesis, whereas overexpression of Wnt ligand in the epidermis increases the number of regenerated hair follicles. These remarkable regenerative capabilities of the adult support the notion that wounding induces an embryonic phenotype in skin, and that this provides a window for manipulation of hair follicle neogenesis by Wnt proteins. These findings suggest treatments for wounds, hair loss and other degenerative skin disorders.

▶ Ito et al show that re-epithelialization occurs when a large open wound is generated in the skin of adult mice, and that when the healed skin is larger than approximately 0.5 cm in diameter, new hair follicles originating from the epidermis form in the center of the wound. The critical event that appears to facilitate wounding-induced folliculogenesis is activation of the Wnt-mediated pathway, an essential factor for normal hair development and cycling. Although there are obvious differences between mouse skin and human skin, the findings will likely inspire new thinking in the management of alopecia.[1]

B. H. Thiers, MD

Reference

1. Chuong CM. New hair from healing wounds. *Nature* 2007;447:265-266.

Generation of germline-competent induced pluripotent stem cells
Okita K, Ichisaka T, Yamanaka S (Kyoto Univ, Japan; Japan Science and Technology Agency, Kawaguchi)
Nature 448:313-317, 2007

We have previously shown that pluripotent stem cells can be induced from mouse fibroblasts by retroviral introduction of Oct3/4 (also called Pou5f1), Sox2, c-Myc and Klf4, and subsequent selection for *Fbx15* (also called *Fbxo15*) expression. These induced pluripotent stem (iPS) cells (hereafter called Fbx15 iPS cells) are similar to embryonic stem (ES) cells in morphology, proliferation and teratoma formation; however, they are different with regards to gene expression and DNA methylation patterns, and fail to produce adult chimaeras. Here we show that selection for *Nanog* expression results in germline-competent iPS cells with increased ES-cell-like gene expression and DNA methylation patterns compared with Fbx15 iPS cells. The four transgenes (*Oct3/4, Sox2, c-myc* and *Klf4*) were strongly silenced in Nanog iPS cells. We obtained adult chimaeras from seven Nanog iPS cell clones, with one clone being transmitted through the germ line to the next generation. Approximately 20% of the offspring developed tumours attributable to reactivation of the *c-myc* transgene. Thus, iPS cells competent for germline chimaeras can be obtained from fibroblasts, but retroviral introduction of c-Myc should be avoided for clinical application.

▶ This report and a report by Wernig et al[1] have generated considerable interest not only in the world of academia but also in the arenas of politics and big business. Two groups of investigators independently and simultaneously showed, using very similar methodology, that cultured murine fibroblasts could be "reprogrammed" to assume the major characteristics of embryonic stem cells. The stimulus to this change included a cocktail of 4 different transcription factor genes delivered to the cells by a retroviral vector. Cells thus successfully induced were identified by their expression of *Nanog*, another transcription factor that is selectively expressed by embryonic stem cells and germ cell tumors. *Nanog* is considered to be a major factor in maintaining the pluripotency of such cells as well as their self-renewal ability; conversely, loss of *Nanog* function results in differentiation of the stem cell into other cell types.

In both studies, the newly minted Nanog-positive cells were extensively examined for their similarities to embryonic stem cells and measured up well, including their ability to form chimeras. However, several of the offspring developed malignancies in which retroviral *c-myc*, 1 of the inducing transcription factor genes, was reactivated. This approach, without substantial modification, would clearly be unsuitable for use in humans. Nevertheless, these data represent a milestone in stem cell research.

Another group of investigators, Takahashi et al,[2] have now also achieved induction of pluripotent stem cells from human fibroblasts, using very similar techniques as those described in the above articles. We eagerly await the next installments in this exciting series.

G. M. P. Galbraith, MD

References

1. Wernig M, Meissner A, Foreman R, et al. *In vitro* reprogramming of fibroblasts into a pluripotent ES-cell-like state. 2007;448:318-324.
2. Takahashi K, Tanabe K, Ohnuki M, et al. Induction of pluripotent stem cells from adult human fibroblasts by defined factors. *Cell*. 2007;131:861-872.

In vitro reprogramming of fibroblasts into a pluripotent ES-cell-like state

Wernig M, Meissner A, Foreman R, et al (Massachusetts Inst of Technology, Cambridge; Massachusetts Gen Hosp, Charlestown; Broad Inst of Harvard and MIT, Cambridge, Mass; et al)
Nature 448:318-324, 2007

Nuclear transplantation can reprogramme a somatic genome back into an embryonic epigenetic state, and the reprogrammed nucleus can create a cloned animal or produce pluripotent embryonic stem cells. One potential use of the nuclear cloning approach is the derivation of 'customized' embryonic stem (ES) cells for patient-specific cell treatment, but technical and ethical considerations impede the therapeutic application of this technology. Reprogramming of fibroblasts to a pluripotent state can be induced *in vitro* through ectopic expression of the four transcription factors Oct4 (also called Oct3/4 or Pou5f1), Sox2, c-Myc and Klf4. Here we show that DNA methylation, gene expression and chromatin state of such induced reprogrammed stem cells are similar to those of ES cells. Notably, the cells—derived from mouse fibroblasts—can form viable chimaeras, can contribute to the germ line and can generate live late-term embryos when injected into tetraploid blastocysts. Our results show that the biological potency and epigenetic state of *in-vitro*-reprogrammed induced pluripotent stem cells are indistinguishable from those of ES cells.

▶ This report and a report by Okita et al[1] have generated considerable interest not only in the world of academia, but also in the arenas of politics and big business. Two groups of investigators independently and simultaneously showed, using very similar methodology, that cultured murine fibroblasts could be "reprogrammed" to assume the major characteristics of embryonic stem cells. The stimulus to this change included a cocktail of 4 different transcription factor genes delivered to the cells by a retroviral vector. Cells thus successfully induced were identified by their expression of *Nanog*, another transcription factor that is selectively expressed by embryonic stem cells and germ cell tumors. *Nanog* is considered to be a major factor in maintaining the pluripotency of such cells as well as their self-renewal ability; conversely, loss of *Nanog* function results in differentiation of the stem cell into other cell types.

In both studies, the newly minted *Nanog*-positive cells were extensively examined for their similarities to embryonic stem cells and measured up well, including their ability to form chimeras. However, several of the offspring developed malignancies in which retroviral *c-myc*, 1 of the inducing transcription factor genes, was reactivated. This approach, without substantial modification, would clearly be unsuitable for use in humans. Nevertheless, these data represent a milestone in stem cell research.

Another group of investigators, Takahashi et al,[2] have now achieved induction of pluripotent stem cells from human fibroblasts, using very similar techniques as those described in the above articles. We eagerly await the next installments in this exciting series.

G. M. P. Galbraith, MD

References

1. Okita K, Ichisaka T, Yamanaka S. Generation of germline-competent induced pluripotent stem cells. *Nature.* 2007;448:313-317.
2. Takahashi K, Tanabe K, Ohnuki M, et al. Induction of pluripotent stem cells from adult human fibroblasts by defined factors. *Cell.* 2007;131:861-872.

Induced Pluripotent Stem Cell Lines Derived from Human Somatic Cells
Yu J, Vodyanik MA, Smuga-Otto K, et al (Genome Ctr of Wisconsin, Madison; Univ of Wisconsin-Madison)
Science 318:1917-1920, 2007

Somatic cell nuclear transfer allows trans-acting factors present in the mammalian oocyte to reprogram somatic cell nuclei to an undifferentiated state. Here we show that four factors (OCT4, SOX2, NANOG, and LIN28) are sufficient to reprogram human somatic cells to pluripotent stem cells that exhibit the essential characteristics of embryonic stem cells. These human induced pluripotent stem cells have normal karyotypes, express telomerase activity, express cell surface markers and genes that characterize human ES cells, and maintain the developmental potential to differentiate into advanced derivatives of all three primary germ layers. Such human induced pluripotent cell lines should be useful in the production of new disease models and in drug development as well as application in transplantation medicine once technical limitations (for example, mutation through viral integration) are eliminated.

▶ This article and an article by Takahashi et al[1] report the landmark observation that human skin cells can be reprogrammed to act like embryonic stem cells.

Yu et al reprogrammed human skin cells obtained from a baby's foreskin, while Takahashi et al[1] used cells taken from adult skin. Both groups used just 4 genes to reprogram the human skin cells, although 2 of the genes used differed from group to group. However, all the genes involved in these studies are considered master regulator genes that turn other genes on and off. Although the scientists reported that the reprogrammed cells behaved very much like human ES cells, they preferred to call them induced pluripotent stem cells. Nevertheless, it is still uncertain whether they really are identical to stem cells produced from embryos. If this does indeed prove to be the case, their use in research would avoid the ethical, political, and practical obstacles of cloning embryos to make stem cells.

B. H. Thiers, MD

Reference

1. Takahashi K, Tanabe K, Ohnuki M, et al. Induction of pluripotent stem cells from adult human fibroblasts by defined factors. *Cell.* 2007;131:861-872.

Induction of Pluripotent Stem Cells from Adult Human Fibroblasts by Defined Factors
Takahashi K, Tanabe K, Ohnuki M, et al (Kyoto Univ, Japan; Japan Science and Technology Agency, Kawaguchi; Gladstone Inst of Cardiovascular Disease, San Francisco)
Cell 131:861-872, 2007

Successful reprogramming of differentiated human somatic cells into a pluripotent state would allow creation of patient- and disease-specific stem cells. We previously reported generation of induced pluripotent stem (iPS) cells, capable of germline transmission, from mouse somatic cells by transduction of four defined transcription factors. Here, we demonstrate the generation of iPS cells from adult human dermal fibroblasts with the same four factors: Oct3/4, Sox2, Klf4, and c-Myc. Human iPS cells were similar to human embryonic stem (ES) cells in morphology, proliferation, surface antigens, gene expression, epigenetic status of pluripotent cell-specific genes, and telomerase activity. Furthermore, these cells could differentiate into cell types of the three germ layers in vitro and in teratomas. These findings demonstrate that iPS cells can be generated from adult human fibroblasts.

▶ This article and an article by Yu et al[1] report the landmark observation that human skin cells can be reprogrammed to act like embryonic stem cells. Yu et al[1] reprogrammed human skin cells obtained from a baby's foreskin, while Takahashi et al used cells taken from adult skin. Both groups used just 4 genes to reprogram the human skin cells, although 2 of the genes used differed from group to group. However, all the genes involved in these studies are considered master regulator genes that turn other genes on and off. Although the scientists reported that the reprogrammed cells behaved very much like human ES cells, they preferred to call them induced pluripotent stem cells. Nevertheless, it is still uncertain whether they really are identical to stem cells produced from embryos. If this does indeed prove to be the case, their use in research would avoid the ethical, political, and practical obstacles of cloning embryos to make stem cells.

B. H. Thiers, MD

Reference

1. Yu J, Vodyanik MA, Smuga-Otto K, et al. Induced pluripotent stem cell lines derived from human somatic cells. *Science*. 2007;318:1917-1920.

DERMATOLOGIC SURGERY AND CUTANEOUS ONCOLOGY

16 Nonmelanoma Skin Cancer

Protective Effect of Hyperpigmented Skin on UV-Mediated Cutaneous Cancer Development
Kato M, Ohgami N, Kawamoto Y, et al (Chubu Univ, Kasugai-shi, Aichi, Japan; Nagoya Univ Graduate School of Medicine, Aichi, Japan; Aichi Med Univ School of Medicine, Japan)
J Invest Dermatol 127:1244-1249, 2007

Recently, we crossed an original haired *RET*-transgenic mouse of line 242 with a hairless mouse and established a hairless *RET-(HL/RET)*-transgenic mouse line (242-hr/hr) with hyperpigmented skin but no tumors. In this study, we examined the effect of hyperpigmented skin in *HL/RET*-transgenic mice on UV irradiation-mediated cutaneous cancer development. UV irradiation to this mouse line never induced melanoma despite the presence of melanoma-inducible transgenic *RET* oncogenes. On the contrary, the hyperpigmented skin efficiently protected UV-mediated squamous carcinoma development in the skin. Probably underlying this result, hyperpigmentation protected the skin from damage and blocked the accompanying signal transduction for tyrosine phosphorylation of multiple cellular proteins and activation/phosphorylation of extracellular signal-regulated, c-Jun N-terminal, and p38 kinases. Thus, we demonstrated hyperpigmentation-mediated *in vivo* protection against UV irradiation-induced skin cancer.

▶ Kato and colleagues present direct evidence of a protective effect of melanin against the development of tumors in mice. The melanin seemed to provide protection against ultraviolet-associated tissue damage as well. Caution is necessary when extrapolating these findings to human skin, because the response of human skin to this type of exposure differs in many ways as compared with that observed in mice.

B. H. Thiers, MD

Central Role of p53 in the Suntan Response and Pathologic Hyperpigmentation

Cui R, Widlund HR, Feige E, et al (Harvard Med School, Boston)
Cell 128:853-864, 2007

UV-induced pigmentation (suntanning) requires induction of α-melanocyte-stimulating hormone (α-MSH) secretion by keratinocytes. α-MSH and other bioactive peptides are cleavage products of pro-opiomelanocortin (POMC). Here we provide biochemical and genetic evidence demonstrating that UV induction of POMC/MSH in skin is directly controlled by p53. Whereas p53 potently stimulates the POMC promoter in response to UV, the absence of p53, as in knockout mice, is associated with absence of the UV-tanning response. The same pathway produces β-endorphin, another POMC derivative, which potentially contributes to sun-seeking behaviors. Furthermore, several instances of UV-independent pathologic pigmentation are shown to involve p53 "mimicking" the tanning response. p53 thus functions as a sensor/effector for UV pigmentation, which is a nearly constant environmental exposure. Moreover, this pathway is activated in numerous conditions of pathologic pigmentation and thus mimics the tanning response.

▶ Previous studies have shown that UV irradiation activates the p53 protein to stimulate transcription of target genes involved in DNA repair. Cui et al noted that mice genetically deficient in p53 failed to tan after UV radiation. They went on to show that the likely mechanism behind this failure to tan involves the ability of p53 to stimulate transcription of the POMC gene in keratinocytes. They suggest that transcription of this gene in sun-exposed epidermal cells leads to increased release of α-MSH, activation of the melanocortin-1 receptor on melanocytes, and ultimately increased melanogenesis. The direct connection between p53, melanocortin signaling, and tanning may provide a photoprotective effect that complements the DNA repair effect of p53.[1] Interestingly, keratinocyte derived β-endorphin is derived from POMC. This could explain the sun-seeking behavior and "tanner's high" that has been reported after natural or artificial UV light exposure.

B. H. Thiers, MD

Reference

1. Barsh G, Attardi LD. A healthy tan? *N Engl J Med.* 2007;356:2208-2210.

An inducible mouse model for skin cancer reveals distinct roles for gain- and loss-of-function *p53* mutations

Caulin C, Nguyen T, Lang GA, et al (Baylor College of Medicine, Houston; Univ of Texas, Houston)

J Clin Invest 117:1893-1901, 2007

Mutations in *ras* and *p53* are the most prevalent mutations found in human nonmelanoma skin cancers. Although some *p53* mutations cause a loss of function, most result in expression of altered forms of p53, which may exhibit gain-of-function properties. Therefore, understanding the consequences of acquiring *p53* gain-of-function versus loss-of-function mutations is critical for the generation of effective therapies for tumors harboring *p53* mutations. Here we describe an inducible mouse model in which skin tumor formation is initiated by activation of an endogenous *K-ras^{G12D}* allele. Using this model we compared the consequences of activating the *p53* gain-of-function mutation *p53^{R172H}* and of deleting the *p53* gene. Activation of the *p53^{R172H}* allele resulted in increased skin tumor formation, accelerated tumor progression, and induction of metastasis compared with deletion of *p53*. Consistent with these observations, the *p53^{R172H}* tumors exhibited aneuploidy associated with centrosome amplification, which may underlie the mechanism by which *p53^{R172H}* exerts its oncogenic properties. These results clearly demonstrate that *p53* gain-of-function mutations confer poorer prognosis than loss of *p53* during skin carcinogenesis and have important implications for the future design of therapies for tumors that exhibit *p53* gain-of-function mutations.

▶ Caulin et al used an inducible mouse model to demonstrate that endogenous *ras* and gain-of-function *p53* mutations cooperate in skin cancer initiation, progression, and metastasis. Their observations confirm that *p53* has potent oncogenic properties and suggest that a better understanding of the mechanisms involved in the interaction between *ras* and *p53* may lead to the development of novel molecules for the prevention and treatment of skin cancer. In an article by Nibbs et al,[1] the investigators found that inhibition of cutaneous inflammation by manipulation of the atypical chemokine receptor D6 suppresses the development of chemically induced skin tumors. The insights provided into cutaneous carcinogenesis by these 2 articles add to our understanding of the role of the immune system in this process.[2]

B. H. Thiers, MD

References

1. Nibbs RJB, Gilchrist DS, King V, et al. The atypical chemokine receptor D6 suppresses the development of chemically induced skin tumors. *J Clin Invest.* 2007;117:1884-1892.
2. Owens DM. p53, chemokines, and squamous cell carcinoma. *J Clin Invest.* 2007;117:1752-1755.

Modeling the Therapeutic Efficacy of p53 Restoration in Tumors

Martins CP, Brown-Swigart L, Evan GI (Univ of California, San Francisco)
Cell 127:1323-1334, 2006

Although restoration of p53 function is an attractive tumor-specific therapeutic strategy, it remains unclear whether p53 loss is required only for transition through early bottlenecks in tumorigenesis or also for maintenance of established tumors. To explore the efficacy of p53 reinstatement as a tumor therapy, we used a reversibly switchable p53 knockin (KI) mouse model that permits modulation of p53 status from wild-type to knockout, at will. Using the well-characterized *Eµ-myc* lymphoma model, we show that p53 is spontaneously activated when restored in established *Eµ-myc* lymphomas in vivo, triggering rapid apoptosis and conferring a significant increase in survival. Nonetheless, reimposition of p53 function potently selects for emergence of p53-resistant tumors through inactivation of p19^{ARF}or p53. Our study provides important insights into the nature and timing of p53-activating signals in established tumors and how resistance to p53 evolves, which will aid in the optimization of p53-based tumor therapies.

▶ There is little doubt that the protein product of the p53 gene is one of the most important molecules in human biology, touching on our growth, health, longevity, and death. It indeed appears to be the "master and commander" of key cellular processes that determine our fate.[1]

B. H. Thiers, MD

Reference

1. Foulkes WD. p53-master and commander. *N Engl J Med.* 2007;357:2539-2541.

Restoration of p53 function leads to tumour regression *in vivo*

Ventura A, Kirsch DG, McLaughlin ME, et al (Massachusetts Inst of Technology, Cambridge; Massachusetts Gen Hosp, Boston; Harvard Med School, Boston)
Nature 445:661-665, 2007

Tumorigenesis is a multi-step process that requires activation of oncogenes and inactivation of tumour suppressor genes. Mouse models of human cancers have recently demonstrated that continuous expression of a dominantly acting oncogene (for example, *Hras*, *Kras* and *Myc*) is often required for tumour maintenance; this phenotype is referred to as oncogene addiction. This concept has received clinical validation by the development of active anticancer drugs that specifically inhibit the function of oncoproteins such as BCR-ABL, c-KIT and EGFR. Identifying additional gene mutations that are required for tumour maintenance may therefore yield clinically useful targets for new cancer therapies. Although loss of p53 function is a common feature of human cancers, it is not known whether sustained inactivation of this or other tumour suppressor pathways is required for tumour maintenance. To explore this issue, we developed a Cre-*loxP*-based strategy to temporally control tumour suppressor gene expression *in vivo*. Here we show that restoring endogenous p53 expression leads to regression of autochthonous lymphomas and sarcomas in mice without affecting normal tissues. The mechanism responsible for tumour regression is dependent on the tumour type, with the main consequence of p53 restoration being apoptosis in lymphomas and suppression of cell growth with features of cellular senescence in sarcomas. These results support efforts to treat human cancers by way of pharmacological reactivation of p53.

▶ Mutation of the p53 tumor suppressor gene and its resultant inactivation is a common mutation in human cancer. Indeed, it has been hypothesized that the pathway that controls this gene may be compromised to some degree in all human cancers. This pathway appears to help the cell respond to DNA damage; such damage activates the p53 protein, which in turn switches on the cell-division cycle to allow for repair. Activation of p53 may also initiate programs that lead to cell death, apoptosis, or primary growth arrest (senescence) if the DNA damage is persistent and severe. Mice lacking p53 activity are highly prone to spontaneous and carcinogen-induced tumors. Conversely, when the p53 gene is stimulated, prompt and impressive regression of established tumors may be noted. Unfortunately, in human beings, therapies that stimulate tumor-suppressing oncogenes may be effective initially, although secondary genetic events often occur that render the tumors resistant to such treatment. Indeed, in an article by Martins et al,[1] reactivation of p53 did induce widespread tumor-cell apoptosis, but this was followed by the rapid reappearance of tumors that progressed despite continued p53 expression, suggesting that secondary resistance can limit the long-term benefit of this approach. Nevertheless, multiple studies, including this one, establish that reactivation of the p53 tumor suppressor gene can be of therapeutic benefit even in established cancers.[2,3]

B. H. Thiers, MD

References

1. Martins CP, Brown-Swigart L, Evan GI. Modeling the therapeutic efficacy of p53 restoration in tumors. *Cell.* 2006;127:1323-1334.
2. Sharpless NE, DePinho RA. Cancer biology: gone but not forgotten. *Nature.* 2007;445:606-607.
3. Xue W, Zender L, Miething C, et al. Senescence and tumour clearance is triggered by p53 restoration in murine liver carcinomas. *Nature.* 2007;445:656-660.

Senescence and tumour clearance is triggered by p53 restoration in murine liver carcinomas

Xue W, Zender L, Miething C, et al (Cold Spring Harbor Lab, NY; Howard Hughes Med Inst, NY; Mem Sloan-Kettering Cancer Ctr, NY)
Nature 445:656-660, 2007

Although cancer arises from a combination of mutations in oncogenes and tumour suppressor genes, the extent to which tumour suppressor gene loss is required for maintaining established tumours is poorly understood. p53 is an important tumour suppressor that acts to restrict proliferation in response to DNA damage or deregulation of mitogenic oncogenes, by leading to the induction of various cell cycle checkpoints, apoptosis or cellular senescence. Consequently, *p53* mutations increase cell proliferation and survival, and in some settings promote genomic instability and resistance to certain chemotherapies. To determine the consequences of reactivating the p53 pathway in tumours, we used RNA interference (RNAi) to conditionally regulate endogenous p53 expression in a mosaic mouse model of liver carcinoma. We show that even brief reactivation of endogenous p53 in p53-deficient tumours can produce complete tumour regressions. The primary response to p53 was not apoptosis, but instead involved the induction of a cellular senescence program that was associated with differentiation and the upregulation of inflammatory cytokines. This program, although producing only cell cycle arrest *in vitro*, also triggered an innate immune response that targeted the tumour cells *in vivo*, thereby contributing to tumour clearance. Our study indicates that p53 loss can be required for the maintenance of aggressive carcinomas, and illustrates how the cellular senescence program can act together with the innate immune system to potently limit tumour growth.

▶ These 3 articles review some tough basic science concepts, but given the relevance of p53 in skin cancer pathophysiology they are certainly relevant to dermatology. Mutation of the p53 tumor suppressor gene and its resultant inactivation is a common mutation in human cancer. Indeed, it has been hypothesized that the pathway that controls this gene may be compromised to some degree in all human cancers. This pathway appears to help the cell respond to DNA damage; such damage activates the p53 protein, which in turn switches on the cell-division cycle to allow for repair. Activation of p53 may also initiate programs that lead to cell death, apoptosis, or primary growth arrest (senescence) if the DNA damage is persistent and severe. Mice lacking p53 activity are highly prone to spontaneous and carcinogen-induced tumors. Conversely, when the p53 gene is stimulated, prompt and impressive regression of established tumors may be noted. Unfortunately, in human beings, therapies that stimulate tumor-suppressing oncogenes may be effective initially, although secondary genetic events often occur that render the tumors resistant to such treatment. Indeed, in an article by Martins et al,[1] reactivation of p53 did induce widespread tumor-cell apoptosis, but this was followed by the rapid reappearance of tumors that progressed despite continued p53 expression, suggesting that secondary resistance can limit the long-term benefit of this approach. Nevertheless, multiple studies, including this one, establish that reactivation of the p53 tumor suppressor gene can be of therapeutic benefit even in established cancers.[2-3]

B. H. Thiers, MD

References

1. Martins CP, Brown-Swigart L, Evan GI. Modeling the therapeutic efficacy of p53 restoration in tumors. *Cell.* 2006;127:1323-1334.
2. Sharpless NE, De Pinho RA. Cancer biology: gone but not forgotten. *Nature.* 2007;445:606-607.
3. Ventura A, Kirsch DG, McLaughlin ME, et al. Restoration of p53 function leads to tumour regression *in vivo. Nature.* 2007;445:661-665.

The atypical chemokine receptor D6 suppresses the development of chemically induced skin tumors
Nibbs RJB, Gilchrist DS, King V, et al (Univ of Glasgow, Scotland; CR-UK Beatson Labs, Glasgow, Scotland)
J Clin Invest 117:1884-1892, 2007

A subset of CC chemokines, acting through CC chemokine receptors (CCRs) 1 to 5, is instrumental in shaping inflammatory responses. Recently, we and others have demonstrated that the atypical chemokine receptor D6 actively sequesters and destroys many of these proinflammatory CC chemokines. This is critical for effective resolution of inflammation in vivo. Inflammation can be protumorigenic, and proinflammatory CC chemokines have been linked with various aspects of cancer biology, yet there is scant evidence supporting a critical role for these molecules in de novo tumor formation. Here, we show that D6-deficient mice have increased susceptibility to cutaneous tumor development in response to chemical carcinogenesis protocols and, remarkably, that D6 deletion is sufficient to make resistant mouse strains susceptible to invasive squamous cell carcinoma. Conversely, transgenic D6 expression in keratinocytes dampens cutaneous inflammation and can confer considerable protection from tumor formation in susceptible backgrounds. Tumor susceptibility consistently correlated with the level of recruitment of T cells and mast cells, cell types known to support the development of skin tumors in mice. These data demonstrate the importance of proinflammatory CC chemokines in de novo tumorigenesis and reveal chemokine sequestration by D6 to be a novel and effective method of tumor suppression.

▶ In an article by Caulin et al,[1] the investigators used an inducible mouse model to demonstrate that endogenous *ras* and gain-of-function *p53* mutations cooperate in skin cancer initiation, progression, and metastasis. Their observations confirm that *p53* has potent oncogenic properties and suggest that a better understanding of the mechanisms involved in the interaction between *ras* and *p53* may lead to the development of novel molecules for the prevention and treatment of skin cancer. Nibbs et al found that inhibition of cutaneous inflammation by manipulation of the atypical chemokine receptor D6 suppresses the development of chemically induced skin tumors. The insights provided into cutaneous carcinogenesis by these 2 articles add to our understanding of the role of the immune system in this process.[2]

B. H. Thiers, MD

References

1. Caulin C, Nguyen T, Lang GA, et al. An inducible mouse model for skin cancer reveals distinct roles for gain- and loss-of-function *p53* mutations. *J Clin Invest.* 2007;117:1893-1901.
2. Owens DM. p53, chemokines, and squamous cell carcinoma. *J Clin Invest.* 2007; 117:1752-1755.

Does solar exposure, as indicated by the non-melanoma skin cancers, protect from solid cancers: Vitamin D as a possible explanation
Tuohimaa P, Pukkala E, Scélo G, et al (Univ of Tampere, Finland; Finnish Cancer Registry, Helsinki; Internatl Agency for Research on Cancer, Lyon, France; et al)
Eur J Cancer 43:1701-1712, 2007

Background.—Skin cancers are known to be associated with sun exposure, whereas sunlight through the production of vitamin D may protect against some cancers. The aim of this study was to assess whether patients with skin cancer have an altered risk of developing other cancers.

Methods.—The study cohort consisted of 416,134 cases of skin cancer and 3,776,501 cases of non-skin cancer as a first cancer extracted from 13 cancer registries. 10,886 melanoma and 35,620 non-melanoma skin cancer cases had second cancers. The observed numbers (O) of 46 types of second primary cancer after skin melanoma, basal cell carcinoma or non-basal cell carcinoma, and of skin cancers following non-skin cancers were compared to the expected numbers (E) derived from the age, sex and calendar period specific cancer incidence rates in each of the cancer registries (O/E = SIR, standardised incidence ratios). Rates from cancer registries classified to sunny countries (Australia, Singapore and Spain) and less sunny countries (Canada, Denmark, Finland, Iceland, Norway, Scotland, Slovenia and Sweden) were compared to each other.

Results.—SIR of all second solid primary cancers (except skin and lip) after skin melanoma were significantly lower for the sunny countries (SIR(S) = 1.03; 95% CI 0.99–1.08) than in the less sunny countries (SIR(L) = 1.14; 95%CI 1.11–1.17). The difference was more obvious after non-melanoma skin cancers: after basal cell carcinoma SIR(S)/SIR(L) = 0.65 (95%CI = 0.58–0.72); after non-basal cell carcinoma SIR(S)/SIR(L)= 0.58 (95%CI = 0.50–0.67). In sunny countries, the risk of second primary cancer after nonmelanoma skin cancers was lower for most of the cancers except for lip, mouth and non-Hodgkin lymphoma.

Conclusions.—Vitamin D production in the skin seems to decrease the risk of several solid cancers (especially stomach, colorectal, liver and gall-bladder, pancreas, lung, female breast, prostate, bladder and kidney cancers). The apparently protective effect of sun exposure against second primary cancer is more pronounced after non-melanoma skin cancers than melanoma, which is consistent with earlier reports that non-melanoma skin cancers reflect cumulative sun exposure, whereas melanoma is more related to sunburn.

▶ The authors conclude that, in sunny countries, high levels of sun exposure, as indicated by the presence of primary skin cancer, have a protective role against internal solid cancers. This protective role was not observed in less sunny countries. The weakness of the study is that it assumes, to the exclusion of all other risk factors, that patients with primary skin cancer have higher levels of sun exposure and higher levels of vitamin D production than do their counterparts without skin cancer. This, clearly, is not true as genetic factors, age, and other variables may influence both conditions. Stated more simply, the presence of skin cancer cannot be considered a proxy for sun exposure; the relationship between the 2 is certainly more complex. Whatever the case, for patients desiring to increase their vitamin D levels, methods other than excessive sun exposure should be encouraged.

B. H. Thiers, MD

A comparison of sunlight exposure in men with prostate cancer and basal cell carcinoma

Rukin NJ, Zeegers MP, Ramachandran S, et al (Keele Univ Med School, Staffordshire, England; Univ Hosp of North Staffordshire, England; Univ of Birmingham, England; et al)
Br J Cancer 96:523-528, 2007

Ultraviolet radiation exposure increases basal cell carcinoma (BCC) risk, but may be protective against prostate cancer. We attempted to identify exposure patterns that confer reduced prostate cancer risk without increasing that of BCC. We used a questionnaire to assess exposure in 528 prostate cancer patients and 442 men with basal cell carcinoma, using 365 benign prostatic hypertrophy patients as controls. Skin type 1 (odds ratio (OR) = 0.47, 95% CI = 0.26–0.86), childhood sunburning (OR = 0.38, 95% CI = 0.26–0.57), occasional/frequent sunbathing (OR = 0.21, 95% CI = 0.14–0.31), lifetime weekday (OR = 0.85, 95% CI = 0.80–0.91) and weekend exposure (OR = 0.79, 95% CI = 0.73–0.86) were associated with reduced prostate cancer risk. Skin type 1 (OR = 4.00, 95% CI = 2.16–7.41), childhood sunburning (OR = 1.91, 95% CI = 1.36–2.68), regular foreign holidays (OR = 6.91, 95% CI = 5.00–9.55) and weekend (OR = 1.17, 95% CI = 1.08–1.27) but not weekday exposure were linked with increased BCC risk. Combinations of one or two parameters were associated with a progressive decrease in the ORs for prostate cancer risk (OR = 0.54–0.25) with correspondingly increased BCC risk (OR = 1.60–2.54). Our data do not define exposure patterns that reduce prostate cancer risk without increasing BCC risk.

▶ Rukin and colleagues show that sunlight exposure patterns seem to correlate with the risk of prostate cancer and BCC. Specifically, increased sunlight exposure seems to reduce prostate cancer risk and increase BCC risk. The authors were unable to define levels of exposure that would reduce prostate risk without increasing the risk of BCC risk. On the basis of current knowledge, it would be unwise to advise a visit to the beach as a reasonable strategy to reduce the risk of prostate cancer.

B. H. Thiers, MD

Quality-of-Life Outcomes of Treatments for Cutaneous Basal Cell Carcinoma and Squamous Cell Carcinoma
Chren M-M, Sahay AP, Bertenthal DS, et al (San Francisco Veterans Affairs Med Ctr and Dept of Veterans Affairs, California; Univ of California, San Francisco)
J Invest Dermatol 127:1351-1357, 2007

Quality of life is an important treatment outcome for conditions that are rarely fatal, such as cutaneous basal cell carcinoma and squamous cell carcinoma (typically called nonmelanoma skin cancer (NMSC)). The purpose of this study was to compare quality-of-life outcomes of treatments for NMSC. We performed a prospective cohort study of 633 consecutive patients with NMSC diagnosed in 1999 and 2000 and followed for 2 years after treatment at a university-based private practice or a Veterans Affairs clinic. The main outcome was tumor-related quality of life 1 to 2 years after therapy, measured with the 16-item version of Skindex, a validated measure. Skindex scores vary from 0 (best) to 100 (worst) in three domains: Symptoms, Emotions, and Function. Treatments were electrodessication and curettage (ED&C) in 21%, surgical excision in 40%, and Mohs surgery in 39%. Five hundred and eight patients (80%) responded after treatment. Patients treated with excision or Mohs surgery improved in all quality-of-life domains, but quality of life did not improve after ED&C. There was no difference in the amount of improvement after excision or Mohs surgery. For example, mean Skindex Symptom scores improved 9.7 (95% CI: 6.9, 12.5) after excision, 10.2 (7.4, 12.9) after Mohs surgery, and 3.4 (−0.9, 7.6) after ED&C. We conclude that, for NMSC, quality-of-life outcomes were similar after excision and Mohs surgery, and both therapies had better outcomes than ED&C.

▶ Many variables need to be considered when evaluating treatments for NMSC. These include recurrence rate, cost-effectiveness, and the improvement in quality of life. In this study, the investigators found that there was no difference between Mohs surgery and excisional surgery in the improvement in tumor-related quality of life. In contrast, the use of electrodesiccation and curettage was not associated with an improvement in quality of life.

P. G. Lang Jr, MD

5% 5-Fluorouracil Cream for the Treatment of Small Superficial Basal Cell Carcinoma: Efficacy, Tolerability, Cosmetic Outcome, and Patient Satisfaction

Gross K, Kircik L, Kricorian G (Skin Surgery Med Group, San Diego, Calif; Physicians Skin Care PLLC, Louisville, Ky; Valeant Pharmaceuticals Internatl, Costa Mesa, Calif)
Dermatol Surg 33:433-440, 2007

Background.—Five percent 5-fluorouracil (5-FU) cream is approved by the FDA for the treatment of superficial basal cell carcinomas but has been underutilized.

Objective.—The objective was to evaluate the efficacy, tolerability, cosmetic outcome, and patient satisfaction of 5% 5-FU in the treatment of superficial basal cell carcinomas.

Materials and Methods.—A total of 29 patients with 31 biopsy-proven superficial basal cell carcinoma lesions on the trunk or limbs were treated with 5% 5-FU cream twice daily for up to 12 weeks. Treatment could be stopped sooner if the lesion was clinically resolved. The lesional site was surgically excised 3 weeks after the end of treatment for histologic evaluation of cure.

Results.—The histologic cure rate was 90% (28/31 lesions cured) and the mean time to clinical cure was 10.5 weeks. 5-FU was generally well tolerated with a good cosmetic outcome—the majority of patients had no pain or scarring and only mild erythema. Patients were generally very satisfied with their treatment.

Conclusion.—Five percent 5-FU is a highly effective and well-tolerated treatment option for superficial basal cell carcinomas offering a generally good cosmetic outcome and high levels of patient satisfaction.

▶ It is impossible to compare data from different studies of different drugs as a result of disparate inclusion and exclusion criteria, inconsistent evaluation criteria, and variability in evaluator judgment. Most useful to dermatologists would be a large blinded study comparing 5-FU and imiquimod for the treatment not only of superficial basal cell carcinomas but of actinic keratoses as well. However, the realities of pharmaceutical marketing suggest that such a study will never occur.

B. H. Thiers, MD

Recurrence rates of primary basal cell carcinoma in facial risk areas treated with curettage and electrodesiccation

Rodriguez-Vigil T, Vázquez-López F, Perez-Oliva N (Univ of Oviedo, Spain)
J Am Acad Dermatol 56:91-95, 2007

Background.—The incidence of basal cell carcinoma (BCC) is increasing. Curettage and electrodesiccation (CE) are not recommended for BCC treatment at medium- and high-risk facial sites. Surgical excision has been proposed as the treatment of choice.

Objective.—We sought to evaluate the cumulative recurrence rate (RR) of primary BCC in facial areas of medium and high risk after CE.

Methods.—This nonrandomized, clinical trial enrolled 257 patients with primary BCC located in medium- and high-risk facial areas, and treated with 4 or 5 cycles of CE by a single operator from a section specializing in BCC CE in a tertiary teaching hospital in Oviedo, Spain. Exclusion criteria for study entry included: recurrent BCC, fibrosing BCC, ill-defined BCC, and BCC larger than 10 mm in diameter (high-risk facial sites) or larger than 15 mm in diameter (medium-risk sites); BCC smaller than 4 mm; and nonbiopsy-proven BCC. BCCs included in the study were from the nose, and paranasal and nasal-labial fold (n = 105); eyelids and canthi (n = 48); perioral areas (n = 12); ears (n = 11); forehead and temples (n = 48); periauricular areas (n = 14); and malar areas and cheeks (n = 19). The primary outcome was recurrence of carcinoma, which was clinically evaluated by at least two observers in consensus. Data were analyzed using both a life table method and Kaplan-Meier analysis. The statistical analysis included best- and worst-case scenarios (which means that all cases lost to follow-up were considered as recurrences).

Results.—The 5-year cumulative non-RR in the best-case scenario was 98.80% (SE 0.70, 95% confidence interval 97.40%-100%); thus, a 5-year cumulative RR of 1.20% was found after CE in our medium- and high-risk BCCs of the face (best case). The 5-year cumulative non-RR in the worst-case scenario was 79.40% (95% confidence interval 78.90%-79.90%); thus, a 5-year cumulative RR of 20.60%.

Limitations.—Retrospective design with a relatively small number of patients lost to follow-up is a study limitation.

Conclusion.—High 5-year cure rates can be obtained after CE of primary, nonfibrosing BCCs of medium- and high-risk areas of the face performed in a specialized section.

▶ Over the years, there has been much controversy regarding the efficacy of CE in the management of BCC of the head and neck. Prior histologic studies have demonstrated persistent BCC in up to one third of cases after CE of tumors in high-risk areas. Although this study was marred by the loss of 50 patients to follow-up, it would suggest that CE, when performed by experienced clinicians and on carefully selected tumors, can provide acceptable cure rates, even for tumors located in medium- and high-risk areas. Although touched on briefly, the cosmetic results were not analyzed in detail.

P. G. Lang Jr, MD

Incomplete Exicision of Basal Cell Carcinoma: Rate and Associated Factors among 362 Consecutive Cases

Farhi D, Dupin N, Palangié A, et al (Université Paris)
Dermatol Surg 33:1207-1214, 2007

Background.—Reported rates of incomplete excision of basal cell carcinoma (BCC) range from 4% to 16.6%.

Objective.—The objective was to assess, in clinical practice, the rate and the factors associated with pathologically reported incomplete excision of BCC.

Methods.—In this retrospective monocentric study, data from all surgically excised BCCs during the year 2004 were computerized. Age, sex, number of BCC excised during the same surgical session, BCC location, pathologic types, and involvement of surgical margins were analyzed.

Results.—Mean age of the 284 patients was 67.4 ± 14.9 (SD) years (range, 27–96 years). A total of 52.7% of the 362 BCCs were located on the face (including nose, 10%; eyelids, 4.2%; lips, 2%; and ears, 2.2%). Incomplete excisions occurred in 10.3% of the cases including 8.6% of positive lateral margins and 2.5% of positive deep margins. In the multivariate analysis, incomplete excision was independently associated with location on the nasal ala ($p<.02$), other parts of the nose ($p=.02$), and inner canthus ($p=.01$) and with infiltrative ($p<.0001$) and multifocal ($p<.0001$) types.

Conclusion.—Pathologically reported incomplete excision rate was comparable to that of other studies and was significantly associated with the location on the face, particularly on the nose and inner canthus, and with infiltrative and multifocal histologic types.

▶ The results of this retrospective study are not particularly surprising and are consistent with previous data. Certainly, for BCC in high-risk areas, Mohs micrographic surgery, or conventional excision with frozen section control are reasonable treatment modalities. The debate continues as to whether incompletely excised BCCs should be immediately re-treated. Recurrence rates after incomplete excision have been reported to range from 26% to 67%, and the recurrence rate is higher after incomplete resection (26%) than after complete resection.[1,2] This suggests that most incompletely excised tumors should indeed be retreated.

B. H. Thiers, MD

References

1. Nagore E, Grau C, Molinero J, Fortea JM. Positive margins in basal cell carcinoma: relationship to clinical features and recurrence risk. A retrospective study of 248 patients. *J Eur Acad Dermatol Venereol.* 2003;17:167-170.

2. Sussman LA, Liggins DF. Incompletely excised basal cell carcinoma: a management dilemma? *Aust N Z J Surg.* 1996;66:276-278.

Treatment of post-transplant premalignant skin disease: a randomized intrapatient comparative study of 5-fluorouracil cream and topical photodynamic therapy

Perrett CM, McGregor JM, Warwick J, et al (Inst of Cell and Molecular Science, London; London Research Labs; Univ of London)
Br J Dermatol 156:320-328, 2007

Background.—Organ transplant recipients (OTR) are at high risk of developing nonmelanoma skin cancer and premalignant epidermal dysplasia (carcinoma in situ/Bowen's disease and actinic keratoses). Epidermal dysplasia is often widespread and there are few comparative studies of available treatments.

Objectives.—To compare topical methylaminolaevulinate (MAL) photodynamic therapy (PDT) with topical 5% fluorouracil (5-FU) cream in the treatment of post-transplant epidermal dysplasia.

Methods.—Eight OTRs with epidermal dysplasia were recruited to an open-label, single-centre, randomized, intrapatient comparative study. Treatment with two cycles of topical MAL PDT 1 week apart was randomly assigned to one area of epidermal dysplasia, and 5-FU cream was applied twice daily for 3 weeks to a clinically and histologically comparable area. Patients were reviewed at 1, 3 and 6 months after treatment. The main outcome measures were complete resolution rate (CRR), overall reduction in lesional area, treatment-associated pain and erythema, cosmetic outcome and global patient preference.

Results.—At all time points evaluated after completion of treatment, PDT was more effective than 5-FU in achieving complete resolution: eight of nine lesional areas cleared with PDT (CRR 89%, 95% CI: 0.52–0.99), compared with one of nine lesional areas treated with 5-FU (CRR 11%, 95% CI: 0.003–0.48) ($P = 0.02$). The mean lesional area reduction was also proportionately greater with PDT than with 5-FU (100% vs. 79% respectively). Cosmetic outcome and patient preference were also superior in the PDT-treated group.

Conclusions.—Compared with topical 5-FU, MAL PDT was a more effective and cosmetically acceptable treatment for epidermal dysplasia in OTRs and was preferred by patients. Further studies are now required to confirm these results and to examine the effect of treating epidermal dysplasia with PDT on subsequent development of squamous cell carcinoma in this high risk population.

▶ The management of precancerous and neoplastic skin lesions in OTRs is often a never-ending and challenging process. The clinician must use a number of modalities to successfully manage these patients. Traditional and new therapies such as topical 5-FU and imiquimod are often ineffective or not well tolerated. Recently topical PDT has shown promise in the management of actinic keratoses (AKs) and superficial carcinomas. In this study, the authors compared the efficacy of topical 5-FU with topical PDT in the management of AKs and carcinoma in situ (CIS) in OTRs. Although topical PDT emerged the winner, a number of observations need to be made. First, the authors used the methyl ester of 5-aminolevulinic acid (5-ALA), which may be more efficacious than 5-ALA. Second, a red light source which penetrates more deeply was used instead of the "Blu Light." Third, the study consisted of only 8 patients. Fourth, with regard to CIS, there was no mention of whether follicular involvement was present. This certainly impacts the response to 5-FU and could likewise impact the response to PDT. Finally, the study was flawed in its design. Topical 5-FU, used twice a day for 3 weeks, may be effective for treating AKs, but it is not going to eradicate many CISs. These lesions often require 12 to 16 weeks of therapy for clearance. Despite these criticisms, PDT does appear to have a role in the management of precancers and cancers of the skin in OTRs. Although the initial pain and tissue reaction may be quite intense, these side effects usually resolve within 1 week, whereas the inflammation induced by topical agents such as 5-FU must be endured for the duration of therapy and longer. This is probably the main advantage of PDT; however, it also obviates the need for the repetitive application of a medication for an extended period.

P. G. Lang Jr, MD

Randomized, double-blind, prospective study to compare topical 5-aminolaevulinic acid methylester with topical 5-aminolaevulinic acid photodynamic therapy for extensive scalp actinic keratosis

Moloney FJ, Collins P (City of Dublin Skin and Cancer Hosp; St Vincent's Univ, Dublin)
Br J Dermatol 157:87-91, 2007

Background.—5-aminolaevulinic acid methylester (MAL) and 5-aminolaevulinic acid (ALA) photodynamic therapy (PDT) are both effective treatment options for actinic keratosis (AK). While MAL is significantly more expensive than ALA, no studies have directly compared their efficacy in the treatment of extensive scalp AK.

Objectives.—To compare the efficacy and adverse effects of MAL-PDT with ALA-PDT in the treatment of scalp AK.

Methods.—Sixteen male patients aged 59–87 years with extensive scalp AK were randomized into a double-blind, split-scalp prospective study. Two treatment fields were defined (right and left frontoparietal scalp) and treated 2 weeks apart. These fields were randomized to receive either MAL or ALA as first or second treatment. MAL cream was applied for 3 h; 20% ALA cream was applied for 5 h. A blinded observer assessed efficacy comparing AK counts before and 1 month after treatment. Pain was assessed using a visual analogue scale at 3, 6, 12 and 16 min.

Results.—Fifteen patients completed treatment to both fields. There was a mean reduction from baseline in AK counts with the use of ALA-PDT of 6.2

± 1.9 compared with 5.6 ± 3.2 with MAL-PDT ($P = 0.588$). All patients experienced pain which was of greater intensity in the ALA-treated side at all time points: 3 min ($P = 0.151$), 6 min ($P = 0.085$), 12 min ($P = 0.012$) and 16 min ($P = 0.029$). Similarly, duration of discomfort post-procedure persisted for longer following treatment with ALA when compared with MAL-PDT ($P = 0.044$).

Conclusions.—This study demonstrates that both ALA-PDT and MAL-PDT result in a significant reduction in scalp AK. There is no significant difference in efficacy. However, ALA-PDT is more painful than MAL-PDT in the treatment of extensive scalp AK.

▶ Several interesting observations can be made from this study. The methylester of 5-ALA has been touted as being more effective than 5-ALA, presumably because of better penetration. However, in this study, no difference in efficacy was noted. In addition, the pain associated with the use of 5-ALA was more intense and prolonged. This could greatly impact patient compliance and acceptance of PDT. It should be noted that a broadband light source (580-740 nm) was utilized for the treatments.

P. G. Lang Jr, MD

Methyl aminolaevulinate–photodynamic therapy: a review of clinical trials in the treatment of actinic keratoses and nonmelanoma skin cancer
Lehmann P (Klinikum der Universität Witten-Herdecke, Wuppertal, Germany)
Br J Dermatol 156:793-801, 2007

Methyl aminolaevulinate–photodynamic therapy (MAL-PDT) has advanced the management of nonmelanoma skin cancer (NMSC), providing a treatment option for actinic keratosis (AK), basal cell carcinoma [both superficial (sBCC) and nodular (nBCC)] and Bowen's disease, with good clinical outcomes, low recurrence rates and enhanced cosmetic acceptability. Excellent results have been reported, with complete responses (CRs) in AK ranging from 69% to 93% at 3 months; CRs in Bowen's disease are 93% at 3 months and 68% at 24 months. In sBCC, CRs range from 85% to 93% at 3 months and are comparable with cryosurgery up to 60 months (75% vs. 74%). In nBCC, CRs range from 75–82% at 3 months to 77% at 60 months. MAL-PDT specifically targets diseased cells, leaving healthy tissue unharmed. This noninvasive treatment option is associated with minimal risk of scarring. Moreover, systemic uptake of MAL is negligible and the local phototoxic reactions that often occur during treatment rapidly heal to produce excellent cosmetic results. The side-effects of therapy, which are predominantly local phototoxic effects (burning, stinging and prickling sensations), are of mild-to-moderate intensity, of short duration and easily managed. Overall, the efficacy and low risk of side-effects afforded by this therapy have resulted in high patient preference in clinical trials. The current evidence base for MAL-PDT in the treatment of AK and NMSC is reviewed in this article.

▶ PDT is increasing in popularity, especially for the treatment of AK. This review summarizes the data available on the use of PDT (MAL as the topical photosensitizer) in the treatment of AK, sBCC and nBCC, and Bowen's disease (BD). The results shown may not be extrapolated to PDT by using aminolevulinic acid (ALA), because MAL may penetrate deeper and be more tumor specific. It may also be less painful. As in other studies, a treatment cycle that includes 2 treatments appears to be more effective. It also appears that a 3-hour incubation period is optimal. Surprisingly, the treatment protocol usually used is one in which the sequential treatments are spaced 1 week apart—a time span during which many patients may not have healed from the initial treatment. One universal observation appears to be that the cosmetic results are generally good to excellent. Not surprisingly, deeper lesions are less likely to be eradicated. Although initial cure rates for a variety of tumors appear to be good, with the passage of time there often is a significant number of recurrences. It is obvious that the author is very enthusiastic about PDT, but this enthusiasm needs to be tempered. Although PDT adds to our armamentarium in the treatment of skin cancer, one needs to be very selective when using this modality.

P G. Lang Jr, MD

Vehicle-controlled, randomized, double-blind study to assess safety and efficacy of imiquimod 5% cream applied once daily 3 days per week in one or two courses of treatment of actinic keratoses on the head
Alomar A, Bichel J, McRae S (Hosp de al Santa Creu i Sant Pau, Barcelona; 3M Medica, Neuss, Germany; 3M Pharmaceuticals, St Paul, Minn)
Br J Dermatol 157:133-141, 2007

Background.—Imiquimod has been investigated as a safe and effective therapeutic option for the treatment of actinic keratosis (AK).

Objectives.—To evaluate imiquimod vs. vehicle applied three times a week for 4 weeks in one or two courses of treatment for AK on the face or balding scalp.

Patients and Methods.—Patients diagnosed with AK were enrolled in this multicentre, vehicle-controlled, double-blind study conducted in Europe. Twenty study centres enrolled a total of 259 patients in this study. Patients applied the study drug for 4 weeks, entered a 4-week rest period and if they did not have complete clearance, they then entered a second course of treatment.

Results.—Patients in the imiquimod group had an overall complete clearance rate of 55.0% (71/129) vs. a rate of 2.3% (3/130) for the vehicle group. There was a high rate of agreement between the clinical assessment and histological findings with respect to AK lesion clearance. At both 8-week posttreatment visits, the negative predictive value of the investigator assessment was 92.2% for clinical assessments vs. histological results.

Conclusions.—A 4-week course of treatment with three times weekly dosing of imiquimod 5% cream, with a repeated course of treatment for those patients who fail to clear after the first course of treatment, is a safe and effective treatment for AK. The overall complete clearance rate (complete clearance after either course 1 or course 2) is comparable to the 16-week treatment regimen, while decreasing drug exposure to the patient and decreasing the overall treatment time.

▶ The authors show that the efficacy of imiquimod cream applied 3 times a week for a 4-week course, with the course being repeated if necessary after a 4-week rest period, is equivalent in efficacy to a continuous 16-week regimen. The intermittent treatment regimen has the advantage of decreased drug exposure and, therefore, decreased cost. Local irritation still does occur and, in fact, may be necessary for a positive treatment response. It is this reviewer's opinion that shorter, more intensive treatment, for example, application every other day or 4 times per week, while associated with a higher incidence of irritation, yields a better therapeutic outcome than a more protracted course of treatment involving less frequent application.

B. H. Thiers, MD

Treatment of Bowen's Disease with Topical 5% Imiquimod Cream: Retrospective Study
Rosen T, Harting M, Gibson M (Baylor College of Medicine)
Dermatol Surg 33:427-432, 2007

Background.—Topical 5% imiquimod cream is an FDA-approved treatment for superficial basal cell carcinomas. It has also been utilized in the treatment of Bowen's disease (squamous cell in situ). The current literature on this subject, however, is scant, and this treatment is only validated by case reports and two small open label studies.

Objective.—The objective was to assess the efficacy of topical 5% imiquimod cream in the treatment of squamous cell in situ in a larger open-label case series.

Methods.—A retrospective study of 49 patients was performed.

Results.—Forty-two of the 49 (86%) patients in the study had a complete response with topical imiquimod. The remaining 7 (14%) failed therapy and required additional treatments. The mean follow-up duration was 19 months, with a range of 1 to 44 months.

Conclusion.—Topical 5% imiquimod cream appears to be clinically beneficial in the treatment of Bowen's disease and should be considered as a treatment option.

▶ This open-label retrospective study evaluated a relatively small number of patients and found topical imiquimod to be effective for the treatment of Bowen's disease. The duration of follow-up was relatively short. In this reviewer's opinion, in the absence of definitive data from large prospective studies, surgical excision will remain the treatment of choice for this condition.

B. H. Thiers, MD

Prolonged Prevention of Squamous Cell Carcinoma of the Skin by Regular Sunscreen Use
van der Pols JC, Williams GM, Pandeya N, et al (Univ of Queensland, Brisbane, Australia; Queensland Inst of Med Research, Brisbane, Australia)
Cancer Epidemiol Biomarkers Prev 15:2546-2548, 2006

Half of all cancers in the United States are skin cancers. We have previously shown in a 4.5-year randomized controlled trial in an Australian community that squamous cell carcinomas (SCC) but not basal cell carcinomas (BCC) can be prevented by regular sunscreen application to the head, neck, hands, and forearms. Since cessation of the trial, we have followed participants for a further 8 years to evaluate possible latency of preventive effect on BCCs and SCCs. After prolonged follow-up, BCC tumor rates tended to decrease but not significantly in people formerly randomized to daily sunscreen use compared with those not applying sunscreen daily. By contrast, corresponding SCC tumor rates were significantly decreased by almost 40% during the entire follow-up period (rate ratio, 0.62; 95% confidence interval, 0.38-0.99). Regular application of sunscreen has prolonged preventive effects on SCC but with no clear benefit in reducing BCC.

▶ Epidemiologic evidence suggests that the exposure profile to UV light differs among patients with BCC and SCC. In general, patients with BCCs give a history of intermittent intense exposure to UV light (a pattern similar to that noted in patients with melanoma), whereas patients with SCCs tend to be outdoor workers who are exposed to UV light on a more regular basis. Van der Pols et al found, perhaps not surprisingly, that the preventive effects of regular sunscreen use differ among the 2 major forms of nonmelanoma skin cancer, with sunscreens being more protective against SCC than with BCC. This result may represent differing pathogenetic pathways for the 2 tumors.

B. H. Thiers, MD

Dietary pattern in association with squamous cell carcinoma of the skin: a prospective study
Ibiebele TI, van der Pols JC, Hughes MC, et al (Queensland Inst of Med Research, Brisbane, Australia; Univ of Queensland, Brisbane, Australia)
Am J Clin Nutr 85:1401-1408, 2007

Background.—The role of diet in the development of skin cancer is inconclusive, and the effect of the combined consumption of foods has never been reported.

Objective.—We prospectively investigated the association between dietary patterns and cutaneous basal cell (BCC) and squamous cell (SCC) carcinoma.

Design.—Principal components analysis of 38 food groups was used to identify dietary patterns in 1360 adults aged 25–75 y who participated in a community-based skin cancer study in Nambour, Australia, between 1992 and 2002. We obtained baseline information about diet, skin color, and sun exposure factors. Multivariate-adjusted relative risks (RRs) for BCC and SCC tumors were estimated by using negative binomial regression modeling.

Results.—Two major dietary patterns were identified: a meat and fat pattern and a vegetable and fruit pattern. The meat and fat pattern was positively associated with development of SCC tumors (RR = 1.83; 95% CI: 1.00, 3.37; P for trend = 0.05) after adjustment for confounders and even more strongly associated in participants with a skin cancer history (RR = 3.77; 95% CI: 1.65, 8.63; P for trend = 0.002) when the third and first tertiles were compared. A higher consumption of the vegetable and fruit dietary pattern appeared to decrease SCC tumor risk by 54% (P for trend = 0.02), but this protective effect was mostly explained by the association with green leafy vegetables. There was no association between the dietary patterns and BCC tumors.

Conclusion.—A dietary pattern characterized by high meat and fat intakes increases SCC tumor risk, particularly in persons with a skin cancer history.

▶ The authors claim to demonstrate that a high intake of meat and fat is associated with an increased risk of developing SCC, even after adjusting for confounding risk factors such as age, sex, skin type, tendency to burn, degree of solar elastosis, history of skin cancer, smoking, and sunscreen use. They do concede that the results do not presume causality. Their data do not suggest an association of dietary patterns with the risk of BCC.

B. H. Thiers, MD

Gene-Drug Interaction at the Glucocorticoid Receptor Increases Risk of Squamous Cell Skin Cancer
Patel AS, Karagas MR, Perry AE, et al (Harvard School of Public Health, Boston; Dartmouth Med School, Lebanon, NH)
J Invest Dermatol 127:1868-1870, 2007

Background.—A rapid increase has been noted in the incidence of nonmelanoma skin cancer (NMSC) among Caucasians in the United States, accounting for more new cases than all other malignancies combined. Although basal cell carcinoma (BCC) is the more common form of NMSC, squamous cell carcinoma (SCC) is more aggressive and often contributes to disease morbidity and mortality. Although NMSC is believed to be induced by UV radiation, certain exposures, including immunosuppressive drugs, can contribute to carcinogenesis. Recent studies have suggested that glucocorticoid-induced immunosuppression may play a role in skin carcinogenesis. Glucocorticoid receptor gene (*NR3C1*) variability has been associated with glucocorticoid hyperresponsiveness, and a common non-coding *Bcl*I restriction fragment length polymorphism has been linked to altered glucocorticoid receptor function, including corticosteroid hyperresponsiveness. The hypothesis that this polymorphism modifies the risk of SCC and BCC associated with glucocorticoid use was tested in a population-based case-control study conducted in New Hampshire.

Methods.—All new cases of NMSC in New Hampshire were identified using an incident survey previously described. Controls were derived from the New Hampshire Department of Transportation and Medicare enrollment lists and were frequency matched to case on the basis of sex and age. Blood samples were obtained for DNA extraction and analysis, and an interview-based questionnaire was used to gather data on sun-exposure histories and other demographic and lifestyle information, including use of glucocorticoids. The study group included 393 controls, 214 SCC, and 443 BCC cases.

Results.—Known risk factors, such as sunburn and skin type, as well as glucocorticoid use were associated with SCC incidence. Among controls, the variant allele (G) frequency was 0.38, and the polymorphism met criteria for Hardy-Weinburg equilibrium. Among SCC cases, glucocorticoid use was associated with increased risk in each genotype strata. The magnitude of the risk increased with the number of gene variant alleles. This trend was not observed among the BCC cases.

Conclusions.—The risk of NMSCs, particularly SCC, is significantly increased by use of long-term immunosuppressive therapy for prevention of allograft rejection.

▶ The association of immunosuppression with skin cancer is well known. Most commonly affected are transplant patients taking drugs, such as cyclosporin and azathioprine that often are combined with glucocorticoids. Some previous studies have suggested an increased risk of SCC in patients taking glucocorticoids alone. Patel et al tested the hypothesis that a polymorphism linked to altered glucocorticoid receptor function may modify the risk of skin cancer, and, indeed, found this to be the case for SCC. This is yet another example of pharmacogenetics having the potential to predict drug responsiveness and, as demonstrated here, potential adverse events.

B. H. Thiers, MD

Expression profile of skin papillomas with high cancer risk displays a unique genetic signature that clusters with squamous cell carcinomas and predicts risk for malignant conversion
Darwiche N, Ryscavage A, Perez-Lorenzo R, et al (American Univ of Beirut, Lebanon; NIH, Bethesda, Md; Pennsylvania State Univ, University Park)
Oncogene 26:6885-6895, 2007

Chemical induction of squamous tumors in the mouse skin induces multiple benign papillomas: high-frequency terminally benign low-risk papillomas and low-frequency high-risk papillomas, the putative precursor lesions to squamous cell carcinoma (SCC). We have compared the gene expression profile of twenty different early low- and high-risk papillomas with normal skin and SCC. Unsupervised clustering of 514 differentially expressed genes ($P<0.001$) showed that 9/10 high-risk papillomas clustered with SCC, while 1/10 clustered with low-risk papillomas, and this correlated with keratin markers of tumor progression. Prediction analysis for microarrays (PAM) identified 87 genes that distinguished the two papilloma classes, and a majority of these had a similar expression pattern in both high-risk papillomas and SCC. Additional classifier algorithms generated a gene list that correctly classified unknown benign tumors as low- or high-risk concordant with promotion protocol and keratin profiling. Reduced expression of immune function genes characterized the high-risk papillomas and SCC. Immunohistochemistry confirmed reduced T-cell number in high-risk papillomas, suggesting that reduced adaptive immunity defines papillomas that progress to SCC. These results demonstrate that murine premalignant lesions can be segregated into subgroups by gene expression patterns that correlate with risk for malignant conversion, and suggest a paradigm for generating diagnostic biomarkers for human premalignant lesions with unknown individual risk for malignant conversion.

▶ Using microarray technology, researchers can simultaneously compare the degree to which hundreds of genes are expressed, that is, converted into proteins. Darwiche et al used microarray technology to identify skin lesions in mice that show a high risk of progression to SCC. They showed that precancerous lesions could be separated into subgroups according to their pattern of gene activity, that is, which genes were turned on and which genes were turned off. A specific pattern of activity, also called the molecular signature, correlated with a high risk for malignant conversion. It is hoped this technique will eventually lead to identification of similar high-risk lesions in humans. Moreover, not only may gene expression analysis of human premalignant lesions serve as a diagnostic biomarker for cancer risk, it also may provide novel therapeutic targets for high-risk lesions.

B. H. Thiers, MD

Squamous cell carcinoma of the nail apparatus: clinicopathological study of 35 cases
Dalle S, Depape L, Phan A, et al (Hôpital de l'Hôtel-Dieu, Lyon, France)
Br J Dermatol 156:871-874, 2007

Background.—Subungual squamous cell carcinoma (SCC) is rare. Its diagnosis is often missed or delayed because the clinical presentation is often atypical and can mimic other conditions such as verruca vulgaris, onychomycosis, trauma-induced nail dystrophy or exostosis.

Objectives.—To define the different clinical presentations and the main pathological features and to evaluate the most appropriate surgical management of subungual SCC.

Methods.—A retrospective review of all the cases of subungual SCC seen in our institution over a 5-year period.

Results.—Thirty-five cases were selected. The spectrum of the clinical features encountered was extremely large including leuconychia, subungual hyperkeratosis, trachonychia, subungual tumoral syndrome, longitudinal erythronychia and melanonychia. Most cases (31 of 35) were invasive. Relapse rate after surgical treatment was low after wide surgical excision (5%) of the nail apparatus or amputation of the digit. However, limited surgical excision led to more frequent relapses (56%).

Conclusions.—Nail apparatus SCC is often misdiagnosed. Most cases are invasive at the time of diagnosis. Wide surgical excision bears a lower risk of relapse. Micrographic surgery should be considered for a better control in cases treated with limited surgical excision.

▶ Squamous cell carcinoma of the nail apparatus is commonly misdiagnosed. Many patients we have seen in our department have initially been misdiagnosed either as onychodystrophy secondary to trauma or fungal nail disease. A careful examination usually will yield clues to the diagnosis, although an adequate surgical biopsy remains the gold standard. Mohs micrographic surgery (MMS) has been proposed to treat this condition; however, the nail is a challenging location because of its unique anatomical and histologic characteristics. Moreover, the use of MMS for nail tumors can be tedious and time consuming, and in the end conservation of a small part of the nail bed may be of little benefit to the patient. In cases with bone infiltration, digital amputation is sometimes recommended. It also must be remembered that metastatic spread can be observed with more aggressive tumors.

B. H. Thiers, MD

Sentinel lymph node biopsy for high risk cutaneous squamous cell carcinoma: Case series and review of the literature
Renzi C, Caggiati A, Mannooranparampil TJ, et al (IDI-IRCSS, Rome; Ospedale Cristo Re, Rome)
EJSO 33:364-369, 2007

Aims.—Cutaneous squamous cell carcinoma (SCC) is the second most common skin cancer. The metastatic potential is generally low. However, there are subgroups of patients at higher risk, for whom sentinel lymph node biopsy (SLNB) might be useful. SLNB might allow the timely inclusion of high risk patients in more aggressive treatment protocols, sparing at the same time node-negative patients the morbidity of potentially unnecessary therapy. Our aim was to introduce the concept of SLNB for patients with high risk cutaneous SCC.

Patients and Methods.—We examined a consecutive series of high risk cutaneous SCC patients undergoing SLNB at our large dermatological hospital, and performed a literature review and pooled analysis of all published cases of SLNB for cutaneous SCC.

Results.—Among the 22 clinically node-negative patients undergoing SLNB at our hospital, one patient (4.5%) showed a histologically positive

TABLE 1.—Positive Sentinel Lymph Node (SLN) Biopsies for Cutaneous SCC Reported in the Literature and Characteristics of Patients with Positive Sentinel Nodes

Study	No. of SLN+ Pts/total Pts Studied (%)	Age of SLN+ Pts	Tumor Location of SLN+ Pts	Tumor Size of SLN+ Pts (cm)	Tumor Depth of SLN+ Pts
Michl, 2003	2/9 (22.2)	52	Presternal	9.0	Subcutis
		78	Lower leg	5.0	Deep dermis
Reschly, 2003	4/9 (44.4)	73	Wrist	4.5	>4 mm
		66	Lower leg	11.0	>4 mm
		41	Clavicle	3.0	>4 mm
		45	Scalp	3.5	>4 mm
Nouri, 2004	1/8 (12.5)	n.a.	Face	n.a.	n.a.
Wagner, 2004	2/11 (18.2)	66	Face	4.5	n.a.
		93	Face	3.0	n.a.
Altinyollar, 2002	3/18 (16.6)	n.a.	Lower lip	>2.0	n.a.
		n.a.	Lower lip	>2.0	n.a.
		n.a.	Lower lip	>2.0	n.a.
Stadelmann, 1997	1/1	72	Wrist	4.0	n.a.
Weisberg, 2000	0/1				
Perez-Naranjo, 2005	0/1				
Ardabili, 2003	0/1				
Yamada, 2004	0/1				
Ozcelik, 2004	0/1				
Renzi[a]	1/22 (4.5)	70	Foot	2.5	>4 mm

SLN = sentinel lymph node; pts = patients; n.a. = not available.
[a]IDI case series.
(Courtesy of Renzi C, Caggiati A, Mannooranparampil TJ, et al. Sentinel lymph node biopsy for high risk cutaneous squamous cell carcinoma: case series and review of the literature. *EJSO.* 2007;33:364-369.)

sentinel node and developed recurrences during follow-up. Sentinel node-negative patients showed no metastases at a median follow-up of 17 months (range: 6–64). The incidence of positive sentinel nodes in previous reports ranged between 12.5% and 44.4% (Table 1). Pooling together patients from the present and previous studies (total 83 patients), we calculated an Odds Ratio of 2.76 (95% CI 1.2–6.5; $p = 0.02$) of finding positive sentinel nodes for an increase in tumor size from <2 cm to 2.1–3 cm to >3 cm.

Conclusions.—Our case series and the pooled analysis support the concept that SLNB can be performed for high risk cutaneous SCC. Prospective multicenter studies are needed to examine the role, utility and cost-effectiveness of SLNB for this population.

▶ Although commonly used in the management of melanoma, the role of SLNB in the management of nonmelanoma skin cancer (NMSC), except for Merkel cell carcinoma, is unclear. Most of the data on the use of the SLNB in the management of NMSC has been derived from studies on SCC. Unfortunately, most of the studies consist of small numbers of patients with short follow-up times. Although these studies support the concept that SLNB is a reliable prognostic indicator, there has been a great deal of variability regarding the incidence of positive SLNBs (Table 1). For this reason, it is difficult to conclude how useful SLNB is in the management of "high risk" SCCs and what patients are suitable candidates for the procedure. This is another small study that examines the role of the SLNB in the management of "high risk" SCCs.

Unfortunately, the conclusions of the authors are similar to those of prior investigators, ie, large multicenter studies will be required to define what constitutes a "high risk" SCC and what role, if any, there is for the use of the SLNB in its management. Similar to our experience, the authors found that the incidence of a positive SLNB was quite low and that it was not possible to predict which patients were at greatest risk.

P. G. Lang, Jr, MD

High-Risk Cutaneous Squamous Cell Carcinoma without Palpable Lymphadenopathy: Is There a Therapeutic Role for Elective Neck Dissection?
Martinez J-C, Cook JL (Duke Univ, Durham, NC)
Dermatol Surg 33:410-420, 2007

Purpose.—The beneficial role of elective neck dissection (END) in the management of high-risk cutaneous squamous cell carcinoma (CSCC) of the head and neck remains unproven. Some surgical specialists suggest that END may be beneficial for patients with clinically node-negative (N0) high-risk CSCC, but there are few data to support this claim. We reviewed the available literature regarding the use of END in the management of both CSCC and head and neck SCC (HNSCC).

Methodology.—The available medical literature pertaining to END in both CSCC and HNSCC was reviewed using PubMed and Ovid Medline searches.

Results.—Many surgical specialists recommend that END be routinely performed in patients with N0 HNSCC when the risk of occult metastases is estimated to exceed 20%; however, patients who undergo END have no proven survival benefit over those who are initially staged as N0 and undergo therapeutic neck dissection (TND) after the development of apparent regional disease. There is a lack of data regarding the proper management of regional nodal basins in patients with N0 CSCC. In the absence of evidence-based data, the cutaneous surgeon must rely on clinical judgment to guide the management of patients with N0 high-risk CSCC of the head and neck.

Conclusions.—Appropriate work-up for occult nodal disease may occasionally be warranted in patients with high-risk CSCC. END may play a role in only a very limited number of patients with high-risk CSCC.

▶ With the advent of the sentinel lymph node biopsy (SLNB), and because most studies have not supported a survival advantage of END in the management of several different malignancies, one must question why one would consider performing an END, especially for a CSCC. On the other hand, there are good data supporting the performance of a parotidectomy when a CSCC invades the parotid gland.

P. G. Lang, Jr, MD

Mohs Micrographic Surgery in the Treatment of Rare Aggressive Cutaneous Tumors: The Geisinger Experience

Thomas CJ, Wood GC, Marks VJ (Geisinger Med Ctr, Danville, Pa)
Dermatol Surg 33:333-339, 2007

Background.—Mohs micrographic surgery (MMS) offers high cure rates and maximum tissue preservation in the treatment of more common cutaneous malignancies, but its effectiveness in rare aggressive tumors is poorly defined.

Objective.—Evaluate the effectiveness of MMS in the treatment of six rare aggressive cutaneous malignancies as seen by Mohs surgeons working at a referral center.

Methods.—Retrospective chart review of 26,000 cases treated with MMS at the Geisinger Medical Center Department of Dermatology during a 16-year period with the following diagnoses: poorly differentiated squamous cell carcinoma (PDSCC), dermatofibrosarcoma protuberans (DFSP), microcystic adnexal carcinoma (MAC), extramammary Paget's disease (EMPD), Merkel cell carcinoma (MCC), and sebaceous carcinoma (SEB CA). Patient demographic data, tumor measurements, treatment characteristics, and marginal recurrence rates were compiled and evaluated.

Results.—The mean numbers of cases identified per year for each tumor type were as follows: PDSCC, 6.19; DFSP, 2.44; MAC, 1.63; and EMPD, 0.63. For PDSCC, 85 cases were available for follow-up with a local recurrence rate of 6% at a mean follow-up time of 45 months. For DFSP, there were 35 cases with no local recurrence at a mean follow-up of 39 months. For MAC, there were 25 cases with a local recurrence rate of 12% at a mean follow-up of 39 months. For EMPD, there were 10 cases with no local recurrences at a mean follow-up of 34 months.

Conclusions.—Collectively, our data on PDSCC, DFSP, MAC, and EMPD, combined with other studies in the literature, show that MMS is the most effective therapy for these rare aggressive cutaneous malignancies.

▶ This is an important study that demonstrates the effectiveness of Mohs surgery in the treatment of aggressive tumors of the skin, some of which are quite uncommon. Unfortunately, only a few cases of MCC and SEB CA were treated. This study also demonstrates that when PDSCC and MAC have previously been treated and recur, they are much more difficult to cure, even with Mohs surgery. This would suggest that adjunctive therapy should be considered in selected cases.

P. G. Lang, Jr, MD

Expression profiles associated with aggressive behavior in Merkel cell carcinoma

Fernández-Figueras M-T, Puig L, Musulén E, et al (Autonomous Univ of Barcelona)
Mod Pathol 20:90-101, 2007

Primary neuroendocrine carcinoma of the skin, or Merkel cell carcinoma, is the most aggressive cutaneous neoplasm. In spite of its similarities to small cell carcinomas from other locations, Merkel cell carcinoma shows many peculiarities probably related to its epidermal origin and the etiologic role of UV radiation. We have immunohistochemically investigated 43 markers on a tissue microarray in which 31 surgically resected Merkel cell carcinomas were represented. Of these, 15 patients remained free of disease after removal, whereas 16 developed metastases. Immunoreactivity was scored according to staining intensity and the percentage of positive cells. We found statistically significant correlations between metastatic tumor spread and overexpression of matrix metalloproteinase (MMP) 7, MMP10/2, tissue inhibitor of metalloproteinase 3, vascular endothelial growth factor (VEGF), P38, stromal NF-kappaB, and synaptophysin. Also detected were statistically significant correlations between the expression levels of MMP7 and VEGF, MMP7 and P21, MMP7 and P38, MMP10/2 and VEGF, P38 and synaptophysin, P38 and P53, and P21 and stromal NF-kappaB. These findings may be helpful in predicting the clinical course of Merkel cell carcinoma and are potentially useful for the development of targeted therapies.

▶ Fernández-Figueras et al attempted to correlate the overexpression of certain cell markers with metastatic potential in patients with Merkel cell carcinoma. In addition to predicting the clinical course of the disease, the authors suggest that these markers might prove to be inviting targets for future therapies for this challenging and aggressive tumor. Like melanoma, Merkel cell carcinoma can be invasive and metastasize. Also like melanoma, early diagnosis and excision appear to offer the best hope for cure.

B. H. Thiers, MD

Prognostic Value of Tumor Thickness in Patients With Merkel Cell Carcinoma

Goldberg SR, Neifeld JP, Frable WJ (Virginia Commonwealth Univ, Richmond)
J Surg Oncol 95:618-622, 2007

Background and Objectives.—Merkel cell carcinoma is an aggressive skin malignancy that often presents with tumor metastases. We hypothesized that tumor thickness might correlate with both regional and metastatic tumor spread and could, therefore, be used as an independent prognostic variable. The purpose of this study was to see if depth of tumor invasion would predict prognosis independent of tumor stage.

Methods.—Data pertaining to clinical presentation, pathology, treatment, and survival were collected for patients diagnosed with Merkel cell carcinoma from 1972 to 2005. Patients were staged according to AJCC guidelines. Pathologic specimens were evaluated for tumor thickness. The relationship between tumor thickness and disease-free survival or overall survival was analyzed using Kaplan–Meier survival analyses.

Results.—Sixty patients were identified. Five-year disease-free survivals for Stages 1, 2, and 3 patients were 20%, 33%, and 0%, respectively. Five-year overall survivals for Stages 1, 2, and 3 patients were 33.3%, 60%, and 16.7%, respectively. There was no correlation between tumor thickness and either disease-free survival or overall survival.

Conclusions.—This study suggests that tumor thickness is not an independent risk factor for survival. Mean tumor thickness did increase with the AJCC stages, but this most likely represents more advanced stage of disease.

▶ The supposed purpose of this study was to determine whether there was a correlation between tumor thickness and disease-free (DFS) and overall survival (OS) in patients with Merkel cell carcinoma (MCC). However, most of the discussion centered on deficiencies in the AJCC staging system for MCC. Moreover, the authors did not go into detail regarding their definition of thickness and how this was determined. Nevertheless, they found no correlation between tumor thickness and DFS and OS. Unlike melanoma, where tumor thickness reflects depth of invasion, in MCC the tumor is already present in the dermis. It is thus already well positioned to invade lymphatics and blood vessels and subsequently metastasize. Clearly, any impact tumor "thickness" might have is overshadowed by the location of the tumor in the dermis and subcutaneous tissue.

P. G. Lang, Jr, MD

Sentinel lymph node mapping for patients with Merkel cell carcinoma—experience of 5 years

Liebau J, Arens A, Schwipper V, et al (Fachklinik Hornheide at the Westfalian Wilhelms Univ, Münster, Germany)
Eur J Plast Surg 29:107-109, 2006

Background.—Merkel cell carcinoma (MCC) is a rare, highly malignant carcinoma of the neuroendocrinologic system first described by Toker in 1972. MCC is a fast-growing, red or blue skin lesion that sometimes occurs with superficial eruptions, frequently on the face of older patients. The local recurrence rate and rate of lymphatic metastases are high (45% to 65%, respectively after 1 year). Retrospective studies of the literature have identified several factors with a prognostic disadvantage, including male sex, localization of the primary tumor to the extremities and trunk, small cell type, age less than 60 years, and metastases at the time of diagnosis. The purpose of the present report was to describe the prognostic factor of sentinel lymph node (SLN) mapping for MCC.

Methods.—From 1986 to 2004, 152 patients with MCC stages 1 to 3 were treated at one clinic. The patients ranged in age from 37 to 96 years, with the average age being 69.3 years. From 1999 to 2004, 12 patients (11 women, 1 man) with MCC stage 1 underwent SLN evaluation in addition to the regular radical tumor resection with a 3-cm margin. Clinical exclusion of lymphatic metastases with ultrasound and staging examinations was performed initially. Head and neck tumors were present in 7 patients, and 4 patients had tumors of the upper extremities. One patient had a tumor of the lower extremity.

Results.—In 9 of the 12 patients, SLN was negative. One patient had a locoregional recurrence, which was resected and treated with postoperative radiotherapy. Locoregional lymphadenectomies were performed in the other 3 patients with positive SLN findings. All 3 patients had regional and systemic metastases in less than 1 year and had to undergo reoperation and/or treatment with radiotherapy or chemotherapy.

Conclusions.—Early diagnosis of MCC is the most important prognostic factor. Additional beneficial factors are being female and having the lesion in the head and neck area. The therapy of choice is radical surgical excision. Careful local and regional control is essential for achievement of long-term survival. The SLN technique is a valuable staging method for detection of metastases before local lymph node dissection. Its value as a prognostic factor has yet to be evaluated.

▶ Previous studies on sentinel lymph node (SLN) biopsy in patients with Merkel cell carcinoma (MCC) have demonstrated that (1) the SLN can be reliably identified, (2) SLN biopsy is useful as a staging tool, and (3) SLN biopsy is useful as a prognostic indicator. The authors of this study and a study by Ortin-Perez and colleagues[1] share their experience in managing their MCC patients using SLN biopsy. Interestingly, neither group used postoperative irradiation, which is thought by many to decrease the incidence of local recurrence. The experience of the two groups is somewhat contrasting, in that in this study recurrent disease developed in patients with a positive SLN biopsy, whereas in the Ortin-Perez et al study such patients uniformly did well, a result that is also inconsistent with previously published studies. There does not appear to be an obvious explanation for this finding.

P. G. Lang, Jr, MD

Reference

1. Ortin-Perez J, van Rijk MC, Valdes-Olmos RA, et al. Lymphatic mapping and sentinel node biopsy in Merkel's cell carcinoma. *EJSO.* 2007;33:119-122.

Lymphatic mapping and sentinel node biopsy in Merkel's cell carcinoma

Ortin-Perez J, van Rijk MC, Valdes-Olmos RA, et al (Univ of Barcelona; The Netherlands Cancer Inst/Antoni van Leeuwenhoek Hosp, Amsterdam; Institut d'Investigacions Biomèdiques August Pi i Sunyer (IDIBAPS), Barcelona)
EJSO 33:119-122, 2007

Aim.—The purpose of this study was to determine the predictive value of lymphatic mapping with selective lymphadenectomy in patients with Merkel's cell carcinoma.

Methods.—Eight patients with biopsy proven Merkel's cell carcinoma underwent sentinel node biopsy. Lymphoscintigraphy was performed the day before surgery following intradermal injection of 74–111MBq of 99mTc-nanocolloid divided into four doses around the biopsy scar. Dynamic and static images were obtained.

Results.—At least one sentinel node was visualized in all patients. The sentinel node was intra-operatively identified with the aid of a hand-held gamma probe in all cases and patent blue dye in six out of eight cases. During surgery, all sentinel nodes were successfully harvested. Metastatic cell deposits were subsequently identified in three patients (37.5%) and they underwent regional lymphadenectomy. No additional involved lymph nodes were identified. No recurrence has been reported in a median follow-up of 4.6 years (range: 8 months–10 years).

Conclusions.—In conclusion, sentinel node biopsy in patients with Merkel's cell carcinoma appears to be a reliable staging technique.

▶ Previous studies on sentinel lymph node (SLN) biopsy in patients with Merkel's cell carcinoma (MCC) have demonstrated that (1) the SLN can be reliably identified, (2) SLN biopsy is useful as a staging tool, and (3) SLN biopsy is useful as a prognostic indicator. The authors of this study and a study by Liebau and colleagues[1] share their experience in managing their MCC patients using SLN biopsy. Interestingly, neither group used postoperative irradiation, which is thought by many to decrease the incidence of local recurrence. The experience of the 2 groups is somewhat contrasting in that in the Liebau et al study[1] recurrent disease developed in patients with a positive SLN biopsy, whereas in the study discussed here, such patients uniformly did well, a result that is also inconsistent with previously published studies. There does not appear to be an obvious explanation for this finding.

P. G. Lang, Jr, MD

Reference

1. Liebau J, Arens A, Schwipper V, Schulz A. Sentinel lymph node mapping for patients with Merkel cell carcinoma—experience of 5 years. *Eur J Plast Surg.* 2006;29:107-109.

Merkel Cell Carcinoma: Assessing the Effect of Wide Local Excision, Lymph Node Dissection, and Radiotherapy on Recurrence and Survival in Early-Stage Disease—Results From a Review of 82 Consecutive Cases Diagnosed Between 1992 and 2004

Jabbour J, Cumming R, Scolyer RA, et al (Sydney Cancer Centre; Univ of Sydney; St Vincent's Hosp, Sydney; et al)
Ann Surg Oncol 14:1943-1952, 2007

Background.—Wide surgical excision, lymph node dissection, and radiotherapy have been used with varying efficacy in the management of early-stage Merkel cell carcinoma.

Methods.—Records of 82 patients with early-stage Merkel cell carcinoma between 1992 and 2004 were reviewed.

Results.—Forty-two patients developed a recurrence, and 44 died during the study period. Twenty-nine patients presented with regional lymph node disease, which was independently associated with diminished survival (hazard ratio [HR], 4.08; 95% confidence interval [CI], 1.55–10.75; P = .005). Lymphadenectomy was independently associated with prolonged disease-free survival (median, 28.5 vs. 11.8 months; HR, .46; 95% CI, .22–.94; P = .034) but not overall survival (P = .25). Margin-negative excision of the primary tumor (60 of 73) was not significantly associated with either prolonged disease-free survival (median, 16 vs. 14 months) or overall survival (median, 54 vs. 34 months). Forty-eight patients received radiotherapy: 36 to the primary site and 31 to the regional lymph nodes. Radiotherapy to both sites was associated with a longer median time to first recurrence (primary site, 24.2 vs. 11.8 months; regional lymph nodes, 46.2 vs. 11.3 months) and survival (primary site, 53.9 vs. 45.7 months; regional lymph nodes, 103.1 vs. 34.2 months). Administration of any radiotherapy was significantly associated with a prolonged time to first recurrence (HR, .39; 95% CI, .20–.75; P = .004) and survival (HR, .39; 95% CI, .18–.82; P = .013) on the Cox regression multivariate analyses.

Conclusions.—Adjuvant radiotherapy to the primary site after surgical excision is recommended in early-stage disease. Involved regional lymph nodes should be treated with radiotherapy with or without lymphadenectomy.

▶ The role or benefit of adjunctive radiation therapy in the management of early-stage Merkel cell carcinoma has been somewhat controversial; however, there have been a number of studies that suggest it enhances local control of disease. The major contribution of this article is the fact that it demonstrates that postoperative radiation to the operative site and regional nodes not only improve disease-free survival but also overall survival.

P. G. Lang, Jr, MD

Photodynamic therapy using a methyl ester of 5-aminolevulinic acid in recurrent Paget's disease of the vulva: A pilot study

Raspagliesi F, Fontanelli R, Rossi G, et al (Istituto Nazionale Tumori, Milan, Italy)
Gynecol Oncol 103:581-586, 2006

Objective.—In the past, treating vulvar Paget's disease through surgery has resulted in a high recurrence rate of the disease. Photodynamic therapy (PDT) using 5-aminolevulinic acid (5 ALA) is an effective treatment for some conditions such as Bowen's disease, subsets of basal cell carcinomas and vulvar carcinoma. Methyl 5-aminolevulinate (MAL) is an ester of 5 ALA that seems to be more effective and produces fewer side effects than 5 ALA. This paper outlines a pilot study designed to test the feasibility of using MAL-PDT in the treatment of recurrent vulvar Paget's disease.

Methods.—5 MAL-PDT was applied for 3 h and than irradiated with red-light (620 nm) using a total light dose of 37 J/cm^2 for a period of 10 min. Patients taking part in the study were treated once every 3 weeks, for a total of three treatments. Vulvar biopsies were obtained before and 1 month after the PDT-treatment.

Results.—Seven patients were enrolled in the study. Four cases had a complete clinical response, and this was pathologically confirmed in two of the cases. The cosmetic outcome was acceptable and the treatment was well tolerated. All the patients developed local edema and mild local pain, controlled with non-steroidal antiinflammatory drugs (NSAIDS). One patient experienced severe pain and a mild local phototoxicity reaction.

Conclusions.—MAL-PDT is a feasible treatment and seems to offer a reliable strategy in the control of vulvar Paget's disease and of its symptoms (Table 1).

▶ Extramammary Paget's disease (EMPD) is a difficult neoplasm to manage. Frequently, treatment is delayed because of misdiagnosis, and by the time the patient is correctly diagnosed, the disease may be quite extensive. Thus, the patient may be inoperable, or the surgery required to render the patient tumor-free may be mutilating and associated with significant morbidity. Consequently, there is a real need for alternative forms of therapy. Surgery remains the treatment of choice; however, routine surgical excision with conventional pathologic examination of the tissue is associated with a significant recurrence rate. Mohs microscopic surgery, with its more exacting margin control, yields much higher cure rates, although it has the drawbacks of considerable discomfort when performed with local anesthesia and can become quite time consuming when multiple stages are required to render the patient tumor free. Superficial destruction often fails because of the extension of tumor along the adnexal structures. This may be 1 reason laser surgery is often unsuccessful. Although not specifically addressed in this article, this could also explain why there were so few complete responses in the study reported here by Raspagliesi et al (Table 1). If topical PDT (TPDT) is being contemplated as a way to treat a patient with EMPD, numerous scouting biopsies should be done to

TABLE 1.—Clinical Characteristics of the Patients With Recurrent EMPD Treated With PDT

Patient	Age	No. Recurrence	Previous Therapy	Site of Last Recurrence	Percent of Involved Area	Diameters (cm)	Size of the Lesion After PDT Applications (cm)			Clinical Response	Histological Control of Response	Follow-up (Months)
							1st	2nd	3rd			
1	55	2	2 Surgical excisions, 4 Laser excisions	Mucosal vulvar	>50%	5 × 4	3 × 3	3 × 1.5	0	CR	NA	5
2	60	8	8 Laser excisions	Cutaneous perianal	<50%	3.5 × 3	3 × 2.5	3 × 1.5	3 × 1.5	NC	POS	4
				Mucosal vulvar		2 × 7	5 × 1.5	5 × 1.5	5 × 1.5	NC	POS	
3	57	1	1 Surgical excision, 3 Laser excisions	Mucosal vulvar	<50%	3.5 × 2	2.5 × 1.5	2 × 1.5	0	CR	NEG	4
4	67	2	2 Surgical excisions	Cutaneous perianal	>50%	1.5 × 1	1 × 0.8	1 × 0.8	0	CR	NEG	4
				Mucosal vulvar		6 × 3	6 × 1.5	3 × 1.5	0	CR	NEG	
5	59	5	2 Surgical excisions, 4 Laser excisions	Cutaneous perianal	>50%	4 × 3	2 × 2	1.5 × 1.2	0	CR	NEG	2
				Mucosal vulvar		5 × 3	2 × 2.5	2 × 1	0	CR	POS	
6	69	2	1 Surgical excision, 2 Laser excisions	Mucosal vulvar	<50%	2.5 × 2.5	1.5 × 1.5	1.5 × 1.5	0	CR	POS	1
7	75	2	1 Laser excision	Cutaneous vulvar	>50%	6 × 3	4 × 2	4 × 1.5	0	PR	POS	1
				Axillar		4.5 × 4	3 × 3	3 × 2.5	0	CR	NA	

PDT: photodynamic therapy; POS: positive; NA: not available; CR: Complete response; PR: partial response; NC: no change.
(Courtesy of Raspagliesi F, Fontanelli R, Rossi G, et al. Photodynamic therapy using a methyl ester of 5-aminolevulinic acid in recurrent Paget's disease of the vulva: a pilot study. *Gynecol Oncol.* 2006;103:581-586. Copyright Elsevier, 2006.)

assess (1) the lateral extent of disease, (2) the extent of adnexal involvement, and (3) the presence of invasive disease or of an underlying adenocarcinoma. If disease is not confined to the epidermis, then alternative forms of therapy should be considered. One form of therapy not mentioned by the authors is the use of imiquimod, which has been successfully used in the management of EMPD. On a cautionary note, imiquimod requires more prolonged treatment and can be associated with severe irritation and discomfort. Therefore, until more data are accumulated, surgery should remain the treatment of choice in a viable surgical candidate, and treatments, such as TPDT, should be reserved for patients who refuse surgery, have inoperable disease, or in whom mutilating surgery would be required for cure. In these circumstances, even when the TPDT is not curative, it appears to provide significant symptomatic relief, especially in the associated pruritus. The major weaknesses of this study are (1) the small number of patients reported and (2) the short duration of follow-up.

P. G. Lang, Jr, MD

The outcomes of patients with positive margins after excision for intra-epithelial Paget's disease of the vulva
Black D, Tornos C, Soslow RA, et al (Memorial Sloan-Kettering Cancer Ctr, New York)
Gynecol Oncol 104:547-550, 2007

Objectives.—Vulvar Paget's disease is a rare neoplasm that usually occurs in postmenopausal women. Treatment with surgical excision can be complicated by extension of microscopic disease in an irregular manner well beyond the visible margins of the lesion. The objective or our study was to analyze the outcomes of patients with primary vulvar intraepithelial Paget's disease who had positive microscopic margins after primary excision.

Methods.—We reviewed the records of all patients with Paget's disease of the vulva treated at our institution from 1/80 to 9/02. Patients whose sample showed stromal invasion or an underlying carcinoma were excluded. Data were collected regarding patient demographics, disease location, treatment, surgical margin status, additional treatment, and clinical outcome.

Results.—The medical records and histopathologic specimens of 28 women with intraepithelial Paget's disease of the vulva were evaluated. Surgical treatment consisted of radical vulvectomy in 3 patients (11%), simple vulvectomy in 18 patients (64%), and wide local excision in the other 7 patients (25%). Of the 20 patients with microscopically positive margins, 14 (70%) developed recurrent disease and the remaining 6 (30%) are disease free. Of the 8 patients with negative margins, 3 (38%) developed disease recurrence and the remaining 5 (63%) are disease free. With a median follow-up of 49 months (range, 3–186 months), there was no correlation between disease recurrence and margin status ($P=0.20$). Of the 17 patients who recurred, 14 (82%) underwent additional surgical excision and 1 patient was treated with Retin-A. The remaining 2 patients refused further treatment and were lost to follow-up. In those patients who underwent surgery for recurrence, between 1 and 3 re-excisions were performed. Of the 15 evaluable patients who were treated for recurrent disease, 12 (80%) had no evidence of persistent disease and 3 (20%) had persistent disease at a median follow-up of 63.7 months (range, 18.5–186 months).

Conclusions.—Microscopically positive margins following surgical excision of vulvar intraepithelial Paget's disease is a frequent finding, and disease recurrence is common regardless of surgical margin status. Long-term monitoring of patients is recommended, and repeat surgical excision is often necessary.

▶ Extramammary Paget's disease is a difficult neoplasm to treat. Because of subclinical spread, it often requires an extensive resection to obtain clear margins. In this study the authors report that the achievement of tumor-free margins has no effect on the incidence of recurrence. Their explanation for this is that the disease is multicentric and clear margins may have little clinical relevance. Furthermore, they report that not all patients with margin involvement have recurrent disease develop, although the length of follow-up is not given. To this reviewer, it is no surprise that some patients with clear margins experience recurrence. Although in some cases this could be due to multicentric disease, it is more likely because of the inadequacy of standard vertical sectioning routinely used in the pathologic examination of excised specimens. This is why Mohs surgery offers a much better chance of cure. Why, not all tumors with margin involvement that recur, can be explained by (1) inadequate follow-up time and (2) postulating that the tumor was actually totally excised, albeit only with several microns of surrounding normal skin. Invasive Paget's disease is associated with a significant risk of metastasis and death; thus, when possible, every attempt to obtain clear margins should be made.

P. G. Lang, Jr, MD

17 Nevi and Melanoma

Dermoscopy report: Proposal for standardization. Results of a consensus meeting of the International Dermoscopy Society
Malvehy J, Puig S, Argenziano G, et al (Hosp Clinic, Barcelona; Second Univ of Naples, Italy; Mem Sloan-Kettering Cancer Ctr; et al)
J Am Acad Dermatol 57:84-95, 2007

Background.—Dermoscopy can assist clinicians in the evaluation and diagnosis of skin tumors. Since dermoscopy is becoming widely accepted and used in the medical community, there is now the need for a standardized method for documenting dermoscopic findings so as to be able to effectively communicate such information among colleagues.

Objectives.—Toward this end, the International Dermoscopy Society embarked on creating a consensus document for the standardization and recommended criteria necessary to be able to effectively convey dermoscopic findings to consulting physicians and colleagues.

Methods.—The Dermoscopy Report Steering Committee created an extensive list of dermoscopic criteria obtained from an exhaustive search of the literature. A preliminary document listing all the dermoscopic criteria that could potentially be included in a standardized dermoscopy report was elaborated and presented to the members of the International Dermoscopy Society Board in two meetings of the Society and subsequently discussed via Internet communications between members and the Steering Committee.

Results.—A consensus document including 10 points categorized as either recommended or optional and a template of the dermoscopy report were obtained. The final items included in the document are as follows: (1) patient's age, relevant history pertaining to the lesion, pertinent personal and family history (recommended); (2) clinical description of the lesion (recommended); (3) the two-step method of dermoscopy differentiating melanocytic from nonmelanocytic tumors (recommended); (4) the use of standardized terms to describe structures as defined by the Dermoscopy Consensus Report published in 2003. For new terms it would be helpful to provide a working definition (recommended); (5) the dermoscopic algorithm used should be mentioned (optional); (6) information on the imaging equipment and magnification (recommended); (7) clinical and dermoscopic images of the tumor (recommended); (8) a diagnosis or differential diagnosis (recommended); (9) decision concerning the management (recommended);

(10) specific comments for the pathologist when excision and histopathologic examination are recommended (optional).

Limitations.—The limitations of this study are those that are intrinsic of a consensus document obtained from critical review of the literature and discussion by opinion leaders in the field.

Conclusions.—Although it may be acceptable for a consulting physician to only state the dermoscopic diagnosis, the proposed standardized reporting system, if accepted and utilized, will make it easier for consultants to communicate with each other more effectively.

▶ This report contains a wealth of information for the dermoscopist along with numerous tables and algorithms that are too lengthy to be reprinted here. Any physician engaged in dermoscopy should certainly consult the original article. Malvehy et al provide guidelines that improve the quality of the dermoscopic examination. They advocate a standardized reporting system to make it easier for physicians to communicate with each other more effectively.

B. H. Thiers, MD

The CASH (color, architecture, symmetry, and homogeneity) algorithm for dermoscopy

Henning JS, Dusza SW, Wang SQW, et al (New York Univ; Army Med Dept Ctr and School, Fort Sam Houston, Tex; Skin and Cancer Associates, Plantation, Fla)
J Am Acad Dermatol 56:45-52, 2007

Background.—The color, architecture, symmetry, and homogeneity (CASH) algorithm for dermoscopy includes a feature not used in prior algorithms, namely, architecture. Architectural order/disorder is derived from current concepts regarding the biology of benign versus malignant melanocytic neoplasms (Fig 2).

Objective.—We sought to evaluate the accuracy of the CASH algorithm.

Methods.—A total CASH score (TCS) was calculated for dermoscopic images of 325 melanocytic neoplasms. Sensitivity, specificity, diagnostic accuracy, and receiver operating characteristic curve analyses were performed by comparing the TCS with the histopathologic diagnoses for all lesions.

Results.—The mean TCS was 12.28 for melanoma, 7.62 for dysplastic nevi, and 5.24 for nondysplastic nevi. These differences were statistically significant ($P < .001$). A TCS of 8 or more yielded a sensitivity of 98% and specificity of 68% for the diagnosis of melanoma.

Limitations.—This is a single-evaluator pilot study. Additional studies are needed to verify the CASH algorithm.

Conclusions.—The CASH algorithm can distinguish melanoma from melanocytic nevi with sensitivity and specificity comparable with other algorithms. Further study is warranted to determine its intraobserver and interobserver correlations.

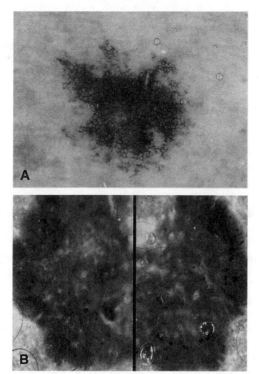

FIGURE 2.—Dermoscopic images showing: architecturally ordered lesion yet asymmetrical in orientation (diagnosis: lentigo simplex) (**A**) and monoaxial symmetric lesion (*black line*) yet markedly architecturally disordered (diagnosis: melanoma) (**B**). (Courtesy of Henning JS, Dusza SW, Wang SW, et al. The CASH [color, architecture, symmetry, and homogeneity] algorithm for dermoscopy. *J Am Acad Dermatol.* 2007;56:45-52. Copyright Elsevier, 2007.)

▶ Several algorithms have been proposed for the use of dermoscopy in evaluating pigmented lesions of the skin. In the current article, Henning et al evaluate the addition of architectural disorder into another scoring system: color, architecture, symmetry and homogeneity (CASH). They found that the CASH algorithm could distinguish benign from malignant melanocytic neoplasms with a level of sensitivity, specificity, and diagnostic accuracy comparable to those with other published dermoscopic algorithms. The CASH algorithm will be subjected to an Internet consensus meeting analysis, an evaluation tool that has been successfully used with other proposed algorithms.[1]

B. H. Thiers, MD

Reference

1. Argenziano G, Soyer HP, Talamini R, et al. Dermoscopy of pigmented skin lesions: results of a consensus meeting via the Internet. *J Am Acad Dermatol.* 2003;48: 679-692.

Melanomas That Failed Dermoscopic Detection: A Combined Clinicodermoscopic Approach for Not Missing Melanoma

Puig S, Argenziano G, Zalaudek I, et al (Hosp Clínic i Provincial de Barcelona; Second Univ of Naples, Italy; Med Univ of Graz, Austria; et al)
Dermatol Surg 33:1262-1273, 2007

Objective.—The objective was to describe the clinical and dermoscopic characteristics of difficult-to-diagnose melanomas (DDM).

Design.—This study was a retrospective analysis of clinical data and dermoscopic images in a series of excised melanomas.

Setting.—Cases were obtained from the database registers of three public hospitals in Barcelona (Spain), Naples (Italy), and Graz (Austria).

Patients.—A total of 97 tumors with a main preoperative diagnosis different from melanoma and without sufficient criteria to be diagnosed clinically and dermoscopically as melanoma were studied. We studied clinical data from the patients and lesions, mean reason for excision, and consensus dermoscopic description of the lesions according to pattern analysis performed by a panel of four dermoscopists to obtain clues that allow these melanomas to be recognized.

Results.—Ninety-three DDMs were evaluated. Three main dermoscopic categories of DDM have been identified: (1) DDMs lacking specific features (16/97), (2) DDMs simulating nonmelanocytic lesions (14/93), and (3) DDMs simulating benign melanocytic proliferations (67/93). The reasons for excision were (1) the subjective history of change referred by the patient (38% of cases), (2) the presence of clinical and/or dermoscopic "hints" for biopsy (33% of cases), and (3) the objective evidence of changes detected by digital dermoscopic follow-up (29% of cases).

Conclusions.—A diagnostic algorithm is proposed not to miss melanoma.

▶ Even the most enthusiastic dermoscopist will admit that the technique is not 100% accurate, and it is estimated that 5% to 10% of melanomas are difficult to diagnose by dermoscopy. Unfortunately, little is known about the clinical and dermoscopic features of these tumors. Puig et al defined DDMs as those tumors that were not thought to be melanomas at the time of excisional biopsy. They sought to analyze the clinical data, dermoscopic characteristics, and the reasons leading to biopsy of these lesions. They found that most of these lesions did have certain clinical or dermoscopic features that aroused suspicion leading to the decision to biopsy. They also proposed certain rules to help identify these features and suggested a diagnostic algorithm to minimize the possibility of misdiagnosing a melanoma. Unfortunately, this was a retrospective study and the real impact on accurate melanoma diagnosis is uncertain.

B. H. Thiers, MD

The impact of total body photography on biopsy rate in patients from a pigmented lesion clinic

Risser J, Pressley Z, Veledar E, et al (Emory Univ, Atlanta, Ga; Atlanta Dept of Veterans Affairs Med Ctr, Ga)
J Am Acad Dermatol 57:428-434, 2007

Background.—Total body cutaneous photography is increasingly being used by dermatologists to monitor patients at risk for the development of melanoma, but limited evidence exists regarding the impact of such photography on melanoma and melanoma-related outcomes.

Objective.—We sought to compare biopsy number in patients with multiple atypical nevi in their first year of care at our pigmented lesion clinic (PLC) between those who received total body skin examination alone and those who received total body skin examination and total body digital photography (TBDP). We sought to identify predictors of biopsy number and number of dysplastic nevi diagnosed in patients with multiple atypical nevi.

Methods.—A chart review was performed of patients attending the PLC during the years 1998 to 2003 to identify the number of biopsies performed in the first year of care. Patient demographics, melanoma risk factors, and melanoma outcome events were also abstracted from the charts.

Results.—The mean number of biopsies performed in patients in their first year of care at the PLC in those who did not receive TBDP was equal to the mean number of biopsies performed in patients who did receive TBDP (0.82 and 0.8, respectively). Linear regression analysis revealed that the interaction term between a lack of both personal history of melanoma and severe dysplastic nevi (-0.930, $P = .005$) has a significant protective effect on the number of biopsies. Similar regression analysis also showed that the interaction term between a lack of both personal history of melanoma and of severe dysplastic nevi (-1.209, $P < .0001$), increasing provider experience (-0.047, $P = .029$), and increased number of biopsies before the initial PLC (-0.028, $P = .050$) have a statistically significant protective effect on the number of dysplastic nevi diagnosed in the first year of PLC. TBDP did not have an effect on the number of biopsies or on the number of dysplastic nevi diagnosed in the first year of care at the PLC.

Limitations.—This study is limited by being retrospective in nature, having a small sample size, and having a short follow-up period.

Conclusion.—Overall, this small retrospective study does not provide evidence that would suggest that TBDP changes provider behavior in caring for patients at high risk for melanoma. Rather, our study supports the fact that a patient's positive history of melanoma and a history of severe dysplastic nevi have the most significant impact on provider biopsy behavior, resulting in a lower threshold to biopsy suggestive lesions.

▶ Risser et al found that the use of TBDP in melanoma-prone patients during a 1-year period did not influence the total number of biopsies performed or the number of dysplastic nevi diagnosed. A personal history of melanoma or a personal history of severe dysplastic nevi was the most significant factor for predicting a biopsy. Moreover, patients without a personal history of melanoma or dysplastic nevi and those seen by more experienced providers were less likely to have a new diagnosis of dysplastic nevi during the study period. The results presented here challenge the assumption that TBDP may be useful in reducing the number of unnecessary biopsies.[1]

B. H. Thiers, MD

Reference

1. Feit N, Dusza S, Marghoob A. Melanomas detected with the aid of total cutaneous photography. *Br J Dermatol.* 2004;150:706-714.

Is 2,3,5-Pyrrolectricarboxylic Acid in Hair a Better Risk Indicator for Melanoma than Traditional Epidemiologic Measures for Skin Phenotype?

Rosso S, for the Helios Working Group (Piedmont Cancer Registry, Turin, Italy; et al)

Am J Epidemiol 165:1170-1177, 2007

This study aims to assess type of melanin as a risk indicator for skin tumors, in a sample of melanoma cases and controls within a larger multicenter study (Helios 2), held in Europe and South America in 2001–2002. In each case and control, the melanin content in hair was assessed by three methods: 1) the amount of 2,3,5-pyrroletricarboxylic acid (PTCA); 2) the absorbance ratio with ultraviolet spectroscopy; and 3) the spectra of near-infrared spectroscopy. Statistical analysis was performed in a Bayesian setting, defining priors for confounders and effect modifiers from the larger study data set. Subjects with values of PTCA of less than 85 ng/mg carried an increased risk (26 vs. seven discordant pairs: odds ratio = 4.4, 95% confidence interval: 1.52, 14.54), adjusted by hair color, eye color, and number of nevi ($n = \geq40$). The absorbance ratio showed a weaker and nonsignificant odds ratio of 1.5. After correction by misclassification, near-infrared spectroscopy was associated with an odds ratio of 2.3 (95% confidence interval: 1.36, 4.22). The amount of PTCA is thus a strong and independent risk indicator for melanoma. Incorporating PTCA determination into epidemiologic studies is therefore recommended.

▶ Using melanin as a risk factor for skin cancer might be simplistic. In fact, several genes control melanin synthesis and function, including those that regulate tyrosine oxidation, those involved in melanosone transport, and those that modulate the signals that activate synthesis. In an effort to identify a more-specific risk factor, the authors' data suggest that a relative lack of eumelanin (measured here by its degradation product, 2,3,5-pyrroletricarboxylic acid [PTCA]) may be an independent risk factor for melanoma. They further speculate that other types of melanin such as pheomelanin may play a less-important role or, at least, cannot be measured with sufficient precision. They argue that the fourfold increased risk of melanoma in patients with low levels of eumelanin (or the more easily

Dispelling the myth of the "benign hair sign" for melanoma
Scope A, Tabanelli M, Busam KJ, et al (Mem Sloan-Kettering Cancer Ctr; Univ of Bologna, Italy; Univ Hosp Geneva)
J Am Acad Dermatol 56:413-416, 2007

Background.—Most melanocytic lesions with hair are benign. Prominent hairs can be observed clinically in approximately 50% of congenital nevi and can be frequently seen in acquired nevi. Although hair is not formally listed among the discriminatory criteria, it is thought that the presence of 1 or more hairs in a melanocytic lesion is confirmatory for the benign nature of the lesion. This belief was dispelled in the following cases of 3 patients in whom melanocytic lesions showed terminal hairs on clinical and dermscopic evaluation, but in which the final diagnosis was invasive melanoma.

Case 1.—Man, 67, was seen for evaluation of a lesion on the right side of the occipital scalp. He denied the existence of any nevi during his early childhood. The lesion consisted of a brown plaque with a central blue nodule. The bluish nodule contained a few visible hairs at its periphery, and the brown plaque was studded with multiple terminal hairs. Histopathologic analysis showed an invasive melanoma not associated with a melanocytic nevus. The epithelium of the infundibular portion of the hair follicle was populated by melanoma cells.

Case 2.—Man, 38, was referred for periodic surveillance of moles. He denied the existence of any nevi during his childhood years and confirmed that all of his nevi had been acquired later in life. His personal history was negative for melanoma, but his family history was notable for melanoma in his mother. In the past, he had multiple moles removed that were found to by dysplastic nevi. On physical examination, the patient had multiple large and irregular nevi on his head, neck, and trunk regions. On the flank he had a hypomelanotic, reddish, firm raised nodule with visible terminal hair follicles. Histopathologic analysis revealed a melanoma arising in association with a dysplastic melanocytic nevus.

Case 3.—Man, 63, was seen with an irregularly shaped pigmented lesion on the abdomen that had been present for several years. He denied having a lesion at this location during childhood. Examination showed a star-shaped, asymmetric, ill-defined multicolored pigmented flat lesion on the abdomen, studded by multiple terminal hairs. Dermoscopy showed a reticular-homogeneous disorganized pattern with a hypopigmented area surrounded by multiple bluish gray dots and granules, suggestive of regression. Hair shafts were not observed in the areas with significant regression. Histologic analysis revealed melanoma with significant regression, not associated with a melanocytic nevus.

Conclusions.—Although most melanocytic lesions that have hair are, in fact, benign, the detection of a hair in a lesion should not overrule other features that are suggestive of a diagnosis of melanoma. Clinical and dermoscopic criteria should guide clinicians to the correct diagnosis.

▶ Many clinicians use the presence of hair in a melanocytic lesion to confirm its benign nature. The authors present 3 cases in which this was not the case. As they correctly point out, the vast majority of melanocytic lesions with hair are, in fact, benign. However, in evaluating pigmented lesions, the presence or absence of hair is only 1 of several criteria that must be assessed, no one of which can be used alone to indicate with certainty the true biological potential of the lesion. Clinical, dermatoscopic, and histologic criteria may be necessary to fully evaluate questionable lesions.

B. H. Thiers, MD

Melanomas arising from naevi and *de novo* melanomas—does origin matter?
Weatherhead SC, Haniffa M, Lawrence CM (Royal Victoria Infirmary, Tyne and Wear, England)
Br J Dermatol 156:72-76, 2007

Background.—It is widely accepted that some melanomas arise from pre-existing naevi, while others appear *de novo*. The proportions involved and the effect of melanoma origin on prognosis is unclear.

Objectives.—To determine whether melanomas reported by the patient to have developed from a pre-existing naevus are associated with a better or worse prognosis compared with those arising *de novo* when adjusted for confounding variables.

Methods.—All patients attending a dedicated melanoma screening clinic between March 1997 and March 2002 were included. The distinction between melanoma arising without any pre-existing lesion (*de novo*) and those derived from a pre-existing lesion (naevus melanoma) was based on patient history. We categorized patients into three groups: those who gave a history of their lesion arising within a pre-existing naevus, those in whom the melanoma developed *de novo* and those in whom no conclusive history could be obtained. We compared prognostic indicators between the naevus and *de novo* melanoma groups.

Results.—Of 8593 patients screened, 377 had a positive diagnosis of melanoma (*in situ* or invasive). Of these 42% had naevus melanomas, 34% new melanomas and 24% were uncertain. Patients presenting with a melanoma arising from a pre-existing naevus had a greater Breslow thickness despite presenting sooner than the *de novo* group, although no significant difference in thickness was found when other prognostic factors were controlled for.

Conclusions.—This prospective study shows that naevi that undergo malignant change may result in melanomas that are thicker and thus potentially have a worse prognosis than *de novo* melanomas. Although our results were not statistically significant when other risk factors were also taken into account, it is possible that a larger study would identify a significant association.

▶ Although the authors found that common acquired nevi that evolve to melanoma tend to yield thicker tumors with a potentially poorer prognosis than do *de novo* melanomas, the results were not statistically significant after adjusting for age, sex, family history, and past medical history of melanoma. Recall bias is clearly the Achilles heel of the study, as an individual's ability to recognize or recall a preexisting mole might be prone to error. Interestingly, however, in the nevus/melanoma group, the patients appeared to present sooner after having noticed that their lesion was changing. Nevertheless, they still had a worse prognosis than did those in the new melanoma group.

B. H. Thiers, MD

Trends in melanoma epidemiology suggest three different types of melanoma

Lipsker D, Engel F, Cribier B, et al (Université Louis Pasteur, Strasbourg, France)
Br J Dermatol 157:338-343, 2007

Background.—It has been suggested that the incidence of thin melanomas but not of thick tumours is rising in fair-skinned populations, although the reason for this discrepancy is not understood.

Objectives.—To describe temporal trends in melanoma epidemiology in a limited part of France in order to confirm this observation and to provide an explanation.

Methods.—This is a retrospective population- and academic centre-based study in which all melanomas diagnosed in the department of the Bas-Rhin, France between January 1980 and December 2004 were included.

Results.—The study included 2094 melanomas diagnosed in 2020 patients. There was a steady increase in incidence of thin (< 1 mm) melanomas, mainly located on the trunk, and to a lesser extent in the head and neck region, in both sexes, and of intermediate (1–2 mm) melanomas in men. The incidence of intermediate melanomas in women and of thick (> 2 mm) melanomas, as well as mortality related to melanoma, remained stable. There was a steady decline of mean and median Breslow thickness. The 12 months median delay to diagnosis of thick tumours was significantly shorter than the 24 months delay to diagnosis of thin tumours.

Conclusions.—Temporal trends suggest the existence of three unrelated types of melanoma: type I, thick melanomas, with stable incidence; type II, thin melanoma with a steady and important increase in incidence, mainly located on the trunk; and type III, melanoma with a slower increase in incidence, mainly located on the head and neck region.

▶ Based on epidemiologic evidence, the authors suggest that there are 3 subtypes of melanoma. One is thicker, grows rapidly, and often is atypical in appearance (amelanotic). Because it is difficult to detect early and does not appear to be increasing in frequency, its existence may explain why mortality caused by melanoma has remained stable or slightly decreased. On the other hand, the subtype of melanoma that accounts for the majority of the observed increase in melanoma is probably caused by intermittent sun exposure. It tends to be thin, slow growing, classical in appearance, and thus subject to early detection. Finally, there is the subtype primarily occurring on the head and neck in the elderly, which again is thin, classical in appearance, and thus easily diagnosed. It is slow growing and its increased incidence reflects an aging population. The authors also note, as has this reviewer, that melanomas in women are no longer predominantly located on the legs, but as in men, are occurring with increased frequency on the trunk, a result perhaps of a change in sun exposure habits.

P. G. Lang Jr, MD

Melanoma in Children and Teenagers: An Analysis of Patients From the National Cancer Data Base

Lange JR, Palis BE, Chang DC, et al (Johns Hopkins Medicine, Baltimore, Md; American College of Surgeons, Chicago; Univ of Alabama School of Medicine, Birmingham)
J Clin Oncol 25:1363-1368, 2007

Purpose.—This study examines the demographics, presentation, and outcomes of children and teenagers with melanoma using a US hospital-based oncology database.

Patients and Methods.—Data from the National Cancer Data Base from 1985 through 2003 were examined for demographics, presentation, and survival of patients aged 1 to 19 years, as well as a comparison group of patients aged 20 to 24 years. Two-sided linear and Pearson χ^2 tests were calculated to examine associations. Proportions were compared using two-sided z tests. Five-year overall observed survival was evaluated using the Kaplan-Meier method and the log-rank test. Cox proportional hazards regression was used to estimate risk of mortality.

Results.—Of 3,158 patients aged 1 to 19 years, 96.3% had cutaneous melanoma, 3.0% had ocular melanoma, and 0.7% had an unknown primary tumor. Cutaneous melanoma in patients aged 1 to 19 years was more common in girls (55.5%) and patients older than 10 years (90.5%). The demographics and presentation of cutaneous melanoma were age related; younger children were significantly more likely to be nonwhite and male and more likely to present with a head and neck primary tumors and with regional or distant metastases (linear χ^2, $P < .001$ for sex, race, and extent of disease). Poorer survival was associated with higher stage and younger age. In contrast to patients aged 20 to 24 years, survival was not related to thickness in patients aged 1 to 19 years with localized invasive melanoma.

Conclusion.—Melanoma in children and teenagers differs from melanoma in young adults in demographics, presentation, and survival. Further investigation is warranted to elucidate possible biologic correlates of the unique aspects of melanoma in children and teenagers.

▶ Although the data for this study were obtained from hospital tumor registries and therefore may not include data from thin melanomas removed in an office-based setting, it nevertheless appears to be the largest reported series of pediatric melanomas. Because hospital tumor registries do not collect information on whether melanomas arise in congenital nevi, we do not know in what percentage of children a congenital nevus was the site of origin of the tumor. Somewhat surprisingly, as seen in Table 2 of the original article, the head and neck was the most common location for melanomas in very young children. Children less than 9 years of age were more likely to present with regional or distant metastases than older children. Fortunately, interferon used as adjunctive therapy after surgery is well tolerated by this young age group. Although tumor thickness is the single most important prognostic factor in all other age groups, this study did not show it to be a prognostic factor in children, suggesting that melanoma may have an inherently different biology and natural history in children. Future understanding of the molecular and genetic aspects of this tumor in children may help in the diagnosis of cases that are pathologically ambiguous and lead to targeted therapies.

S. Raimer, MD

The association between residential pesticide use and cutaneous melanoma
Fortes C, Mastroeni S, Melchi F, et al (Istituto Dermopatico dell'Immacolata (IDI-IRCCS), Rome)
Eur J Cancer 43:1066-1075, 2007

Occupational pesticide exposure has been linked to cutaneous melanoma in epidemiological studies. We studied the association between cutaneous melanoma and the residential use of pesticides. This is a case-control study of cutaneous melanoma (287 incident cases; 299 controls). Data on pesticide use was obtained with a standardised interview. An increased risk of melanoma was found for high use (≥ 4 times annually) of indoor pesticides (odds ratio (OR) = 2.18; 95% confidence intervals (CI) 1.07–4.43) compared to low use (≤ 1 times annually), after adjustment for sex, age, education, sun exposure and pigmentary characteristics. Subjects exposed for 10 years or more had two and a half times the risk (OR = 2.46; 95% CI 1.23–4.94) of those exposed for less than 10 years. A dose response was observed for the intensity of pesticides use ($p_{trend} = 0.027$). The results indicate that residential pesticide exposure may be an independent risk factor for cutaneous melanoma.

▶ The authors cite previous studies that suggest a link between pesticides and increased melanoma risk, and they investigate the association between residential pesticide exposure and cutaneous melanoma. The results indicated that residential pesticide exposure may be an independent risk factor for cutaneous melanoma. Further studies are clearly needed to confirm this finding.

B. H. Thiers, MD

Gene Expression Signatures for Tumor Progression, Tumor Subtype, and Tumor Thickness in Laser-Microdissected Melanoma Tissues
Jaeger J, Koczan D, Thiesen H-J, et al (Max Planck Inst for Molecular Genetics, Berlin; Univ of Rostock, Germany)
Clin Cancer Res 13:806-815, 2007

Purpose.—To better understand the molecular mechanisms of malignant melanoma progression and metastasis, gene expression profiling was done of primary melanomas and melanoma metastases.

Experimental Design.—Tumor cell–specific gene expression in 19 primary melanomas and 22 melanoma metastases was analyzed using oligonucleotide microarrays after laser-capture microdissection of melanoma cells. Statistical analysis was done by random permutation analysis and support vector machines. Microarray data were further validated by immunohistochemistry and immunoblotting.

Results.—Overall, 308 genes were identified that showed significant differential expression between primary melanomas and melanoma metastases (false discovery rate≤0.05). Significantly overrepresented gene ontology categories in the list of 308 genes were cell cycle regulation, mitosis, cell communication, and cell adhesion. Overall, 47 genes showed up-regulation in metastases. These included *Cdc6, Cdk1, septin 6, mitosin, kinesin family member 2C, osteopontin,* and *fibronectin.* Down-regulated genes included *E-cadherin, fibroblast growth factor binding protein,* and *desmocollin 1* and *desmocollin 3, stratifin/14-3-3σ,* and the chemokine *CCL27.* Using support vector machine analysis of gene expression data, a performance of >85% correct classifications for primary melanomas and metastases was reached. Further analysis showed that subtypes of primary melanomas displayed characteristic gene expression patterns, as do thin tumors (≤1.0 mm Breslow thickness) compared with intermediate and thick tumors (>2.0 mm Breslow thickness).

Conclusions.—Taken together, this large-scale gene expression study of malignant melanoma identified molecular signatures related to metastasis, melanoma subtypes, and tumor thickness. These findings not only provide deeper insights into the pathogenesis of melanoma progression but may also guide future research on innovative treatments.

▶ Jaeger et al used oligonucleotide microarrays to analyze the expression of 22,283 probe sets from laser microdissected tissues harvested from 41 primary melanomas and melanoma metastases. They were able to identify 389 probe sets (representing 308 different genes) that show significant differential expression between the 2 disease stages. They were able to create a predictive diagnostic model to discriminate primary tumors from metastases with greater than 85% accuracy. The results show that melanoma metastasis represents a specific biological stage of tumor progression with a particular gene pattern. Upregulated genes in metastatic lesions were consistent with current pathogenic concepts of tumor progression and may serve as targets for innovative treatment approaches. The authors suggest future studies to analyze whether gene expression patterns in primary melanomas may have predictive value and whether gene expression patterns in metastases may be useful for monitoring treatment in clinical trials.

B. H. Thiers, MD

Down-Regulation of Pro-Apoptotic Genes is an Early Event in the Progression of Malignant Melanoma
Jensen EH, Lewis JM, McLoughlin JM, et al (H Lee Moffitt Cancer Ctr and Research Inst, Tampa, Fla; University of Minnesota Medical School, Minneapolis; Univ of South Alabama, Mobile)
Ann Surg Oncol 14:1416-1423, 2007

Introduction.—Down-regulation of apoptosis genes has been implicated in the development and progression of malignant melanoma. We used cDNA microarray to evaluate pro-apoptotic gene expression comparing normal skin to melanoma (thin and thick), nodal disease and distant metastases.

Methods.—Twenty-eight specimens including skin ($n = 1$), thin melanoma ($n = 6$), thick melanoma ($n = 7$), nodal disease ($n = 6$), and distant metastases ($n = 8$), were harvested at the time of resection from 16 individuals. RNA was isolated and microarray analysis utilizing the Affymetrix GeneChip (54,000 genetic elements, U133A+B . . . levels) was performed. Mean level of expression was calculated for each gene within a sample group. Expression profiles were then compared between tissue groups. Student's *t*-test was used to determine variance in expression between groups.

Results.—We reviewed the expression of 54,000 genetic elements, of which 2,015 were found to have significantly altered expression. This represents 1,602 genes. Twenty-two pro-apoptotic genes were found to be down-regulated when compared to normal skin. Overall reduction was evaluated comparing normal skin to metastases with a range of 3.31–64.04-fold-decrease. When comparing the tissue types sequentially, the greatest fold-decrease in gene expression occurred when comparing skin to all melanomas (thin and thick) ($p = 0.011$). Subset analysis comparing normal skin to thin melanoma or thick melanoma, revealed the greatest component of overall reduction at the transition from thin to thick lesions ($p = 0.003$).

Conclusion.—Sequential down-regulation of pro-apoptotic genes is associated with the progression of malignant melanoma. The greatest fold-decrease occurs in the transformation from thin to thick lesions.

▶ Jensen and colleagues have identified a group of genes that are involved in the cellular apoptosis pathway and that are downregulated during the progression of primary melanoma to metastatic melanoma. The findings support a central role for the loss of apoptotic mechanisms in melanoma evolution and spread. Significant genetic alterations are observed and correlate with the clinical progression from stage I disease to stage II disease. The downregulation of proapoptotic genes has been described in other cancers as well.

B. H. Thiers, MD

Overexpression of Akt converts radial growth melanoma to vertical growth melanoma
Govindarajan B, Sligh JE, Vincent BJ, et al (Emory Univ School of Medicine, Atlanta, Ga; Vanderbilt Univ Med Ctr, Nashville, Tenn; Loyola Univ Health System, Chicago; et al)
J Clin Invest 117:719-729, 2007

Melanoma is the cancer with the highest increase in incidence, and transformation of radial growth to vertical growth (i.e., noninvasive to invasive) melanoma is required for invasive disease and metastasis. We have previously shown that p42/p44 MAP kinase is activated in radial growth melanoma, suggesting that further signaling events are required for vertical growth melanoma. The molecular events that accompany this transformation are not well understood. Akt, a signaling molecule downstream of PI3K, was introduced into the radial growth WM35 melanoma in order to test whether Akt overexpression is sufficient to accomplish this transformation. Overexpression of Akt led to upregulation of VEGF, increased production of superoxide ROS, and the switch to a more pronounced glycolytic metabolism. Subcutaneous implantation of WM35 cells overexpressing Akt led to rapidly growing tumors in vivo, while vector control cells did not form tumors. We demonstrated that Akt was associated with malignant transformation of melanoma through at least 2 mechanisms. First, Akt may stabilize cells with extensive mitochondrial DNA mutation, which can generate ROS. Second, Akt can induce expression of the ROS-generating enzyme NOX4. Akt thus serves as a molecular switch that increases angiogenesis and the generation of superoxide, fostering more aggressive tumor behavior. Targeting Akt and ROS may be of therapeutic importance in treatment of advanced melanoma.

▶ This is a fascinating study that helps elucidate the mechanism for invasive disease in melanoma. Recent research has clearly shown that tumor cells in vertical growth phase melanoma are quite different from those tumors limited to the radial growth phase. Govindarajan et al demonstrate that the signaling molecule Akt may play a key role in the transformation of melanoma to an aggressive, vertical growth phase. Possible mechanisms of action include its ability to confer resistance to apoptotic stimuli and its ability to inactivate potential tumor suppressor genes.[1,2] Previous studies have confirmed Akt expression in advanced human melanomas.[3]

B. H. Thiers, MD

References

1. Majewski N, Nogueira V, Bhaskar P, et al. Hexokinase-mitochrondria interaction mediated by Akt is required to inhibit apoptosis in the presence or absence of Bax and Bak. *Mol Cell.* 2004;16:819-830.
2. Arbiser JL, Kau T, Konar M, et al. Solenopsin, the alkaloidal component of the fire ant (*Solenopsis invicta*), is a naturally occurring inhibitor of phosphatidylinositol-3-kinase signaling and angiogenesis. *Blood.* 2006;109:560-565.
3. Dai DL, Martinka M, Li G. Prognostic significance of activated Akt expression in melanoma: a clinicopathologic study of 292 cases. *J Clin Oncol.* 2005;23:1473-1482.

Monoclonal Antibody 4C5 Immunostains Human Melanomas and Inhibits Melanoma Cell Invasion and Metastasis

Stellas D, Karameris A, Patsavoudi E (Technological Educational Inst of Athens, Greece; Hellenic Pasteur Inst, Athens, Greece; Veterans Administration Hosp [NIMTS], Athens, Greece)
Clin Cancer Res 13:1831-1838, 2007

Purpose.—Tumor cell metastasis constitutes a major problem in the treatment of cancer. Because the cure rate of metastatic tumors is very low, new therapeutic approaches are needed. Heat shock protein 90 (HSP90) is a molecular chaperone that is recognized as a new target for the treatment of cancer. Here, we examine the value of a monoclonal antibody (mAb) against HSP90, mAb 4C5, as a potential marker in malignant melanomas. Moreover, we investigate the possibility to use mAb 4C5 as an inhibitor of melanoma cell invasion and metastasis.

Experimental Design.—Paraffin blocks of formalin-fixed human melanoma tumor tissues were used to prepare tissue microarrays. The B16 F10 melanoma cell line was used in all the *in vitro* experiments. To assess melanoma cell invasion, the wound-healing assay and the Matrigel invasion assay were applied. To evaluate the effect of mAb 4C5 on tumor metastasis, we used an experimental model of metastatic melanoma.

Results.—Immunohistochemical studies done on a panel of malignant melanomas showed positive immunostaining with mAb 4C5 in all cases. mAb 4C5 inhibits B16 F10 cell invasion by binding to surface HSP90 because it is not internalized. mAb 4C5 significantly inhibits melanoma metastasis in C57BL/6 mice inoculated with B16 F10 cells.

Conclusions.—mAb 4C5 could be potentially used as a novel specific marker for malignant melanomas. mAb 4C5 inhibits melanoma cell invasion *in vitro* by binding to cell surface HSP90 expressed on B16 F10 melanoma cells. Finally, this antibody significantly inhibits melanoma metastasis, thus rendering it a potential therapeutic agent for the treatment of cancer metastasis.

▶ Stellas et al present data to suggest that mAb 4C5 may be a novel specific marker for malignant melanoma. They also show that mAb 4C5 inhibits invasion in a melanoma cell line by binding to cell surface HSP90. Additionally, in an experimental metastatic model, mAb 4C5 significantly inhibits melanoma metastasis. They conclude that mAb 4C5 may have therapeutic potential for the treatment of cancer metastasis. Humanization of mAb 4C5 will facilitate studies of this antibody in human melanoma.

B. H. Thiers, MD

Phase I/II study of topical imiquimod and intralesional interleukin-2 in the treatment of accessible metastases in malignant melanoma
Green DS, Bodman-Smith MD, Dalgleish AG, et al (St George's Univ of London)
Br J Dermatol 156:337-345, 2007

Background.—Patients with metastatic skin disease in malignant melanoma can be difficult to treat effectively, often requiring repeated treatments with different modalities in an attempt to control their disease. Treatment of nonsurgically resectable melanoma deposits is unsatisfactory, as they are often multiple and recurring. Anecdotal evidence from individual use of imiquimod in superficial metastases and intralesional interleukin (IL)-2 in subcutaneous deposits suggests that the combination may be more effective in bulky subcutaneous disease.

Objectives.—To investigate the combination of topical imiquimod and, for selected lesions, intralesional IL-2, to treat a small cohort of patients with accessible melanoma metastases resistant to other treatments.

Methods.—Thirteen patients were recruited: all had evidence of multiple cutaneous and/or subcutaneous metastases. Imiquimod was applied to the metastases on a daily basis for 4 weeks, before the introduction of intralesional IL-2. This was injected up to three times a week, into selected lesions, with 0.1 mL injected per lesion at a concentration of 3.6 MIU mL^{-1}, a total of 1 mL being given at each session. The treated lesions were assessed individually at intervals of 3 months.

Results.—Thirteen patients were treated, with 10 being eligible for assessment. In total, 182 lesions were treated: 137 purely cutaneous lesions and 41 subcutaneous lesions. Overall, a clinical response was seen in 92 lesions (50.5%) with 74 (40.7%) of these being a complete response (CR) with 91% of the CRs being in the cutaneous lesions. New lesions did appear during the treatment course; however, patients with cutaneous disease experienced a marked slowing of the appearance of new cutaneous lesions. No cutaneous lesions that responded reappeared on cessation of treatment.

Conclusions.—The combination of imiquimod and IL-2 is effective in controlling this mixed cutaneous and subcutaneous disease, and is well tolerated. Imiquimod alone is often enough to elicit a response in purely cutaneous lesions. The addition of intralesional IL-2 increases the response rates in subcutaneous lesions, and in otherwise refractory cutaneous lesions.

▶ Current methodologies to manage patients with metastatic melanoma emphasize the importance of the immune response against the tumor. Green et al studied whether topical application of the immunomodulatory drug imiquimod, in conjunction with intralesional IL-2 injections, could have a beneficial therapeutic effect. In this early-phase study, they found evidence of efficacy with minimal toxicity. There was a significant palliative benefit to some patients in whom conventional therapies were no longer appropriate or acceptable. A larger, multicenter trial is necessary to confirm the results.

B. H. Thiers, MD

Non-Radical Diagnostic Biopsies Do Not Negatively Influence Melanoma Patient Survival

Molenkamp BG, Sluijter BJR, Oosterhof B, et al (VU Univ Med Ctr, Amsterdam)
Ann Surg Oncol 14:1424-1430, 2007

Background.—In fair-skinned Caucasian populations both the incidence and mortality rates of cutaneous melanoma have been increasing over the past decades. With adjuvant therapies still being under investigation, early detection is the only way to improve melanoma patient survival. The influence of incisional biopsies on melanoma patient survival has been discussed for many years. This study investigates both the influence of diagnostic biopsy type and the presence of residual tumor cells in the re-excision specimen on disease free and overall survival.

Methods.—After (partial) removal of a pigmented skin lesion 471 patients were diagnosed with stage I/II melanoma and underwent re-excision and a sentinel node biopsy. All patients were followed prospectively, mean follow up >5 years. Patients were divided according to their diagnostic biopsy type (wide excision biopsy, narrow excision biopsy, excision biopsy with positive margins and incisional biopsy) and the presence of residual tumor cells in their re-excision specimen. Survival analysis was done using Cox's proportional hazard model adjusted for eight important confounders of melanoma patient survival.

Results.—The diagnostic biopsy was wide in 279 patients, narrow in 109 patients, 52 patients underwent an excision biopsy with positive margins and 31 patients an incisional biopsy. In 41 patients residual tumor cells were present in the re-excision specimen. Both the diagnostic biopsy type and the presence of tumor cells in the re-excision specimen did not influence disease free and overall survival of melanoma patients.

Conclusions.—Non-radical diagnostic biopsies do not negatively influence melanoma patient survival.

▶ Although there has been some difference of opinion regarding the effect of biopsy technique on the prognosis of patients with cutaneous melanoma, the consensus has been that incomplete removal (provided the lesion is subsequently completely excised) has no adverse effect. This study confirms this opinion. Although incomplete removal may not affect prognosis, an argument for an excisional biopsy is that it allows for better staging of the lesion, which impacts decision making in planning for definitive treatment.

P. G. Lang, Jr, MD

Sentinel lymph node status in melanoma: a valuable prognostic factor?
Topar G, Eisendle K, Zelger B, et al (Innsbruck Med Univ, Austria)
Br J Dermatol 154:1080-1087, 2006

Background.—Sentinel lymph node (SLN) biopsy is advocated as the standard of care for patients with primary melanoma. It is a procedure with few side-effects and provides valuable staging information about the regional lymphatics.

Objectives.—To investigate the prognostic value of SLN biopsy and to compare it with that of other known risk factors in primary melanoma.

Methods.—One hundred and forty-nine patients with primary melanomas (tumour thickness >1.0 mm) underwent SLN biopsy between May 1998 and April 2004 at our department. This report summarizes the follow-up data of this cohort until October 2004.

Results.—SLN biopsies of 49 of 149 patients (33%) revealed micrometastatic disease. Of all clinical and histological criteria, only the clinical type of primary melanoma (11 of 19 patients with acrolentiginous melanomas) and the Clark level were predictive for SLN positivity. Progression was observed in 22 patients (15%). It was significantly associated with ulceration of the primary tumour, tumour thickness, clinical type and localization of the primary tumour, female sex and older age. In contrast, SLN positivity was not significantly associated with a higher risk of progression (eight of 49 SLN-positive vs. 14 of 100 SLN-negative patients; $P = 0.807$). Twelve of 149 patients (8%) died because of melanoma in the follow-up period. Significant criteria for death were ulceration of the tumour, clinical type and localization of the primary tumour, but not SLN positivity.

Conclusions.—A high percentage of positive SLNs was observed in the patients with melanoma in our study (33%). The fractions of patients both with progressive disease and with tumour-related death were not significantly higher in patients with positive SLN than in those with negative SLN. We therefore conclude that the SLN status is not a reliable prognostic factor for progression of melanoma.

▶ In contrast to most other studies, the data presented here suggest that there is no correlation among disease prognosis, survival, and sentinel lymph node (SLN) status. Why this is the case is not clear but several observations can be made. First, the number of patients included is not large, although 149 patients are not insignificant. Moreover, there were other findings that are not in keeping with previous studies; for example, there was no correlation among SLN positivity, tumor thickness, and the presence of ulceration. Instead, the Clark level of invasion, which has only been shown to be of significance for lesions less than 1 mm thick, was shown to be 1 of 2 criteria associated with SLN positivity. Finally, SLN positivity and prognosis strongly correlated with a specific histologic subtype: acrolentiginous (ALM) melanoma. This would indicate that this study included a significant number of patients with very thick ALMs, since other studies have shown that histologic subtypes of melanoma, when analyzed by tumor thickness, do not differ in biological behavior, the 1 exception, perhaps, being desmoplastic melanoma. Apparently there was only 1 false-negative SLN biopsy; this probably would not account for the observed results. It also seems unlikely that in the SLN-negative group of patients, all tumors would bypass the nodal basin or only present with satellite lesions, even though by previously set forth criteria, they should have been SLN positive. Although the explanation for these authors' observations remains unclear at this time, judgment should be reserved until more data accumulate that either support or refute their findings.

P. G. Lang, Jr, MD

Identification of High-Risk Patients Among Those Diagnosed With Thin Cutaneous Melanomas

Gimotty PA, Elder DE, Fraker DL, et al (Univ of Pennsylvania School of Medicine, Philadelphia)
J Clin Oncol 25:1129-1134, 2007

Purpose.—Most patients with melanoma have microscopically thin (≤ 1 mm) primary lesions and are cured with excision. However, some develop metastatic disease that is often fatal. We evaluated established prognostic factors to develop classification schemes with better discrimination than current American Joint Committee on Cancer (AJCC) staging.

Patients and Methods.—We studied patients with thin melanomas from the US population-based Surveillance, Epidemiology, and End Results (SEER) cancer registry (1988 to 2001; n = 26,291) and those seen by the University of Pennsylvania's Pigmented Lesion Group (PLG; 1972 to 2001; n = 2,389; Philadelphia, PA). AJCC prognostic factors were thickness, anatomic level, ulceration, site, sex, and age; PLG prognostic factors also included a set of biologically based candidate prognostic factors. Recursive partitioning was used to develop a SEER-based classification tree that was validated using PLG data. Next, a new PLG-based classification tree was developed using the expanded set of prognostic factors.

Results.—The SEER-based classification tree identified additional criteria to explain survival heterogeneity among patients with thin, nonulcerated lesions; 10-year survival rates ranged from 89.1% to 99%. The new PLG-based tree identified groups using level, tumor cell mitotic rate, and sex. With survival rates from 83.4% to 100%, it had better discrimination.

Conclusion.—Prognostication and related clinical decision making in the majority of patients with melanoma can be improved now using the validated, SEER-based classification. Tumor cell mitotic rate should be incorporated into the next iteration of AJCC staging.

▶ Prognostic trees have always seemed cumbersome and confusing. Moreover, their application to clinical practice remains questionable. The prognostic tree proposed by these authors seems no different. It has frequently been demonstrated that thin melanomas, which are Clark level IV or greater or which are ulcerated are more likely to metastasize. The authors of this article contend that if other variables are added to the equation, an even more discriminating and accurate prognostic model can be developed. These added variables include age, anatomical site, sex, vertical growth phase, regression, mitotic rate, and the presence of tumor-infiltrating lymphocytes. Although surely the authors are correct, there are many questions that need to be addressed, including the availability and reproducibility of some of the histologic criteria and whether the authors' formula can be easily applied on a daily basis.

P. G. Lang, Jr, MD

Factors associated with a high tumour thickness in patients with melanoma

Baumert J, Plewig G, Volkenandt M, et al (Ludwig-Maximilian-Univ, Munich; GSF-Inst of Epidemiology, Neuherberg, Germany; Rheinische Friedrich-Wilhelm-Univ, Bonn, Germany)
Br J Dermatol 156:938-944, 2007

Background.—Prognosis of patients with melanoma is strongly associated with tumour thickness at time of diagnosis. Therefore, knowledge of patient characteristics and behaviour associated with a high tumour thickness is essential for the development and improvement of melanoma prevention campaigns.

Objectives.—The present study aimed to identify sociodemographic, clinical and behavioural factors associated with high tumour thickness according to Breslow.

Methods.—The study population consisted of 217 patients with histologically proven primary invasive cutaneous melanomas seen at the Department of Dermatology and Allergology at the Ludwig-Maximilian-

University Munich, Germany, between January 1999 and January 2001. Personal interviews were conducted by two physicians to obtain information on sociodemographic characteristics and on patients' knowledge of melanoma symptoms, sun behaviour, delay in diagnosis and related factors. Multivariate linear and logistic regression analysis with stepwise variable selection was used to identify risk groups with a high tumour thickness. To assess possible effect modifications, interaction terms were included in the regression analysis.

Results.—The median tumour thickness was 0.8 mm (interquartile range 0.5–1.6). Fifty-seven patients (26%) had tumour thickness >1.5 mm. In a multivariate linear regression analysis, patients living alone and patients with a low educational level showed a significantly greater tumour thickness. The relation of melanoma knowledge to tumour thickness was modified by the melanoma subtype: whereas lack of melanoma knowledge led to an increased tumour thickness for the subtypes superficial spreading melanoma, lentigo maligna melanoma and unspecified malignant melanoma, no significant effect was estimated for the subtypes nodular melanoma (NM) and acrolentiginous melanoma (ALM). Sex, age, self-detection of melanoma, patient delay and professional delay were not significantly associated with the tumour thickness in multivariate linear regression. Similar results were found in multivariate logistic regression.

Conclusions.—An increased tumour thickness was found in subjects living alone and having a low educational level. These subjects should be targeted in future prevention campaigns in a more focused way. Further efforts are necessary to improve knowledge and earlier detection of melanoma subtypes NM and ALM.

▶ Baumert et al sought to examine factors associated with patient and provider delay in the diagnosis of melanoma. They sought to identify factors associated with a high and therefore prognostically unfavorable tumor thickness. They found a surprising association between greater tumor thickness and patients living alone, an association that has not previously been reported. There also seemed to be an inverse relationship between the level of knowledge about melanoma and tumor thickness. Better educational campaigns would address the latter issue, whereas targeting selected demographic groups should be beneficial as well.

B. H. Thiers, MD

Sentinel Lymph Node Biopsy for Atypical Melanocytic Lesions with Spitzoid Features

Gamblin TC, Edington H, Kirkwood JM, et al (Univ of Pittsburgh School of Medicine, Pa; UPMC Montefiore Hosp, Pittsburgh, Pa)
Ann Surg Oncol 13:1664-1670, 2006

Introduction.—Sentinel lymph node biopsy (SLNB) is routinely used as a staging procedure for melanomas, however may also assist in understanding the biology of atypical and controversial spitzoid melanocytic skin lesions.

Methods.—Five hundred and forty-nine sentinal lymph node excisions were performed over a 5-year period. Fourteen patients with controversial melanocytic lesions were identified and of these ten underwent SLNB. The histology of the primary skin lesion and corresponding sentinal lymph nodes were evaluated and correlated with outcome.

Results.—Thickness of the primary melanocytic lesion ranged from 1.22 to 4 mm. Fifty percent of patients were less than 17 years of age. Ten patients underwent SLNB and three cases (30%) displayed metastatic disease in the SLNB specimen. All three patients were under 17 years of age and all underwent completion axillary dissection. One completion axillary dissection had an additional node with metastasis on routine H&E and immunohistochemical staining. No capsular invasion was seen. All three cases with metastatic disease received adjuvant systemic therapy and remain disease free at 29, 49 and 57 months follow-up. All patients with a negative SLNB remain disease free at mean follow-up of 28.1 months (range: 13–40 months).

Conclusion.—Our results confirm that some of these spitzoid lesions metastasize to regional lymph nodes and SLNB is a valuable adjunct tool in staging these lesions. However, molecular studies and a prolonged follow-up are needed to determine whether these lesions, especially those occurring in children are comparable to stage matched overt melanoma in adults.

▶ Atypical melanocytic lesions with spitzoid features are problematic from a management standpoint. This is compounded by the fact that melanoma is uncommon in children. Although only a small number of patients are reported, this study adds to mounting evidence that suggests a role for SLNB in the diagnosis and management of these lesions. Previous studies have demonstrated a high incidence of SLN positivity in these patients; however, many of them appear to do quite well.

P. G. Lang, Jr, MD

Ultrasonography and Fine-needle Aspiration Cytology in the Preoperative Evaluation of Melanoma Patients Eligible for Sentinel Node Biopsy
van Rijk MC, Teertstra HJ, Peterse JL, et al (The Netherlands Cancer Inst/ Antoni van Leeuwenhoek Hosp, Amsterdam)
Ann Surg Oncol 13:1511-1516, 2006

Background.—Ultrasonography with fine-needle aspiration cytology (FNAC) has proven to be a valuable diagnostic tool in the preoperative workup of patients with breast cancer or penile cancer eligible for sentinel lymph node biopsy. The aim of this study was to evaluate the use of this technique in the initial assessment of patients with primary cutaneous melanoma.

Methods.—A total of 107 patients with cutaneous melanoma eligible for sentinel node biopsy with clinically negative nodes were studied prospectively. Patients underwent ultrasonography of potentially involved basins and FNAC in case of a suspicious lymph node. The sentinel node procedure was omitted in patients with tumour-positive lymph nodes in lieu of lymph node dissection.

Results.—Ultrasonography with FNAC correctly identified disease preoperatively in two of the 107 patients (2%). Thirteen of the 22 patients (59%) with a suspicious node on ultrasonographic imaging but a tumour-negative fine-needle aspirate were shown to have involved nodes. Of the 85 patients with ultrasonographically normal nodes, 25 (29%) were shown to have metastases. Of the total of 43 involved basins, 16 contained metastases > 2 mm and 25 ≤ 2 mm.

Conclusions.—In our hands, the sensitivity and specificity of preoperative ultrasonography to detect lymph node involvement in patients with melanoma are 34% and 87%, respectively. In combination with FNAC, this is 4.7% and 100%, respectively. This yield is insufficient for this technique to be used as a routine diagnostic tool in the selection of patients eligible for sentinel node biopsy.

▶ Investigators continue to look for ways to avoid sentinel lymph node biopsy (SLNB) and yet reliably detect microscopic disease in regional lymph nodes. Studies using positron emission tomography (PET) scanning have shown that this highly sensitive imaging technique cannot replace SLNB in the detection of subclinical nodal disease. In 2 investigations, US was used in conjunction with FNAC to detect microscopic disease in regional lymph nodes. This group from The Netherlands was able to detect subclinical disease in only 2% of patients, whereas a group from Germany[1] had a success rate of 16%, and the consensus appeared to be that this approach could not replace lymphatic mapping and SLNB. Why such a discrepancy existed between the 2 studies is unclear, but possible explanations include a difference in machines used, a difference in experience, and a difference in criteria for determining what constituted a suspicious node. Although this US and FNAC will not replace SLNB, if the higher percentage of detection of subclinical disease could be validated, then this approach might be selectively deployed to spare some patients SLNB and allow the surgeon to proceed directly to a therapeutic node dissection.

P. G. Lang, Jr, MD

Reference

1. Voit C, Kron M, Scháfer G, et al. Ultrasound-guided fine needle aspiration cytology prior to sentinel lymph node biopsy in melanoma patients. *Ann Surg Oncol.* 2006;13:1682-1689.

Ultrasound-guided Fine Needle Aspiration Cytology prior to Sentinel Lymph Node Biopsy in Melanoma Patients

Voit C, Kron M, Scháfer G, et al (Humboldt Univ, Berlin; Univ of Ulm, Germany; Memorial Sloan-Kettering Cancer Ctr)
Ann Surg Oncol 13:1682-1689, 2006

Background.—Sentinel lymph node biopsy (SLNB) allows early detection of metastases, thereby enabling early treatment in melanoma patients likely to benefit from adjuvant therapies. This prospective study analyzes the possible benefits of additional ultrasound (US) and fine needle aspiration cytology (FNAC) of sentinel nodes (SN) prior to SLNB.

Method.—Over a 2-year period 127 melanoma patients with 151 SN were scheduled for SLNB. All SN were initially identified with lymphoscintigraphy, then identified and evaluated by US and the cells aspirated for cytology (FNAC). US findings and FNAC results were compared to surgical findings.

Results.—Of 127 patients, 114 had one SN each, 12 had two, and one had three. In vivo US achieved a sensitivity of 79% (95% CI: 62–91%) and a specificity of 72% (95% CI: 62–81%). FNAC showed a sensitivity of 59% (95% CI: 41–76%) and a specificity of 100% (95% CI: 95–100%). The combination of these two in vivo methods achieved an overall sensitivity of 82% (95% CI: 65–93%) and an overall specificity of 72% [95% CI: 62–81%].

Conclusion.—Combined US and FNAC provides important information prior to SLNB in that both procedures identify metastases in the lymph nodes (sensitivity > 80%). Patients with positive FNAC may proceed directly to complete lymph node dissection (cLND) instead of having initial SLNB. Thus, combined US and FNAC may prevent unnecessary anesthesia and surgical management as well reduce costs. In our study 16% (19/121) fewer SLNB procedures were carried out, subsequently replaced by cLND. For patients with a negative combination of in vivo US and FNAC, SLNB remains the best diagnostic option.

▶ Investigators continue to look for ways to avoid sentinel lymph node biopsy (SLNB) and yet reliably detect microscopic disease in regional lymph nodes. Studies using positron emission tomographic (PET) scanning have shown that this highly sensitive imaging technique cannot replace SLNB in the detection of subclinical nodal disease. In 2 investigations, US was used in conjunction with FNAC to detect microscopic disease in regional lymph nodes. One group from The Netherlands[1] was able to detect subclinical disease in only 2% of patients, whereas this group from Germany had a success rate of 16%, and the consensus appeared to be that this approach could not replace lymphatic mapping and SLNB. Why such a discrepancy existed between the 2 studies is unclear, but possible explanations include a difference in machines used, a difference in experience, and a difference in criteria for determining what constituted a suspicious node. Although this US and FNAC will not replace SLNB, if the higher percentage of detection of subclinical disease could be validated, then this approach might be selectively deployed to spare some patients SLNB and allow their surgeon to proceed directly to a therapeutic node dissection.

P. G. Lang, Jr, MD

Reference

1. van Rijk MC, Teertstra HJ, Peterse JL, et al. Ultrasonography and fine-needle aspiration cytology in the preoperative evaluation of melanoma patients eligible for sentinel node biopsy. *Ann Surg Oncol.* 2006;13:1511-1516.

Diagnosis and Treatment of Interval Sentinel Lymph Nodes in Patients with Cutaneous Melanoma
Carling T, Pan D, Ariyan S, et al (Yale Univ School of Medicine, New Haven, Conn)
Plast Reconstr Surg 119:907-913, 2007

Background.—Interval sentinel lymph nodes in patients with melanoma are occasionally found outside conventional nodal basins. In this study, the authors examined the frequency, location, and incidence of nodal metastasis of such interval nodes in a large cohort of patients with primary cutaneous melanoma.

Methods.—Between September of 1997 and February of 2003, 374 consecutive patients at the Yale Cancer Center Melanoma Unit underwent sentinel lymph node biopsy for primary cutaneous melanoma with a Breslow thickness of at least 1.0 mm and/or Clark IV or greater histologic dermal invasion. All patients underwent preoperative lymphoscintigraphy to map the lymphatic drainage for the primary lesion and intraoperative confirmation, and biopsy was performed on all sentinel lymph nodes identified.

Results.—Unequivocal interval sentinel lymph nodes were identified in eight of 374 patients (2.1 percent). Three of these eight patients had metastatic spread to the interval sentinel nodes. In four of the eight patients, the interval sentinel lymph node was not located in the anticipated lymphatic pathway between the primary tumor and the sentinel lymph node basin.

Conclusions.—Interval sentinel nodes seem as likely to contain micrometastatic disease as those in the expected sentinel lymph node basin. Half of the subjects displayed interval sentinel lymph nodes that were not in the anticipated lymphatic pathway between the primary tumor and the sentinel lymph node basin. These findings suggest that adequate preoperative lymphoscintigraphy and intraoperative recognition of interval nodes are of paramount importance in the treatment of melanoma.

▶ The data confirm previous studies that have demonstrated the importance of identifying interval or aberrant sentinel lymph nodes in patients with cutaneous melanoma. These may be the only site of nodal spread and may either lie in the pathway to the regional nodes (eg, epitrochlear nodes) or in an aberrant or unpredicted location. Their detection is enhanced by scanning larger areas during lymphatic mapping and may be dependent on the type of colloid used.

P. G. Lang, Jr, MD

Tumor-Induced Sentinel Lymph Node Lymphangiogenesis and Increased Lymph Flow Precede Melanoma Metastasis
Harrell MI, Iritani BM, Ruddell A (Fred Hutchinson Cancer Research Ctr, Seattle; Univ of Washington, Seattle)
Am J Pathol 170:774-786, 2007

Lymphangiogenesis is associated with human and murine cancer metastasis, suggesting that lymphatic vessels are important for tumor dissemination. Lymphatic vessel alterations were examined using B16-F10 melanoma cells implanted in syngeneic C57Bl/6 mice, which form tumors metastasizing to draining lymph nodes and subsequently to the lungs. Footpad tumors showed no lymphatic or blood vessel growth; however, the tumor-draining popliteal lymph node featured greatly increased lymphatic sinuses. Lymph node lymphangiogenesis began before melanoma cells reached draining lymph nodes, indicating that primary tumors induce these alterations at a distance. Lymph flow imaging revealed that nanoparticle transit was greatly increased through tumor-draining relative to nondraining lymph nodes. Lymph node lymphatic sinuses and lymph flow were increased in mice implanted with unmarked or with foreign antigen-expressing melanomas, indicating that these effects are not due to foreign antigen expression. However, tumor-derived immune signaling could promote lymph node alterations, as macrophages infiltrated footpad tumors, whereas lymphocytes accumulated in tumor-draining lymph nodes. B lymphocytes are required for lymphangiogenesis and increased lymph flow through tumor-draining lymph nodes, as these alterations were not observed in mice deficient for B cells. Lymph node lymphangiogenesis and increased lymph flow through tumor-draining lymph nodes may actively promote metastasis via the lymphatics.

▶ In previous studies, Harrell et al demonstrated lymph node lymphangiogenesis in mice with metastatic B-cell lymphoma.[1] This suggested that the lymph node itself could promote lymphatic dissemination of such tumors. In the current investigation, they used the B16-F10 metastatic melanoma model to examine whether alterations occur in the lymphatic vessels of lymph nodes in mice developing metastatic disease. It had previously been shown that footpad injection of tumor cells produced metastatic melanoma in draining lymph nodes and ultimately the lungs. Here, Harrell et al identified extensive lymph node lymphangiogenesis and increased lymph flow through the lymph nodes draining the B16 melanomas, suggesting that tumor-derived signals promote these changes and contribute to tumor dissemination.

B. H. Thiers, MD

Reference

1. Ruddell A, Mezquita P, Brandvold KA, Farr A, Iritani BM. B lymphocyte-specific c-Myc expression stimulates early and functional expansion of the vasculature and lymphatics during lymphomagenesis. *Am J Pathol.* 2003;163:2233-2245.

Sentinel node staging of primary melanoma by the "10% rule": pathology and clinical outcomes
Emery RE, Stevens JS, Nance RW, et al (Oregon Health & Science Univ, Portland)
Am J Surg 193:618-622, 2007

Background.—Surgical staging of clinically node-negative primary melanoma involves identification and removal of "sentinel" lymph nodes (SLNs). Although some suggest removal of only the "hottest" SLN, the "10% rule" dictates that nodes are removed until the background count is 10% or less of the count of the "hottest" node.

Methods.—To determine the utility of the 10% rule, a university database of clinically node-negative melanomas surgically staged by using this rule was examined.

Results.—Twenty-two of 177 cases (12.5%; 15% of T2 and T3 lesions) were SLN positive. Among the SLN-positive cases, use of the rule resulted in removal of 21 additional nodes, 7 of which contained tumor. In 3 cases (14%), the positive SLN was not the "hottest" node. At 49 months of mean follow-up time, overall survival was 63% for SLN-positive patients versus 92% for SLN-negative patients ($P = .01$).

Conclusions.—Sentinel node staging of melanoma by the 10% rule provides significant prognostic information and a modest increase in tumor detection compared with removal of only the "hottest" node.

▶ This "refinement" of the sentinel lymph node biopsy (SLNB) technique not only increases the likelihood of detecting a positive SLN but also decreases the likelihood of a false-negative SLNB. Although there may be some increase in morbidity rate, any associated side effects appear to resolve within 6 months. As correctly stated by the authors, the "hottest" node is not always the positive one.

P. G. Lang, Jr, MD

Natural History of Melanoma in 773 Patients with Tumor-Negative Sentinel Lymph Nodes

Zogakis TG, Essner R, Wang H-j, et al (St John's Health Ctr, Santa Monica, Calif)
Ann Surg Oncol 14:1604-1611, 2007

Background.—A tumor-negative sentinel lymph node (SLN) does not preclude recurrence of melanoma. We hypothesized that certain patient-related and tumor factors are predictive of a worse outcome in these patients.

Methods.—Disease-free survival (DFS), overall survival (OS), and recurrence patterns were retrospectively analyzed in 773 patients who underwent lymphatic mapping and SLN biopsy for primary cutaneous melanoma at our institution between 1995 and 2002, and who had tumor-negative SLNs by standard pathological analysis. Patient sex, age, tumor site and thickness, ulceration status, Clark level, and histology were evaluated for their influence on outcome by univariate and multivariate Cox regression analysis and classification and regression tree analysis.

Results.—DFS and OS at 5 years were 88% and 93%, respectively. Sixty-nine (8.9%) of 773 patients developed recurrence. Three-year OS was lower in patients with distant recurrence (17.1%) than in those with local/regional recurrence (55.5%). By multivariate analysis, primary tumor thickness ($P <$ .0001), site on head/neck versus trunk ($P =$ .0093) versus extremity ($P =$ .0042), and ulceration status ($P =$ .0024) were independently significant for DFS; primary tumor thickness ($P =$ .0106) and ulceration status ($P =$ .0001) also were independently significant for OS. Classification and regression tree analysis demonstrated DFS was shortest in patients who had ulcerated tumors >2 mm.

Conclusions.—Melanoma will recur in approximately 9% of patients with tumor-negative SLNs. Patients with thick, ulcerated melanomas on the head or neck have the highest risk for recurrence. This group should be followed closely for recurrence and considered for adjuvant therapy.

▶ Although the status of the sentinel lymph node biopsy (SLNB) in patients with cutaneous melanoma is a strong predictor of disease-free and overall survival, patients with a negative SLNB do not experience a 100% survival rate. In this study of 773 patients with a negative SLNB, approximately 9% experienced a recurrence. Recurrence was most common at a distant site. Recurrence of disease correlated with an older age (>60 years), Clark level and tumor thickness, location of the tumor on the head and neck, the presence of ulceration, and a nonsuperficial spreading melanoma histology. Of these variables, tumor thickness, the presence of ulceration, and location of the tumor on the head and neck were the most important in determining disease-free and overall survival. Tumors larger than 2 mm thick were especially likely to recur. The implications of this study are that patients with a negative SLNB but who have a tumor that is located on the head and neck, is ulcerated, or is larger than 2 mm thick need to be monitored more closely for recurrent disease.

P. G. Lang, Jr, MD

Survival Analysis and Clinicopathological Factors Associated With False-Negative Sentinel Lymph Node Biopsy Findings in Patients with Cutaneous Melanoma

Nowecki ZI, Rutkowski P, Nasierowska-Guttmejer A, et al (M Sklodowska-Curie Mem Cancer Ctr and Inst of Oncology, Warsaw)
Ann Surg Oncol 13:1655-1663, 2006

Background.—We analyzed the outcomes and factors associated with false-negative (FN) results of sentinel lymph node (SLN) biopsy findings in patients with cutaneous melanoma. SLN biopsy failure rate was defined as nodal recurrence in the biopsied regional basin without previous local or in-transit recurrence.

Methods.—Between April 1997 and December 2004, a total of 1207 patients with cutaneous melanoma with a median Breslow thickness of 2.4 mm underwent SLN biopsy by preoperative and intraoperative lymphoscintigraphy combined with dye injection. In 228 cases, we found positive SLNs; of these, 220 underwent completion lymph node dissection (CLND). Median follow-up was 3 years.

Results.—The SLN biopsy failure rate was 5.8% (57 of 979 SLN negative). Median time to occurrence of FN relapse after SLN biopsy was 16 months (range, 3–74 months). The FN SLN biopsy results correlated with primary tumor thickness >4 mm ($P = .0012$), primary tumor ulceration ($P = .0002$), primary tumor level of invasion Clark stage IV/V ($P = .0005$), and nodular melanoma histological type ($P = .0375$). Five-year overall survival, calculated from the date of primary tumor excision, in the FN group was 53.7%, which was not statistically significantly worse than the CLND group (56.8%; $P = .9$). The FN group was characterized by a higher ratio of two or more metastatic nodes and extracapsular involvement of lymph nodes after LND compared with the CLND group ($P < .0001$ and $P < .0001$, respectively). Additional detailed pathological review of FN SLN revealed metastatic disease in 14 patients, which decreased the SLN biopsy failure rate to 4.4% (43 of 979).

Conclusions.—Survival of patients with FN results of SLN biopsy does not differ statistically significantly from that of patients undergoing CLND, although it is slightly lower. The SLN biopsy failure rate is approximately 5.0% in long-term follow-up and is associated mainly with the same factors that indicate a poor prognosis in primary melanoma.

▶ This article is significant from several standpoints. First, it validates the reliability of the SLNB when performed by experienced surgeons (FN rate of 5.8%; when immunohistochemical analysis is used to assess the removed node(s), the FN rate decreases to 4.4%). Second, it characterizes patients with FN SLNB findings; that is, such patients are more likely to have thicker tumors and tumors that are ulcerated. However, the authors do not explain why these characteristics might be associated with a FN SLNB. Finally, it is interesting to note that these patients seem to have the same survival as patients with a positive SLNB who undergo a CLND and those with clinically positive nodes who undergo a therapeutic node dissection.

P. G. Lang, Jr, MD

Detection of tyrosinase mRNA in the sentinel lymph nodes of melanoma patients is not a predictor of short-term disease recurrence
Tatlidil C, Parkhill WS, Giacomantonio CA, et al (Capital District Health Authority, Halifax, NS, Canada)
Mod Pathol 20:427-434, 2007

Sentinel lymph node evaluation has enabled identification of patients with cutaneous melanoma who might benefit from elective regional lymph node dissection. Sentinel nodes are currently assessed by histologic and reverse transcription polymerase chain reaction (RT–PCR) evaluation for melanocyte-specific markers. The clinical significance of positive findings by RT–PCR in the absence of histologic evidence of metastasis (HIS[NEG]/PCR[POS]) remains unclear. Examination of 264 lymph nodes from 139 patients revealed histopathologic positivity in 34 patients (24.5%), in which 26 also demonstrated simultaneous RT–PCR positivity (HIS[POS]/PCR[POS]. Of 35 HIS[NEG]/PCR[POS] patients (25.2%), five also had nodal capsular nevi. In total, capsular nevi were detected in 13 patients (9.4%). A total of 70 patients (50.4%) had negative sentinel nodes by both histopathology and RT–PCR (HIS[NEG]/PCR[NEG]). Over a median follow-up of 25 months, local and/or systemic recurrence developed in 31 patients (22.3%). Recurrence rates were similar among patients with histopathologic evidence of sentinel lymph node metastasis, irrespective of RT–PCR status (HIS[POS]/PCR[POS]) 62%; HIS[POS]/PCR[NEG] 75%). In contrast, only 10% of HIS[NEG]/PCR[NEG] patients developed recurrence, significantly less than those in either HIS[POS] group ($P<0.0001$). Recurrence in the HIS[NEG]/PCR[POS]/CN[NEG] group (7.7%) was comparable to that in HIS[NEG]/PCR[NEG] patients and significantly lower than that in either HIS[POS] group ($P<0.0001$). The only independent prognostic factors identified by multivariate analysis were the Breslow thickness of the primary tumour and histopathologic positivity of sentinel nodes. Our findings support previous observations that histopathologic evidence of metastatic melanoma in sentinel lymph nodes is an independent predictor of disease recurrence. In contrast, detection of tyrosinase mRNA by RT–PCR alone does not appear to increase the likelihood of short-term disease recurrence.

▶ How to manage patients with a sentinel lymph node biopsy (SLNB) positive only by PCR for tyrosinase mRNA has been an area of concern and controversy. Early data suggested such patients had a prognosis intermediate between those with a positive SLNB by routine staining and immunohistochemical analysis and those with an SLNB negative by both immunohistochemical analysis and PCR. In this study, the authors found that PCR positivity alone did not affect survival or the incidence of disease recurrence. Suggested reasons for this observation include (1) a lack of specificity of the molecular markers used, and/or (2) lack of a critical volume of melanoma cells that must be present for disease progression to occur. Interestingly, there were patients who were positive by immunohistochemical analysis but negative by PCR. The major weaknesses of this study were (1) the small number of patients in each subgroup and (2) the relatively short duration of follow-up.

P. G. Lang, Jr, MD

Sentinel lymph node biopsy in melanoma: a micromorphometric study relating to prognosis and completion lymph node dissection
Debarbieux S, Duru G, Dalle S, et al (Hotel Dieu, Lyon, France; Université Claude Bernard Lyon 1, Villeurbanne, France; Centre Hospitalier Lyon Sud, Oullins, France)
Br J Dermatol 157:58-67, 2007

Background.—Sentinel lymph node (SLN) positivity has been found to be strongly associated with a poor prognosis in melanoma.

Objectives.—This large referral centre study was conducted: (i) to confirm the powerful prognostic value of SLN biopsy (SLNB); (ii) to correlate patient prognosis to the micromorphometric features of SLN metastasis in SLN-positive patients; and (iii) to correlate these micromorphometric features to the likelihood of positive completion lymph node dissection (CLND).

Patients and Methods.—SLNB was performed in 455 cases of primary melanoma between January 1999 and December 2004; for patients with positive SLN, the following micromorphometric features were registered: size of the largest metastasis (two diameters), depth of metastasis, number of millimetric slices involved, maximum number of metastases on a single section, presence of intracapsular lymphatic invasion and extracapsular spread. Kaplan–Meier survival curves were compared with the log-rank test; multivariate analysis was performed using a Cox regression model. Dependence of CLND status on micromorphometric features of SLN was assessed by the χ^2 test and predictive values of the different features were evaluated by multivariate analysis using a logistic regression model.

Results.—A positive SLN was identified in 98 of our 455 cases. Survival was significantly shorter in SLN-positive patients than in SLN-negative patients. Extracapsular invasion was found to be an independent prognostic factor of disease-free survival; ulceration of the primary and the maximum diameter of the largest metastasis were identified as independent predictive factors of disease-specific survival. Age and the lowest diameter of the largest metastasis were identified as independent predictive criteria of positive CLND, whereas depth of metastasis was not. Positivity of CLND was not significantly associated with a worse prognosis.

Conclusions.—Our study confirms the previously demonstrated strong prognostic value of SLNB. It also confirms the relationship between tumour burden in the SLN (evaluated by the maximum diameter of the largest metastasis) and clinical outcome. We point out a new micromorphometric feature of SLN, which seems to be predictive of CLND status: the lowest diameter of the largest metastasis.

▶ In patients with a positive sentinel lymph node biopsy (SLNB) who subsequently undergo a complete node dissection (CND), only 20% will have involvement of nonsentinel lymph nodes (NSLN). In an effort to spare 80% of patients from undergoing an unnecessary CND, investigators have attempted to identify variables that might reliably predict involvement of NSLNs. As this article demonstrates, the findings have been variable and often are not reproducible. Moreover, when subjected to multivariate analysis, what appears to be significant may become insignificant. In recent years a number of investigators have attempted to stage the SLN using a number of morphometric features in hopes of predicting which patients might benefit from CND. Based on this approach, these authors add their own observations to the already existing array of conflicting results. In their study, age and the shortest diameter of the largest metastasis predicted positivity of NSLNs, extracapsular spread correlated with the disease-free survival rate, and ulceration of the primary tumor and the maximum diameter of the largest metastasis correlated with disease-specific survival rate. Interestingly, positivity of the NSLNs did not impact prognosis.

P. G. Lang, Jr, MD

Age as predictor in patients with cutaneous melanoma submitted to sentinel lymph node biopsy
Caracò C, Marone U, Botti G, et al (Natl Cancer Inst, Naples, Italy)
EJSO 32:970-973, 2006

Aims.—To analyse the age as prognostic factor exploring the melanoma database at the National Cancer Institute in Naples.

Methods.—Three hundred and ninety-nine patients with cutaneous melanoma were treated with sentinel lymph node biopsy from 1996 to 2003 at the National Cancer Institute of Naples. The results were analysed with particular attention to the overall survival among patients younger or older than 50 years of age.

Results.—No differences were recorded between the younger and older group in terms of the identification rate and incidence of metastases. The analyses of disease-free survival and overall survival showed a significantly more favourable outcome in younger patients. The 5-year overall survival and the 5-year disease free survival were 81.8% vs. 68.0% and 76.3% vs. 59.1% for the younger and older group, respectively.

Conclusions.—The results suggest that in the management of cutaneous melanoma, age might be considered as prognostic factor both for disease free survival and overall survival.

▶ This article appears to suggest that patients with cutaneous melanoma who are older than 50 years have a worse prognosis even though the incidence of a positive sentinel lymph node biopsy (SLNB) is no greater than in such patients younger than 50 years. However, these patients were more likely to be males and were more likely to have thicker lesions and ulcerated lesions, all factors known to affect prognosis even in the presence of a positive SLNB. Moreover, there is no mention as to whether younger patients were less apt to have involvement of the nonsentinel lymph nodes, another factor that could impact prognosis. Additional studies and more careful analysis of the data are required before the true impact of age on prognosis can be fully assessed in patients with cutaneous melanoma.

P. G. Lang, Jr, MD

Prediction of metastases in melanoma patients with positive sentinel node: Histological and molecular approach

Tsutsumida A, Furukawa H, Hata S, et al (Hokkaido Univ, Sapporo, Japan)
J Dermatol 34:31-36, 2007

It is now established that sentinel node (SN) biopsy is a minimally-invasive procedure that accurately indicates the regional nodal status. In our institute, 14 consecutive patients had only one node micrometastases after elective lymph node dissection or positive SN for primary cutaneous melanoma. These 14 patients could be clearly divided into two groups: (i) patients who developed distant metastases or in-transit metastases (metastasized group); and (ii) and patients who remains free from metastases (non-metastasized group). The purpose of this study was to identify the histological and molecular factors that might predict the further dissemination beyond the SN. We assessed the maximum depth from the capsule to the deepest melanoma cells and the maximum diameter of melanoma nests in the lymph nodes as histological parameters and also evaluated the quantitative expression of tyrosinase mRNA as a molecular approach. The mean maximum depth and the maximum diameter were significantly smaller in the metastasized group than those in the non-metastasized group. Tyrosinase mRNA expression was strongly correlated with the histological tumor burden. Tyrosinase mRNA expression was higher in the former group than that in the latter group but there were no significant differences between them. Melanoma patients with small micrometastases (<0.5 mm deep, <1 mm in diameter) and a low level of tyrosinase mRNA had less chances for hematogenous metastases via lymph nodes.

▶ Although this study contains only a few patients, it confirms prior studies that have shown that staging a positive sentinel lymph node provides additional prognostic information. The depth of penetration of the melanoma into the lymph node and the size of the metastatic deposit predict which tumors are more likely to recur and which patients are less likely to survive.

P. G. Lang, Jr, MD

Regional Nodal Metastatic Disease Is the Strongest Predictor of Survival in Patients with Thin Vertical Growth Phase Melanomas: A Case for SLN Staging Biopsy in These Patients

Karakousis GC, Gimotty PA, Czerniecki BJ, et al (Univ of Pennsylvania, Philadelphia; VA Hosp, Philadelphia)

Ann Surg Oncol 14:1596-1603, 2007

Background.—The benefit of sentinel lymph node (SLN) biopsy for patients with thin (≤1.0 mm) melanomas, even for prognostic value, is controversial. This may partly result from the relatively small number and short follow-up of SLN-positive patients in this group. Previously, we have shown that clinical regional nodal metastatic disease (RNMD) serves as a good surrogate for SLN positivity. Here, we use RNMD as a validated surrogate for SLN positivity and examine its prognostic value in a large pre-SLN group of patients with thin vertical growth phase (VGP) lesions who would today commonly be offered SLN biopsy in our practice.

Methods.—Between 1972 and 1991, 472 patients with thin VGP melanomas with at least 10 years' follow-up were eligible for the study. Kaplan-Meier survival curves were computed for patients with and without RNMD. A multivariate Cox model and classification tree analysis were used to evaluate clinical and histopathologic predictors of survival.

Results.—Sixty-seven patients (14.2%) developed recurrence, 53.7% of whom developed RNMD. Forty-five patients (9.5%) experienced melanoma-related deaths (MRD). The most statistically significant predictor of MRD was RNMD (hazard ratio [HR] 13.5, $P < .0001$). Thickness (HR 10.5, $P = .004$), axial location (HR 4.6, $P = .001$), and age >60 years (HR 2.7, $P = .005$) additionally were independently associated with an increased risk of MRD. RNMD patients demonstrated a 44.4% 10-year disease-specific mortality.

Conclusions.—RNMD was the most statistically significant factor associated with MRD in patients with thin VGP lesions. This supports the prognostic use of SLN biopsy in this group, recognizing that additional factors, including thickness, axial location, and older age were independently associated with a worse survival outcome.

▶ The therapeutic value of the sentinel lymph node biopsy (SLNB) in the management of cutaneous melanoma (CM) remains controversial. This is especially true for patients with lesions less than 1 mm thick. Criteria used to select such patients for SLNB have included a Clark level IV/V, the presence of mitoses, the presence of ulceration, and the presence of a VGP. In this study of patients with thin melanomas with a VGP, the authors found that age (> 60 years), thickness, and an axial location were of prognostic significance, whereas ulceration and the Clark level were not. However, the strongest prognostic indicator was metastasis to the regional nodes, suggesting at least a prognostic role for SLNB in patients with VGP thin melanomas.

P. G. Lang, Jr, MD

Sentinel lymph node biopsy in patients with thick (= 4 mm) melanoma: a single-centre experience
Cecchi R, Buralli L, Innocenti S, et al (Pistoia Hosp, Italy; Lucca Hosp, Italy)
J Eur Acad Dermatol Venereol 21:758-761, 2007

Background and Objective.—Lymphatic mapping/sentinel lymph node biopsy (LM/SLNB) have become routine techniques for staging the regional lymph nodes in early stage melanoma, yet their role in the management of thick (= 4 mm) melanoma is debated. The aim of the present study is to review our experience with LM/SLNB in a series of patients with thick primary melanoma, to evaluate its utility in this melanoma subset.

Patients and Methods.—Thirty patients (18 men and 12 women; mean age 70.6 years; median 75 years) with thick primary melanoma underwent LM/SLNB, using both radioisotope and blue dye. The statistical tests were performed by using SAS software for Windows, version 8.2.

Results.—The primary tumour sites were head/neck ($n = 5$; 16.6%), trunk ($n = 10$; 33.3%), and extremities ($n = 15$; 50%). Tumour thickness ranged from 4 to 17 mm (mean 5.14 mm; median 4.5 mm). Ulceration was observed in 23 (76.6%) tumours. Eleven patients (36.6%) had at least a positive sentinel lymph node (SLN). The mean follow-up was 27.3 months (median 26 months; range 5–63 months). Patients without SLN metastases had a 5-year disease-free survival rate of 78.9%, vs. 18.2% for patients with SLN metastases ($P = 0.0121$ by log rank test). The 5-year overall survival rate for patients without SLN metastases was 89.5%, whereas patients with SLN metastases had a 5-year overall survival rate of 36.4% ($P = 0.0272$ by log rank test).

Conclusion.—Our retrospective analysis indicates that the SLN status is predictive of recurrence and survival in patients with thick melanoma, and LM/SLNB should be routinely performed in this subset of melanoma patients.

▶ Clinicians have often questioned the advisability of performing lymphatic mapping and sentinel lymph node biopsy (SLNB) in patients with cutaneous melanomas >4 mm thick. This study reaffirms the prognostic significance of SLNB in patients with thick melanomas. Those patients with a negative SLNB have a better disease-free and overall survival rate than those with a positive SLNB. Thus, it is a worthwhile procedure in these patients. A question that might be raised is whether complete node dissection is justified in these patients, although one could argue that it helps to provide regional control of disease.

P. G. Lang, Jr, MD

Size of sentinel node metastases predicts other nodal disease and survival in malignant melanoma

Pearlman NW, McCarter MD, Frank M, et al (Univ of Colorado Health Sciences Ctr, Denver)
Am J Surg 192:878-881, 2006

Background.—A positive sentinel lymph node (SLN) biopsy is an indication for completion lymph node dissection (CLND) in malignant melanoma; however, most CLNDs are negative. We hypothesized SLN metastatic size of ≤2 mm would predict CLND status and prognosis.

Methods.—We evaluated 80 consecutive patients undergoing CLND for positive SLNs over a 10-year period. Incidence of positive nonsentinel nodes and survival were compared for patients with SLN metastases ≤2 mm and >2 mm.

Results.—Of 504 patients undergoing SLN biopsy, 49 patients had SLN deposits ≤2 mm and a 6% incidence of positive CLNDs. Five-year survival was 85%, essentially the same as negative SLN biopsies. In contrast, 31 had SLN metastases >2 mm, a 45% incidence of addition disease at CLND, and 5-year survival of 47% ($P < .0001$).

Conclusion.—An SLN metastatic cut point of 2 mm is an efficient predictor of CLND status and survival in malignant melanoma (Table 3).

▶ Only 15% to 20% of patients with a positive SLNB for melanoma have involvement of nonsentinel lymph nodes (NSLNs); thus, many of them undergo an unnecessary (CLND). There have been many studies that have examined histologic variables as well as staging of the SLN in an effort to determine which patients might benefit from CLND. Although many of these investigations have been unrewarding, staging of the SLN appears to offer some promise. In breast cancer, if the patient has metastasis less than 2 mm in size, this is considered to be a micrometastasis and CLND is thought not to be necessary. These patients also appear to do better than their counterparts with macro-

TABLE 3.—Extent of Eventual Total Nodal Disease According to Size of Sentinel Node Metastases

	Micrometastasis ≤2 mm (%)	Macrometastasis >2 mm (%)
N	49	31
Nodal metastasis on CLND	3 (6)	14 (45)
More than one positive SLN	2 (4)	2 (6)
Total number of nodal metastasis		
1	46 (94)	17 (55)
2	1 (2)	8 (26)
3	1 (2)	3 (10)
>3	1 (2)	3 (10)

scopic (>2 mm) metastases. In this study, staging the SLNB on the basis of the size of the metastasis appeared to predict involvement of NSLNs (Table 3) and correlated with survival. However, other studies have not confirmed this. Moreover, patients with positive SLNs received biochemotherapy, a treatment that could have influenced the outcome. Unanswered questions include the effect of multiple node involvement by deposits less than 2 mm in size or the effect of multiple deposits less than 2 mm in size in a single node. Finally, the number of patients studied was small, and many important clinical and histological variables of the primary lesion were not available.

P. G. Lang, Jr, MD

Inguinal node dissection for melanoma in the era of sentinel lymph node biopsy
Sabel MS, Griffith KA, Arora A, et al (Univ of Michigan Comprehensive Cancer Ctr, Ann Arbor)
Surgery 141:728-735, 2007

Background.—With the introduction of sentinel lymph node (SLN) biopsy for melanoma, inguinal lymph node dissections (ILND) are more commonly performed for microscopic disease than for clinically palpable disease. We sought to examine the effect this change has on the morbidity of the operation.

Methods.—A retrospective review was performed of all patients who underwent an ILND for melanoma between October 1997 and April, 2006. Clinical and pathologic data were collected and correlated by multivariate analysis with the incidence of a major wound complication.

Results.—We identified 212 patients, 132 who underwent an ILND for a positive SLN and 80 for clinically palpable disease. Age, sex, and body mass index (BMI) were similar in both groups. Patients with clinically palpable disease had a significantly greater number of involved nodes (3.0 vs 1.96, $P = .0013$), more often had ≥4 involved nodes (29% vs 9%, $P < .001$), and a greater incidence of extranodal extension (47% vs 5%, $P < .001$). Of the 212 patients, 41 (19%) had a significant wound complication. This complication was significantly higher among patients with clinical disease compared to patients with a positive SLN (28% vs 14%, $P = .02$). Only BMI (odds ratio of 1.1) and the indication for the procedure (odds ratio of 2.2) were independent predictors of a major wound complication. Lymphedema occurred in 30% of the patients and was only significantly associated with clinical disease (41% vs 24%, $P = .025$). With a median follow-up of 2 years, regional recurrence was not significantly greater in patients with clinically palpable disease (13% vs 9%, $P =$ not significant [ns]), although this result was possibly due to the significantly greater rate of distant recurrence (49% vs 18%, $P < .001$) and death (48% vs 21%) in these patients.

Conclusions.—Patients undergoing an ILND for a positive SLN have a significantly lower risk of postoperative complication or lymphedema than do patients undergoing ILND for clinically palpable disease. There is a benefit in regard to the morbidity of treatment in surgically staging melanoma patients by SLN biopsy and preventing ILND for palpable disease.

▶ Inguinal lymph node dissection traditionally has been associated with significant morbidity, including wound infection, wound dehiscence, and lymphedema. Controversy exists whether sentinel lymph node biopsy (SLNB) followed by complete node dissection (CND) offers any survival advantage over a "wait and see" approach in patients with cutaneous melanoma. However, this study clearly demonstrates that: (1) SLNB followed by CND has a lower incidence of complications than a therapeutic node dissection, and (2) a "wait and see" approach is associated with a higher incidence of distal recurrence of disease and a higher mortality rate.

P. G. Lang, Jr, MD

Morbidity after inguinal sentinel lymph node biopsy and completion lymph node dissection in patients with cutaneous melanoma
de Vries M, Vonkeman WG, van Ginkel RJ, et al (Univ Med Ctr Groningen, The Netherlands; Groningen Univ, The Netherlands)
EJSO 32:785-789, 2006

Background.—Aim of the study was to assess the short-term and long-term morbidity after inguinal sentinel lymph node biopsy (SLNB) with or without completion groin dissection (GD) in patients with cutaneous melanoma.

Methods.—Between 1995 and 2003, 127 inguinal SLNBs were performed for cutaneous melanoma. Sixty-six patients, median age 50 (18–77) years, met the inclusion criteria and were studied. Short-term complications were analysed retrospectively, while long-term complications were evalu-

---

TABLE 2.—Complications After SLNB Alone and After SLNB with Groin Dissection Compared to Complications After Groin Dissection Alone

	Year	No. of Patients	Wound Infection (%)	Seroma (%)	Wound Necrosis (%)	Postoperative Bleeding (%)	Lymph Edema (%)
Present study[a] SLNB	2006	52	2	2	0	2	6[b]
Groin dissection Present study[a] SLNB/GD	2006	14	29	7	7	7	64[b]
Tonouchi et al.[15]	2004	20	24	32	?	4	40[c]
Karakousis and Driscoll[19]	1994	205	16	?	8	?	40[c]
Beitsch and Balch[16]	1992	177	11	6	0	3	44[c]
Baas et al.[11]	1992	151	9	17	3	0	20[c]

[a] University Medical Center Groningen.
[b] Slight lymphedema in all cases (volume difference, 6.5–20%).
[c] No further specifications into slight/moderate/severe.
(Courtesy of de Vries M, Vonkeman WG, van Ginkel RJ, et al. Morbidity after inguinal sentinel lymph node biopsy and completion lymph node dissection in patients with cutaneous melanoma. *EJSO*. 2006;32:785-789.)

ated using volume measurement and range of motion measurement of the lower extremities.

Results.—Fifty-two patients underwent SLNB alone (SLNB group) and 14 patients underwent completion groin dissection after tumour-positive SLNB (SLNB/GD group). Morbidity after SLNB alone: wound infections ($n=1$), seroma ($n=1$), postoperative bleeding ($n=1$), erysipelas ($n=1$), and slight lymphedema 6% ($n=3$). Morbidity after SLNB/GD: wound infections ($n=4$), seroma ($n=1$), wound necrosis ($n=1$), postoperative bleeding ($n=1$), and slight lymphedema 64% ($n=9$). There were differences between the two groups in the total number of short-term complications ($p<0.001$), volume difference ($p<0.001$), flexion ($p=0.009$), and abduction ($p=0.011$) limitation of the hip joint.

Conclusion.—Inguinal SLNB is accompanied with a low complication rate. However, SLNB followed by groin dissection is associated with an increased risk of wound infection and slight lymphedema (Table 2).

▶ Historically, GD has been associated with significant morbidity, especially with lymphedema. However, much of these data have come from the old literature and may be based on a different patient population than is currently treated; that is, patients in the old literature often had a large tumor burden. This article and an article by Essner et al[1] address 2 different surgical teams' approach to the management of potential metastatic melanoma to the groin area. In both studies' patients, lymphatic mapping and SLNB play a major role in management and in determining which patients require GD, thus sparing many of them unnecessary surgery and morbidity. Although both groups perform superficial node dissections in patients with a positive SLNB, their approach to determining who undergoes a deeper dissection appears to vary. In Essner et al's group,[1] the status of Cloquet's node determines whether a deep dissection is done, whereas in de Vries et al's group, a deep dissection is usually done for all patients with a positive SLNB. Although all agree that a superficial dissection is indicated in patients with a positive SLNB, there is some controversy regarding the additional value of a deep dissection, and only more controlled studies and additional data will resolve the controversy. Although there is increased morbidity, in the form of infection and lymphedema, associated with GD, this appears to be much less than anticipated on the basis of the old literature, and the morbidity associated with an SLNB is low (Table 2).

P. G. Lang, Jr, MD

Reference

1. Essner R, Scheri R, Kavanaugh M, Torisu-Itakura H, Wanek LA, Morton DL. Surgical management of the groin lymph nodes in melanoma in the era of sentinel lymph node dissection. *Arch Surg.* 2006;141:877-884.

Morbidity and prognosis after therapeutic lymph node dissections for malignant melanoma

van Akkooi ACJ, Bouwhuis MG, van Geel AN, et al (Erasmus Univ Med Ctr, Rotterdam, The Netherlands)
EJSO 33:102-108, 2007

Melanoma patients with clinically evident regional lymph node metastases are treated with therapeutic lymph node dissections (TLNDs). The aim of this study was to evaluate morbidity and mortality following TLND in our institution. Moreover, disease-free (DFS) and overall (OS) survival were evaluated and factors that influence prognosis after TLND were assessed.

Between 1982 and 2005, 236 patients underwent a TLND. Patients, who received a palliative LND or a sentinel node procedure, were not included. The median Breslow thickness was 2.4 mm. Ulceration was present in 23% of patients and unknown in 66%. 37 patients had unknown primary tumors. There were 129 ilio-inguinal, 50 axillary and 61 cervical dissections performed. 37% of the patients experienced at least one operation related complication. The most frequently seen complications were wound infections/necrosis and chronic lymph edema. Ilio-inguinal dissection patients experienced significantly more complications and a longer duration of hospitalization compared to axillary or cervical patients. The duration of hospitalization has been reduced in recent years from 12 to 5 days. The mean follow-up was 29 months. Kaplan–Meier estimated 5-year regional control was 79%, 5-year DFS was 19% and 5-year OS was 26%. The number of positive lymph nodes, the site of the primary tumor and extra capsular extension (ECE) were independent prognostic factors for DFS and only site and ECE for OS.

TABLE 2.—The Distribution of the Types of Complications According to Dissection Type

Type of Complication	Ilio-inguinal (N = 129)	Axillary (N = 50)	Cervical (N = 61)	Total (N = 240)
Short term				
Wound infection/necrosis	37 (29%)	3 (6%)	2 (3%)	42 (18%)
Seroma	25 (20%)	6 (12%)	–	31 (13%)
Postoperative bleeding	3 (2%)	1 (2%)	2 (3%)	6 (3%)
Transient nerve damage	–	1 (2%)	2 (3%)	3 (1%)
Pulmonary embolism	2 (2%)	–	–	2 (1%)
Urinary tract infection	2 (2%)	–	1 (2%)	3 (1%)
Others*	2 (2%)	–	–	2 (1%)
Long term				
Chronic lymph Edema	39 (30%)	1 (2%)	–	40 (17%)
Permanent nerve damage	–	–	5 (8%)	5 (2%)
Inguinal hernia	1 (1%)	–	–	1 (1%)
Stiff shoulder syndrome	–	1 (2%)	–	1 (1%)

*Included one postoperative bowel obstruction, which was conservatively treated. And one ureter transsection, which was treated with re-implantation of the ureter.

(Courtesy of van Akkooi ACJ, Bouwhuis MG, van Geel AN, et al. Morbidity and prognosis after therapeutic lymph node dissections for malignant melanoma. *EJSO*. 2007;33:102-108.)

In conclusion, TLND for stage III melanoma is accompanied with considerable short-term complications, and can achieve regional control and potential cure in approximately one in every four patients (Table 2).

▶ Experience has taught us that therapeutic ilioinguinal node dissections are associated with higher complication rates than similar dissections for axillary and cervical disease (Table 2). Although TLND provides good regional disease control, the long-term survival rate in these patients (26% in the current study) is poor.

P. G. Lang, Jr, MD

The unexpected sites of melanoma regional recurrences
Shoaib T, Stewart DA, MacKie RM, et al (Royal Infirmary, Glasgow, Scotland)
J Plast Reconstr Aesthetic Surg 59:955-960, 2006

Sentinel node biopsy is a means of identifying nodal involvement in melanoma and lymphoscintigraphy identifies unpredictable sites of melanoma sentinel nodes in up to 25% of cases. Whilst there is a dearth of recent publications in this area, it nevertheless remains an interesting observation that unpredictable sites of sentinel nodes are so common as to be accepted as normal. This study was performed to determine if this high rate of unpredictable lymphatic drainage was reflected in clinical practice, where therapeutic lymph node dissections were performed for pathologically confirmed regional disease.

Methods.—Patients undergoing regional lymph node dissections for histologically proven malignant melanoma were identified from a computer database. Patient details were analysed from case records.

Results.—Two hundred and forty-three case records were examined and 237 were suitable for analysis. The site of the primary was the head and neck in 50 (21%), trunk in 73 (31%), upper limb in 27 (11%) and lower limb in 87 (37%). In 15 cases (6%), the first site of regional disease was unpredictable. In these 15 cases, the site of the primary was the head and neck in two, trunk in 11, upper limb in one and lower limb in one. In 37 cases (16%), a subsequent site of nodal recurrence was unpredictable. Clinicians should be aware that patients with melanomas, particularly of the trunk, especially those in whom a therapeutic nodal dissection has been performed, may have nodal disease at unpredictable sites. However, unexpected sites of regional disease are not as common as sentinel node biopsy would suggest. Guidelines for lymph node examination in cutaneous melanoma are suggested based on these findings.

▶ Previous studies on lymphoscintigraphy have demonstrated a significant discordance between the classic teachings on lymphatic drainage and the actual location of the nodal basin that drains the anatomical site involved by melanoma. In this study, which took a "wait-and-see" approach to following up patients with cutaneous melanoma, the regional nodes predicted by classical teachings to be the site of metastasis were, indeed, often the site of regional spread. Only the trunk demonstrated a significant discordance (13%). The authors could not explain easily this finding. However, this observation would suggest that either the sentinel lymph node identified by lymphoscintigraphy is often incorrect or that the authors are experts in predicting the site of nodal metastasis. Prior data would not support the first theory, and one must wonder why these authors are so adept at predicting the site of nodal disease. Their findings require further validation and elucidation.

P. G. Lang, Jr, MD

Routine use of FDG-PET scans in melanoma patients with positive sentinel node biopsy
Horn J, Lock-Andersen J, Sjøstrand H, et al (Roskilde County Hosp, Denmark; Univ of Copenhagen, Denmark)
Eur J Nucl Med Mol Imaging 33:887-892, 2006

Purpose.—Positron emission tomography (PET) scanning is an efficient and well-known diagnostic tool in various malignant disorders. However, the utility of PET as a clinical routine screening procedure for the detection of subclinical metastases in stage III melanoma patients has not yet been established.

Methods.—Thirty-three patients with cutaneous malignant melanoma and subclinical lymph node metastases diagnosed by sentinel node biopsy (SNB) were submitted to ^{18}F-fluoro-2-deoxy-D-glucose (FDG) whole-body PET scanning within 100 days after SNB and wide local excision. Before PET scanning, patients were screened conventionally and found to be without evidence of further dissemination. Positive PET scan findings were evaluated by computed tomography scanning, magnetic resonance imaging and ultrasonography. Biopsy was performed whenever possible. The median follow-up was 15 months (range 6–39 months).

Results.—Nine patients (27%) had a positive PET scan performed after SNB and WLE. On verification, four cases (12%) were found to be true positive for melanoma metastasis and were thus upgraded from stage III to stage IV. Furthermore, one patient (3%) had another primary malignancy (prostate carcinoma), and two (6%) were found to have non-malignant lesions. Two PET-positive patients (6%) refused further investigations. In one case (3%) the PET scan was false negative. Twenty-three (69%) PET scans were true negative.

Conclusion.—In a number of stage III melanoma patients with positive SNB, postoperative whole-body FDG-PET scanning revealed further melanoma dissemination not found by conventional screening methods and thus identified these cases as stage IV. Relevant therapy can accordingly be instituted earlier on the basis of FDG-PET scanning.

▶ It would appear reasonable and prudent to screen patients with cutaneous melanoma and a positive sentinel lymph node (SLNB) for systemic disease before proceeding with a complete node dissection (CND), although there are those who might argue that a CND will provide local control and decrease subsequent morbidity. In this study, 12% of patients with a positive SLNB who underwent a total body PET scan had evidence of systemic disease. In patients with a positive PET scan the median time for survival was 12 months. There were both false-positive and false-negative scans and several patients with negative PET scans went on to die from metastatic disease. Unfortunately, this study was marred by (1) the small number of patients; (2) the fact that a significant number of patients with a positive SLNB did not participate; and (3) the fact that several patients with a positive PET scan refused further investigation. Nonetheless, this study still provides evidence that in patients with a positive SLNB, studies such as total-body PET scanning, CT scanning of the chest, MRI of the brain, or total-body CT/PET scanning should be considered, preferably before the performance of a CND.

P. G. Lang, Jr, MD

18 Lymphoproliferative Disorders

Usefulness of flow cytometry in the diagnosis of mycosis fungoides
Oshtory S, Apisarnthanarax N, Gilliam AC, et al (Ireland Cancer Ctr of Univ Hospitals of Cleveland/Case Western Reserve Univ, Ohio)
J Am Acad Dermatol 57:454-462, 2007

Background.—The pathologic evaluation of mycosis fungoides (MF) is a challenging area in dermatopathology.

Objective.—We sought to determine the usefulness of flow cytometry for the diagnosis of MF from skin biopsy specimens.

Methods.—Skin biopsy specimens from 22 patients with a clinical suggestion for MF were evaluated by 4-color flow cytometry. The results were correlated with the International Society for Cutaneous Lymphoma (ISCL) MF diagnostic score and molecular studies for T-cell receptor gene rearrangement.

Results.—A T-cell abnormality by flow cytometry was identified in all 11 patients with diagnostic ISCL scores whereas the 7 patients with either subdiagnostic ISCL scores or reactive histology showed no phenotypic abnormality by flow cytometry. In all, 10 of 11 patients with diagnostic skin biopsy specimens for MF had T-cell receptor gene rearrangements by polymerase chain reaction. Gene rearrangements were not detected in the subdiagnostic group.

Limitations.—Small study size was a limitation.

Conclusion.—Flow cytometry of skin biopsy specimens is a sensitive method for detecting abnormalities in MF and should be considered part of the routine workup of patients with a clinical suggestion of MF.

▶ The original staging system for cutaneous T-cell lymphoma (CTCL) was originally published in 1975, with a revised version forthcoming in 1979. Incorporated in an update presented by Olsen et al,[1] is a quarter century of advances in the areas of molecular biology, immunohistochemistry, and imaging, as well as new data on prognostic variables that affect staging. Olsen et al did not incorporate flow cytometry, although Oshtory et al argue for its diagnostic usefulness in patients suspected of having MF. The new staging and classification system also recognizes the fact that neither non-MF/non-SS subtypes of CTCL share the same T or N stages nor have the same prognosis as these 2 conditions; thus, the new classification system excludes these variants. Finally, the new system incorporates involvement of the blood, which is a major prognostic factor for patients with MF and SS. Future revisions to the classification and staging system will likely incorporate factors related to histopathology (eg, the importance of folliculotropic patterns or large cell transformation) and the presence or absence of T- cell receptor gene rearrangements, the prognostic importance of which is as yet uncertain.

B. H. Thiers, MD

Reference

1. Olsen E, Vonderheid E, Pimpinelli N, et al; ISCL/EORTC. Revisions to the staging and classification of mycosis fungoides and Sézary syndrome: a proposal of the International Society for Cutaneous Lymphomas (ISCL) and the cutaneous lymphoma task force of the European Organization of Research and Treatment of Cancer (EORTC). *Blood.* 2007;110: 1713-1722.

Revisions to the staging and classification of mycosis fungoides and Sézary syndrome: a proposal of the International Society for Cutaneous Lymphomas (ISCL) and the cutaneous lymphoma task force of the European Organization of Research and Treatment of Cancer (EORTC)
Olsen E, for the ISCL/EORTC (Duke Univ Med Ctr, Durham, NC; et al)
Blood 110:1713-1722, 2007

The ISCL/EORTC recommends revisions to the Mycosis Fungoides Cooperative Group classification and staging system for cutaneous T-cell lymphoma (CTCL). These revisions are made to incorporate advances related to tumor cell biology and diagnostic techniques as pertains to mycosis fungoides (MF) and Sézary syndrome (SS) since the 1979 publication of the original guidelines, to clarify certain variables that currently impede effective interinstitution and interinvestigator communication and/or the development of standardized clinical trials in MF and SS, and to provide a platform for tracking other variables of potential prognostic significance. Moreover, given the difference in prognosis and clinical characteristics of the non-MF/non-SS subtypes of cutaneous lymphoma, this revision pertains specifically to MF and SS. The evidence supporting the revisions is discussed as well as recommendations for evaluation and staging procedures based on these revisions.

▶ The original staging system for cutaneous T-cell lymphoma (CTCL) was originally published in 1975, with a revised version forthcoming in 1979. Incorporated in the update presented by Olsen et al, is a quarter century of advances in the areas of molecular biology, immunohistochemistry, and imaging, as well as new data on prognostic variables that affect staging. Olsen et al did not incorporate flow cytometry, although in an article by Oshtory et al,[1] the investigators argue for its diagnostic usefulness in patients suspected of having

MF. The new staging and classification system also recognizes the fact that neither non-MF/non-SS subtypes of CTCL share the same T or N stages nor have the same prognosis as these 2 conditions; thus, the new classification system excludes these variants. Finally, the new system incorporates involvement of the blood, which is a major prognostic factor for patients with MF and SS. Future revisions to the classification and staging system will likely incorporate factors related to histopathology (eg, the importance of folliculotropic patterns or large cell transformation) and the presence or absence of T-cell receptor gene rearrangements, the prognostic importance of which is as yet uncertain.

B. H. Thiers, MD

Reference

1. Oshtory S, Apisarnthanarax N, Gilliam AC, Cooper KD, Meyerson HJ, et al. Usefulness of flow cytometry in the diagnosis of mycosis fungoides. *J Am Acad Dermatol.* 2007;57:454-462.

Does adjuvant alpha-interferon improve outcome when combined with total skin irradiation for mycosis fungoides?
Roberge D, Muanza T, Blake G, et al (McGill Univ, Montreal)
Br J Dermatol 156:57-61, 2007

Background.—Patients with mycosis fungoides (MF) experience frequent disease recurrences following total skin electron irradiation (TSEI) and may benefit from adjuvant therapy.

Objectives.—To review the McGill experience with adjuvant alpha-interferon (IFN) in the treatment of MF.

Methods.—From 1990 to 2000, 50 patients with MF were treated with TSEI: 31 with TSEI alone and 19 with TSEI + IFN. Median TSEI dose was 35 Gy. In the TSEI + IFN group, IFN was given subcutaneously at 3×10^6 units three times per week starting 2 weeks prior to start of TSEI, continued concurrently with the radiation and for an additional 12 months following TSEI. The TSEI alone group included 16 men and 15 women with a median age of 61 years (range 31–84). The TSEI + IFN group included 14 men and five women with a median age of 51 years (range 24–83). Clinical stage was IA, IB, IIA, IIB, III and IVA in 2, 9, 4, 8, 1 and 7 patients of the TSEI group and 0, 3, 3, 7, 4 and 2 patients of the TSEI + IFN group.

Results.—Median follow up for living patients was 70 months. All patients responded to treatment. Complete response (CR) rate was 65% following TSEI and 58% following TSEI + IFN (P = 0.6). Median overall survival (OS) was 61 months following TSEI and 38 months following TSEI + IFN (P = 0.4). Acute grade II–III dermatitis was seen in all patients. Fever, chills or myalgia were seen in 32% of patients treated with TSEI + IFN.

Conclusions.—Concurrent IFN and TSEI is feasible, with acceptable toxicity. Even when controlling for disease stage, the addition of IFN did not appear to increase CR rate, disease-free survival or OS.

▶ The authors sought to assess the response rate of mycosis fungoides patients treated with adjuvant interferon alfa in addition to total skin electron beam irradiation (TSEI). Although TSEI is known to produce high response rates, relapses are the norm, even in early-stage patients. Unfortunately, the addition of interferon did not appear to increase the complete response rate, the duration of the complete response, disease-free survival, or overall survival. Hence, the authors no longer recommend interferon alfa as an adjuvant therapy for mycosis fungoides patients treated with TSEI.

B. H. Thiers, MD

Phase IIB Multicenter Trial of Vorinostat in Patients With Persistent, Progressive, or Treatment Refractory Cutaneous T-Cell Lymphoma
Olsen EA, Kim YH, Kuzel TM, et al (Duke Univ, Durham, NC; Stanford Univ, Calif; Northwestern Univ, Chicago; et al)
J Clin Oncol 25:3109-3115, 2007

Purpose.—To evaluate the activity and safety of the histone deacetylase inhibitor vorinostat (suberoylanilide hydroxamic acid) in persistent, progressive, or recurrent mycosis fungoides or Sézary syndrome (MF/SS) cutaneous t-cell lymphoma (CTCL) subtypes.

Patients and Methods.—Patients with stage IB-IVA MF/SS were treated with 400 mg of oral vorinostat daily until disease progression or intolerable toxicity in this open-label phase IIb trial (NCT00091559). Patients must have received at least two prior systemic therapies at least one of which included bexarotene unless intolerable. The primary end point was the objective response rate (ORR) measured by the modified severity weighted assessment tool and secondary end points were time to response (TTR), time to progression (TTP), duration of response (DOR), and pruritus relief ($\geq$ 3-point improvement on a 10-point visual analog scale). Safety and tolerability were also evaluated.

Results.—Seventy-four patients were enrolled, including 61 with at least stage IIB disease. The ORR was 29.7% overall; 29.5% in stage IIB or higher patients. Median TTR in stage IIB or higher patients was 56 days. Median DOR was not reached but estimated to be $\geq$ 185 days (34+ to 441+). Median TTP was 4.9 months overall, and 9.8 months for stage IIB or higher responders. Overall, 32% of patients had pruritus relief. The most common drug-related adverse experiences (AE) were diarrhea (49%), fatigue (46%), nausea (43%), and anorexia (26%); most were grade 2 or lower but those grade 3 or higher included fatigue (5%), pulmonary embolism (5%), thrombocytopenia (5%), and nausea (4%). Eleven patients required dose modification and nine discontinued due to AE.

Conclusion.—Oral vorinostat was effective in treatment refractory MF/SS with an acceptable safety profile.

▶ Vorinostat (Zolinza®) is the newest systemic agent approved by the Food and Drug Administration (FDA) for the treatment of CTCL. It is a histone deacetylase inhibitor that is usually administered in a dose of 400 mg/day. It appears to be quite effective at relieving pruritus, although the objective response rate is quite low. Thus, it is primarily a palliative agent rather than a remittable agent for the disease. Common side effects that require monitoring include thrombocytopenia and diarrhea.

B. H. Thiers, MD

Natural History and Outcome in Systemic AA Amyloidosis
Lachmann HJ, Goodman HJB, Gilbertson JA, et al (Royal Free and Univ College Med School, London)
N Engl J Med 356:2361-2371, 2007

Background.—Deposition of amyloid fibrils derived from circulating acute-phase reactant serum amyloid A protein (SAA) causes systemic AA amyloidosis, a serious complication of many chronic inflammatory disorders. Little is known about the natural history of AA amyloidosis or its response to treatment.

Methods.—We evaluated clinical features, organ function, and survival among 374 patients with AA amyloidosis who were followed for a median of 86 months. The SAA concentration was measured serially, and the amyloid burden was estimated with the use of whole-body serum amyloid P component scintigraphy. Therapy for inflammatory diseases was administered to suppress the production of SAA.

Results.—Median survival after diagnosis was 133 months; renal dysfunction was the predominant disease manifestation. Mortality, amyloid burden, and renal prognosis all significantly correlated with the SAA concentration during follow-up. The risk of death was 17.7 times as high among patients with SAA concentrations in the highest eighth, or octile, ($\geq$155 mg per liter) as among those with concentrations in the lowest octile (<4 mg per liter); and the risk of death was four times as high in the next-to-lowest octile (4 to 9 mg per liter). The median SAA concentration during follow-up was 6 mg per liter in patients in whom renal function improved and 28 mg per liter in those in whom it deteriorated ($P<0.001$). Amyloid deposits regressed in 60% of patients who had a median SAA concentration of less than 10 mg per liter, and survival among these patients was superior to survival among those in whom amyloid deposits did not regress ($P=0.04$).

Conclusions.—The effects of renal dysfunction dominate the course of AA amyloidosis, which is associated with a relatively favorable outcome in patients with SAA concentrations that remain in the low-normal range (<4 mg per liter).

▶ Lachmann et al present data that challenge the widespread perception that amyloidosis is an inexorably progressive disease. They show that AA amyloid deposits often regress and that survival is prolonged in patients who maintain low values of the circulating AA amyloid fibril precursor SAA. Dember et al[1] present a new treatment for the condition, the management of which has historically been quite frustrating.[2] Eprodisate appears to target the amyloid formation that may lead to severe organ dysfunction. Although AA amyloidosis usually presents with proteinuria, the period of latency between the onset of inflammation and clinical signs of the disease is often quite prolonged. Dermatologists need to remember that skin lesions can occur in primary amyloidosis, and a high index of suspicion is warranted when examining suspected cases.

B. H. Thiers, MD

References

1. Dember LM, Hawkins PN, Hazenberg BP. Eprodisate for the treatment of renal disease in AA amyloidosis. N Engl J Med. 2007;356:2349-2360.
2. Rajkumar SV, Gertz MA. Advances in the treatment of amyloidosis. N Engl J Med. 2007;356:2413-2415.

Eprodisate for the Treatment of Renal Disease in AA Amyloidosis

Dember LM, for the Eprodisate for AA Amyloidosis Trial Group (Boston Univ School of Medicine, Boston; et al)
N Engl J Med 356:2349-2360, 2007

Background.—Amyloid A (AA) amyloidosis is a complication of chronic inflammatory conditions that develops when proteolytic fragments of serum amyloid A protein (SAA) are deposited in tissues as amyloid fibrils. Amyloid deposition in the kidney causes progressive deterioration in renal function. Eprodisate is a member of a new class of compounds designed to interfere with interactions between amyloidogenic proteins and glycosaminoglycans and thereby inhibit polymerization of amyloid fibrils and deposition of the fibrils in tissues.

Methods.—We performed a multicenter, randomized, double-blind, placebo-controlled trial to evaluate the efficacy and safety of eprodisate in patients with AA amyloidosis and kidney involvement. We randomly assigned 183 patients from 27 centers to receive eprodisate or placebo for 24 months. The primary composite end point was an assessment of renal function or death. Disease was classified as worsened if any one of the following occurred: doubling of the serum creatinine level, reduction in creatinine clearance by 50% or more, progression to end-stage renal disease, or death.

Results.—At 24 months, disease was worsened in 24 of 89 patients who received eprodisate (27%) and 38 of 94 patients given placebo (40%, P=0.06); the hazard ratio for worsening disease with eprodisate treatment was 0.58 (95% confidence interval, 0.37 to 0.93; P=0.02). The mean rates of decline in creatinine clearance were 10.9 and 15.6 ml per minute per 1.73 m² of body-surface area per year in the eprodisate and the placebo groups, respectively (P=0.02). The drug had no significant effect on progression to end-stage renal disease (hazard ratio, 0.54; P=0.20) or risk of death (hazard ratio, 0.95; P=0.94). The incidence of adverse events was similar in the two groups.

Conclusions.—Eprodisate slows the decline of renal function in AA amyloidosis.

▶ Lachmann et al[1] present data that challenge the widespread perception that amyloidosis is an inexorably progressive disease. They show that AA amyloid deposits often regress and that survival is prolonged in patients who maintain low values of the circulating AA amyloid fibril precursor SAA. Dember et al present a new treatment for the condition, the management of which has historically been quite frustrating.[2] Eprodisate appears to target the amyloid formation that may lead to severe organ dysfunction. Although AA amyloidosis usually presents with proteinuria, the period of latency between the onset of inflammation and clinical signs of the disease is often quite prolonged. Dermatologists need to remember that skin lesions can occur in primary amyloidosis, and a high index of suspicion is warranted when examining suspected cases.

B. H. Thiers, MD

References

1. Lachmann HJ, Goodman HJ, Gilbertson JA. Natural history and outcome in systemic AA amyloidosis. *N Engl J Med.* 2007;356:2361-2371.
2. Rajkumar SV, Gertz MA. Advances in the treatment of amyloidosis. *N Engl J Med.* 2007;356:2413-2415.

High-Dose Melphalan versus Melphalan plus Dexamethasone for AL Amyloidosis
Jaccard A, for the Myélome Autogreffe (MAG) and Intergroupe Francophone du Myélome (IFM) Intergroup (Centre Hospitalier Universitaire, Limoges, France; et al)
N Engl J Med 357:1083-1093, 2007

Background.—High-dose chemotherapy followed by autologous hematopoietic stem-cell transplantation has been reported to provide higher response rates and better overall survival than standard chemotherapy in immunoglobulin-light-chain (AL) amyloidosis, but these two strategies have not been compared in a randomized study.

Methods.—We conducted a randomized trial comparing high-dose intravenous melphalan followed by autologous hematopoietic stem-cell rescue with standard-dose melphalan plus high-dose dexamethasone in patients with AL amyloidosis. Patients (age range, 18 to 70 years) with newly diagnosed AL amyloidosis were randomly assigned to receive intravenous high-dose melphalan plus autologous stem cells or oral melphalan plus oral high-dose dexamethasone.

Results.—Fifty patients were enrolled in each group. The results were analyzed on an intention-to-treat basis, with overall survival as the primary end point. After a median follow-up of 3 years, the estimated median overall survival was 22.2 months in the group assigned to receive high-dose melphalan and 56.9 months in the group assigned to receive melphalan plus high-dose dexamethasone ($P=0.04$). Among patients with high-risk disease, overall survival was similar in the two groups. Among patients with low-risk disease, there was a nonsignificant difference between the two groups in overall survival at 3 years (58% in the group assigned to receive high-dose melphalan vs. 80% in the group assigned to receive melphalan plus high-dose dexamethasone; $P=0.13$).

Conclusions.—The outcome of treatment of AL amyloidosis with high-dose melphalan plus autologous stem-cell rescue was not superior to the outcome with standard-dose melphalan plus dexamethasone.

▶ In AL amyloidosis, amyloid deposits accumulate in vital organs, leading to progressive disability and death. Depending on the extent of organ involvement, life expectancy ranges from a few years to less than 6 months for patients with severe cardiomyopathy. This study compared high-dose melphalan with standard-dose melphalan plus high-dose dexamethasone for patients with AL amyloidosis. Median survival was significantly longer in the latter group than in the former. No significant difference in response rates was noted in the 2 groups. The authors suggest that treatment-related mortality rates may have skewed the results.

B. H. Thiers, MD

19 Miscellaneous Topics in Dermatologic Surgery and Cutaneous Oncology

Electronic Templates versus Dictation for the Completion of Mohs Micrographic Surgery Operative Notes
Cowan DA, Sands MB, Rabizadeh SM, et al (Johns Hopkins Univ, Baltimore)
Dermatol Surg 33:588-595, 2007

Background.—Operative notes can be generated electronically by manual input of the entire note, free-form oral dictation, or using either an electronic template or a template for dictation. There are few studies that have directly compared these modalities in terms of speed, accuracy, and completeness.

Objective.—The objective was to determine whether electronic templates are more efficient and reduce errors compared to free-form oral dictation for the completion of Mohs micrographic surgery operative notes.

Methods.—Operative notes for 110 consecutive Mohs micrographic surgery cases were completed either by oral dictation or by electronic template. The time to dictate or complete the template was recorded for each note. Notes were subsequently edited, recording the number and type of errors as well as the time required to edit each note.

Results.—Compared with dictation, operative notes completed with the electronic template had fewer errors (5.8% vs. 81%), took less time to complete (175.5 seconds vs. 240.0 seconds), took less time to review and edit (41.6 seconds vs. 201.1 seconds), and were completed and signed in a more timely fashion (0.115 days vs. 20.7 days).

Conclusion.—Electronic templates are a more accurate and rapid method compared to free-form oral dictation for the completion of Mohs micrographic surgery operative notes and have the advantage of being immediately available to review and sign.

▶ Many younger Mohs surgeons use an electronic template to generate operative notes. The perceived advantages include efficiency, cost savings, and a reduction in errors. In this study, the authors validate these advantages. Electronic notes, when compared to dictation, required less time to edit, were more error free, and saved the cost of transcription. Moreover, the notes were immediately available for signing, which potentially could facilitate billing.

P. G. Lang, Jr, MD

Perioperative Management of Anticoagulant Therapy during Cutaneous Surgery: 2005 Survey of Mohs Surgeons
Kirkorian AY, Moore BL, Siskind J, et al (Mount Sinai School of Medicine, New York)
Dermatol Surg 33:1189-1197, 2007

Background.—The perioperative management of anticoagulation and antiplatelet therapy is a controversial topic in the field of dermatologic surgery. Dermasurgeons must weigh the risk of bleeding against the risk of thrombotic complications when deciding how to manage perioperative anticoagulation.

Objective.—Our aim is to present a summary of current practice in anticoagulation management perioperatively during cutaneous surgery. We compare our results to those found in a similar survey in 2002.

Methods and Materials.—A questionnaire surveying current practice in perioperative management of anticoagulant therapy was mailed to 720 dermasurgeons.

Results.—Thirty-eight percent of dermasurgeons responded to the questionnaire. Of the responding physicians, 87% discontinue prophylactic aspirin therapy, 37% discontinue medically necessary aspirin, 44% discontinue warfarin, 77% discontinue nonsteroidal anti-inflammatory drugs (NSAIDs), and 77% discontinue vitamin E therapy perioperatively at least some of the time. Although clopidogrel was not surveyed, 78 physicians included comments about the management of this agent.

Conclusion.—Dermasurgeons were more likely to continue medically necessary aspirin and warfarin in 2005 compared to 2002, with the most dramatic shift evident in the management of warfarin. They were more likely to discontinue prophylactic aspirin, NSAIDs, and vitamin E. Surgeons were concerned about bleeding with the antiplatelet agent clopidogrel. More evidence-based medicine is necessary to set guidelines for the management of anticoagulation and antiplatelet therapy perioperatively.

▶ As stated by the authors, the standard of care appears to be the continuation of medically necessary anticoagulant and antiplatelet therapy during Mohs surgery. The safety of discontinuing anticoagulation in low-risk cardiac patients is yet to be demonstrated; indeed, the number of thrombotic events reported by those surveyed was quite worrisome. To minimize the risk of bleeding, meticulous surgical technique is mandatory when operating on anti-coagulated patients. More evidence-based data are needed to determine guidelines for the management of anticoagulant therapy in surgical patients. Even more problematic are over-the-counter herbal supplements, such as gar-lic, ginkgo biloba, and ginseng, all of which are known to have antiplatelet activity.

B. H. Thiers, MD

Should eye protection be worn during dermatological surgery: prospective observational study

Birnie AJ, Thomas KS, Varma S (Queen's Med Centre, Nottingham, England; Univ of Nottingham, England)
Br J Dermatol 156:1258-1262, 2007

Background.—There is a potential risk of infection with blood-borne vi-ruses if a doctor receives a blood splash to a mucous membrane. The quan-tification of facial contamination with blood has never been documented in the context of dermatological surgery.

Objectives.—(i) To identify the number of facial blood splashes that occur during skin surgery and to identify the procedures that present higher risks for the operator and assistant. (ii) To assess the provision of eye protection and attitudes to its use in dermatological surgery in the U.K.

Methods.—(i) Prospective, observational study in the skin surgery suite of a U.K. teaching hospital assessing 100 consecutive dermatological surgery procedures, plus 100 consecutive operations in which an assistant was pres-ent. Primary outcome: number of face-mask visors with at least one blood splash. Secondary outcomes: to identify if any of the following variables in-fluenced the occurrence of a blood splash: grade of operator, site and type of procedure, and the use of electrocautery. (ii) A postal survey of all U.K.-based members of the British Society of Dermatological Surgery (BSDS) was conducted assessing facilities available and the attitudes of U.K.-based clini-cians to the use of face masks during surgery.

Results.—(i) In 33% of all surgical procedures there was at least one facial splash to the operator (range 1–75) and in 15% of procedures the assistant received at least one splash (range 1–11). Use of monopolar electrocautery was significantly less likely to result in splashes to the mask compared with bipolar electrocautery [odds ratio (OR) 0.04; 95% confidence interval (CI) 0.01–0.19]. Compared with the head/neck, operations on the body were sig-nificantly more likely to result in splashes to the mask (OR 6.52) (95% CI 1.7–25.07). The type of procedure and the status of the operator did not have a bearing on the likelihood of receiving a splash to the mask. (ii) From the survey, 33 of 159 (20.8%) of BSDS members had no face masks available and 54 of 159 (34.0%) did not wear any facial protection while operating. The majority (53.5%) thought they received a splash in ≤ 1% of procedures.

Conclusions.—There is a substantial risk of a splash of blood coming into contact with the face during dermatological surgery for both the operator and assistant, regardless of the procedure. The risk of receiving a blood splash to the face may be substantially underestimated by U.K.-based dermatologists. The use of protective eyewear is advisable at all times, but particularly when using bipolar electrocautery, or when operating on high-risk individuals.

▶ With more physicians performing dermatological surgery and with the increasing prevalence of HIV and hepatitis C infections, the transmission of infectious particles during surgery has become a subject of great concern. This study suggests that blood splashes to the face occur more commonly than realized, even with minor procedures, such as a punch biopsy. Although the surgeon is more likely to be splashed, the assistant is also at significant risk. A lack of experience, the use of bipolar cautery, and, possibly, performing surgery of the head and neck appear to be associated with an increased risk of being splashed. The lack of awareness that blood splashes on the face are common, coupled with the fact that many physicians do not use a face mask and eye protection, could potentially translate into a significant occupational hazard and health problem. Unfortunately, there is no way to predict how many of these splashes would have affected the mucous membranes and been of clinical significance. Nevertheless, there are 2 reasons physicians performing dermatological surgery should wear masks with eye shields: (1) the prevention of the acquisition of serious infectious diseases and (2) prevention of the transmission of infections to patients.

P. G. Lang, Jr, MD

A Novel Technique Using a Rotation Flap for Repairing Adjacent Surgical Defects
McGinness JL, Parlette HL III (Univ of Virginia, Charlottesville)
Dermatol Surg 32:272-275, 2006

Background.—The incidence of head and neck carcinomas continues to rise. Surgical excision is a frequently used method for removing these carcinomas. It is not uncommon to have multiple skin carcinomas present at the same time or in close proximity to each other. Therefore, surgeons can be presented with the challenge of repairing adjacent surgical defects while avoiding unacceptable wound closure tension and distortion of neighboring structures.

Objective.—The presentation of a novel method for repairing adjacent surgical defects with a rotation flap.

Materials.—Standard excision tray.

Conclusion.—We present a novel method for repairing adjacent surgical defects with a rotation flap. Surgeons are presented with adjacent surgical defects and challenged to find the repair option that will give the most optimal cosmetic result. The options for closing small adjacent surgical defects include making the defects a single large defect for primary closure, full thickness skin grafting, primary closure of each defect separately, flap coverage, secondary intention healing, or any combination of these. The use of a single rotation flap to cover two adjacent surgical defects provides the surgeon with a convenient and cosmetically acceptable option that avoids unacceptable wound tension and does not distort neighboring structures.

▶ In patients with a history of multiple skin cancers, it is not unusual to treat simultaneously 2 cancers that lie in close proximity to each other. In such situations, several options are available for closing the defects: (1) excising the intervening island of skin, resulting in 1 larger wound that is closed primarily; (2) utilization of a Burrow's advancement flap; and (3) the option presented here, which is the rotation or transposition of the intervening island of tissue into 1 of the adjacent defects and closing the remaining defect primarily. I have used this option on many occasions and can testify to its reliability and good cosmesis.

P. G. Lang, Jr, MD

The punch and graft technique: a novel method of surgical treatment for chondrodermatititis nodularis helicis
Rajan N, Langtry JAA (Sunderland Royal Hosp, England; Royal Victoria Infirmary, Newcastle upon Tyne, England)
Br J Dermatol 157:744-747, 2007

Background.—Chondrodermatitis nodularis helicis (CDNH) is a painful inflammatory condition affecting the helix of the ear. Several surgical treatments are described in the literature, with different cure rates and cosmetic outcomes.
Objectives.—To determine the cure rate of a novel method of surgical treatment, the 'punch and graft' technique, for CDNH and to compare this with reported techniques.
Methods.—Twenty-three lesions in 22 patients over a period of 7 years and 4 months were treated with the punch and graft technique, which is described.
Results.—A cure rate of 83% was obtained. The patients were followed up for a period of 1–86 months and cosmetic results were good.
Conclusions.—The punch and graft technique is a novel method for surgical treatment of CDNH, with results comparable with those of existing methods.

▶ In my experience, to cure a patient with CDNH, it is usually necessary to remove the damaged cartilage. This can be easily achieved by a deep shave biopsy and curettage. However, this can result in a contour defect. To avoid this complication, the authors of this study used a full-thickness skin graft, harvested with the same punch biopsy instrument used to excise the lesion. It should be noted that fat was left on the graft. A number of patients did experience recurrence. In some instances this could have been due to incomplete removal of the diseased cartilage, a problem avoided by curetting the base following shave excision.

P. G. Lang, Jr, MD

A New Surgical Technique for the Correction of Pincer Nail Deformity

Mutaf M, Sunay M, Işik D (Gaziantep Univ, Turkey)
Ann Plast Surg 58:496-500, 2007

Background.—Pincer nail is a rare deformity characterized by transverse overcurvature of the nail that increases distally. Many conservative and surgical treatment modalities have been recommended, but there is not a worldwide accepted technique for long lasting treatment of this deformity yet.

Purpose.—A new surgical technique for the treatment of pincer nail deformity is described.

Material and Method.—In this procedure, after the osteophyte located on the dorsal surface of the distal phalanx is removed to provide a flat surface for the nail bed, the distal part of the nail bed is enlarged in a transverse direction by using a modified 5-flap z-plasty technique. Over 2 years, this technique has been performed on 15 toes in 8 patients.

Results.—In all patients, the deformity was eliminated successfully with no recurrence in 2 years of follow up. The growing nail turned back into its natural form and all clinical signs and symptoms of the pincer nail deformity were relieved.

Conclusions.—Widening and flattening the nail bed provide a long-lasting effective treatment of the pincer nail deformity with an excellent esthetic result. Pain and episodes of infection is relieved perfectly with this new technique (Fig 2).

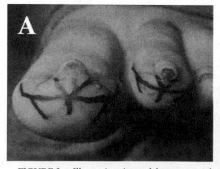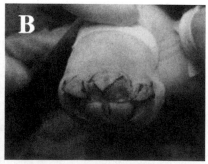

FIGURE 2.—Illustrative views of the case no. 1 for surgical technique. A, A modified z-platy with a considerably lengthened central limb toward the paraungual region is designed on the tip of the affected toe. B, After tourniquet application and digital page, the incisions are done and the skin flaps are elevated. (Courtesy of Mutaf M, Sunay M, Işik D. A new surgical technique for the correction of pincer nail deformity. *Ann Plast Surg.* 2007;58:496-500.)

▶ Pincer nail deformity can be quite painful, and its pathogenesis is unclear. To date, treatment has been less than ideal. The surgical technique described here is novel and is based on the known anatomical deformity (Fig 2A, 2B). For those performing nail surgery, it is an article that should be read.

P. G. Lang, Jr, MD

The Vein Hook Successfully Used for Eradication of Steatocystoma Multiplex
Lee S-J, Choe YS, Park BC, et al (Kyung Pook Natl Univ Hosp, Daegu, Korea)
Dermatol Surg 33:82-84, 2007

Background.—Steatocystoma multiplex is characterized by the formation of the numerous cutaneous cysts in the exposed area leaving some cosmetic problems for the patients. Only surgical excision has been effective, and its several variations were done with limited success. Because the patients usually have many cysts, excision of cysts was tedious for the doctors and left scars on the patients.

Method.—Five patients agreeing to participate in this experiment were selected. The vein hook used for ambulatory phlebectomy was employed to eradicate the cysts. The skin was incised approximately 2 to 3 mm in length. Then the mosquito forceps removed the cysts by gently squeezing or hooking the inner or outer cyst wall. By completely removing tissue around the cyst, recurrence was able to be prevented.

Result.—It took approximately 1 minute to excise one cyst completely, it left no hypertrophic scars except for transient postinflammatory hyperpigmentation, and it had no recurrences for 14 to 30 months on five patients.

Conclusion.—The use of this instrument is very simple and time-saving, providing excellent success rate with favorable cosmetic results. It can be a good alternative for eradication of the cysts in steatocystma multiplex.

▶ Steatocystoma multiplex is another benign condition for which there is no ideal treatment. In this novel approach, a vein hook is introduced through a small incision and is used to extirpate the cyst wall. In the 1 case illustrated, the results appear to be good. According to the authors, recurrences are uncommon.

P. G. Lang, Jr, MD

Periorbital Syringoma: A Pilot Study of the Efficacy of Low-Voltage Electrocoagulation
Al Aradi IK (Al-Sabah Hosp, Kuwait)
Dermatol Surg 32:1244-1250, 2006

Background.—Management of periorbital syringomas is problematic and avoided by many inexperienced physicians. The medical literature presently prefers CO_2 laser resurfacing to many other modalities, but the subject of electrosurgery has not been well explored.

Objectives.—To evaluate the clinical efficacy of electrocoagulation at low voltages in treating periorbital syringomas.

Materials and Methods.—Twenty cases were collected during the period of 2002 through 2005. All cases were photographed before treatment with a dual-frequency 4-MHz radiofrequency device (Surgitron, Ellman International, Inc., Hewlett, NY) at a power of 1 to 2 in electrocoagulation mode. Six-week follow-up visits were scheduled to discuss occurrences and expectations, observe treatment effects, and apply further electrosurgery if needed.

Results.—Clinical improvement increased with each subsequent treatment session. All patients scored either moderate or marked clinical improvement by their final visits, with 60% (11/18) revealing a marked clinical improvement (i.e., >70% clearance). The most common encountered adverse effects consisted of periorbital burning, swelling, redness, and pigmentary changes.

Conclusion.—Low-voltage electrocoagulation is an effective therapy for periorbital syringoma and should be considered when treating this difficult condition. To our knowledge, this is the first study utilizing electrocoagulation for removal of syringomas.

▶ This article represents another approach to the management of periorbital syringomas. Low-voltage electrocoagulation, without the benefit of local anesthesia, was used to treat 18 patients. Only a few clinical examples are illustrated, and in this reviewer's opinion the results are modest at best. Moreover, the frequency of recurrence is not mentioned.

P. G. Lang, Jr, MD

The Treatment of Syringomas by CO_2 Laser Using a Multiple-Drilling Method
Park HJ, Lee D-Y, Lee J-H, et al (Sungkyunkwan Univ, Seoul, Korea)
Dermatol Surg 33:310-313, 2007

Background.—Syringomas are relatively common benign adnexal tumors, predominantly developing in middle-aged women. They frequently involve the periorbital areas and cause cosmetic problems. Up to now, various treatment modalities such as electrodesiccation, laser ablation, cryosurgery, and some chemical peelings have been tried. All of them, however, have the possibilities of frequent recurrences and postoperative complications such as scarring or pigmentary changes.

Objectives.—The objective of this study was to determine the effectiveness of a multiple-drilling method in the treatment of syringomas.

Methods.—We tried a new multiple-drilling method using CO_2 laser for 11 patients having syringomas. Clinical improvement and complications were evaluated by medical records and pre- and postlaser photograph review.

Results.—All patients had good or excellent cosmetic results. No complications, such as scarring, erythema, and pigmentary changes, were observed.

Conclusion.—The multiple-drilling method by CO_2 laser might be an alternative to gain good cosmetic results without complications if applied repeatedly.

▶ Benign tumors and conditions such as syringomas, trichoepitheliomas, and xanthelasma are not easily treated. Overly aggressive treatment can lead to complications such as scarring, hypopigmentation, and ectropion. Moreover, incomplete destruction can lead to recurrence. In this article, the authors describe their approach to the management of syringomas using a super pulsed CO_2 laser. Several examples of outcomes are shown. The results in 2 patients seem good; however, the third patient appears to have scarring (see Fig 2 in original article). In addition, there is no long-term follow-up; thus, it is not possible to determine if any of the treated lesions recurred.

P. G. Lang, Jr, MD

Early Results and Feasibility of Incompetent Perforator Vein Ablation by Endovenous Laser Treatment
Proebstle TM, Herdemann S (Univ of Heidelberg, Germany)
Dermatol Surg 33:162-168, 2007

Background.—Dissection of incompetent perforator veins even when using the subfascial endoscopic perforator surgery technique is associated with substantial side effects.

Objective.—The objective was to evaluate the feasibility of endovenous laser ablation of incompetent perforator veins.

Patients and Methods.—A 940-nm diode laser and a Nd:YAG laser with 1,320 nm were used with laser fibers of 600 μm diameter. Perforators were accessed by ultrasound-guided puncture using 16- and 18-gauge cannulas, respectively. Fiber tips were placed below the fascia with at least 1-cm distance from the deep vein system. After administration of perivascular local anesthesia, laser energy was delivered in a pulsed fashion using laser power in the range between 5 and 30 W.

Results.—A total of 67 perforators were treated. Except one vein, all others were occluded at Day 1 after treatment. With 1,320 nm at 10 W, a median of 250 J (range, 103–443 J) was delivered resulting in significantly reduced posttreatment diameters to a mean of 69 ± 23% ($p=.0005$). With 940 nm at 30 W, a median of 290 J (range, 90–625 J) was administered, showing no significant posttreatment diameter reduction. Side effects were moderate.

Conclusion.—Ultrasound-guided endovenous ablation of incompetent perforators is safe and feasible.

▶ The successful management of venous disease often requires the use of several different modalities and/or techniques. In this study, the authors looked at the effectiveness of endovenous laser ablation (EVLA) of incompetent perforators (IP). Their findings demonstrate that EVLA can be used to treat IPs and that the 1320- nm Nd:YAG laser may be more effective than the 940-nm diode laser. Once these findings are confirmed, it will be important to know how this technique will be integrated into the management of venous disease.

P. G. Lang, Jr, MD

Molecular Markers in Patients with Chronic Wounds to Guide Surgical Debridement

Brem H, Stojadinovic O, Diegelmann RF, et al (Columbia Univ College of Physicians and Surgeons, New York; Hosp for Special Surgery of Weill Cornell College of Medicine, New York; Virginia Commonwealth Univ, Richmond; et al)
Mol Med 13:30-39, 2007

Chronic wounds, such as venous ulcers, are characterized by physiological impairments manifested by delays in healing, resulting in severe morbidity. Surgical debridement is routinely performed on chronic wounds because it stimulates healing. However, procedures are repeated many times on the same patient because, in contrast to tumor excision, there are no objective biological/molecular markers to guide the extent of debridement. To develop bioassays that can potentially guide surgical debridement, we assessed the pathogenesis of the patients' wound tissue before and after wound debridement. We obtained biopsies from three patients at two locations, the nonhealing edge (prior to debridement) and the adjacent, nonulcerated skin of the venous ulcers (post debridement), and evaluated their histology, biological response to wounding (migration) and gene expression profile. We found that biopsies from the nonhealing edges exhibit distinct pathogenic morphology (hyperproliferative/hyperkeratotic epidermis; dermal fibrosis; increased procollagen synthesis). Fibroblasts deriving from this location exhibit impaired migration in comparison to the cells from adjacent nonulcerated biopsies, which exhibit normalization of morphology and normal migration capacity. The nonhealing edges have a specific, identifiable, and reproducible gene expression profile. The adjacent nonulcerated biopsies have their own distinctive reproducible gene expression profile, signifying that particular wound areas can be identified by gene expression profiling. We conclude that chronic ulcers contain distinct subpopulations of cells with different capacity to heal and that gene expression profiling can be utilized to identify them. In the future, molecular markers will be developed to identify the nonimpaired tissue, thereby making surgical debridement more accurate and more efficacious.

▶ Brem et al used gene expression profiling to characterize candidate areas for surgical debridement of chronic wounds. The expression profile appeared to correlate with fibroblast cell migration capacity, and subpopulations of cells within the wound and cells at different locations exhibited an altered capacity to manifest a healing response. The gene expression patterns seemed to correlate with wound location and cellular responses, leading the authors to suggest that such expression patterns might be useful as a tool for guiding surgical debridement. Because the number of patients studied was small, it would be helpful to see these findings confirmed in a larger group of individuals.

B. H. Thiers, MD

Dressings for venous leg ulcers: systematic review and meta-analysis
Palfreyman S, Nelson EA, Michaels JA (Northern Gen Hosp, Sheffield, England; Univ of Leeds, England)
BMJ 335:244, 2007

Objective.—To review the evidence of effectiveness of dressings applied to venous leg ulcers.

Design.—Systematic review and meta-analysis.

Data sources.—Hand searches of journals and searches of electronic databases, conference proceedings, and bibliographies up to April 2006; contacts with dressing manufacturers for unpublished studies.

Studies reviewed.—All randomised controlled trials that evaluated dressings applied to venous leg ulcers were eligible for inclusion. Data from eligible studies were extracted and summarised independently by two reviewers using a data extraction sheet. Methodological quality was assessed independently by two reviewers.

Results.—The search strategy identified 254 studies; 42 of these fulfilled the inclusion criteria. Hydrocolloids were no more effective than simple low adherent dressings used beneath compression (eight trials; relative risk for healing with hydrocolloid 1.02, 95% confidence interval 0.83 to 1.28). For other comparisons, insufficient evidence was available to allow firm conclusions to be drawn. None of the dressing comparisons showed evidence that a particular class of dressing healed more ulcers. Some differences existed between dressings in terms of subjective outcome measures and ulcer healing rates. The results were not affected by the size or quality of trials or the unit of randomisation. Insufficient data were available to allow conclusions to be drawn about the relative cost effectiveness of different dressings.

Conclusions.—The type of dressing applied beneath compression was not shown to affect ulcer healing. The results of the meta-analysis showed that applying hydrocolloid dressings beneath compression produced no benefit in terms of ulcer healing compared with applying simple low adherent dressings. No conclusive recommendations can be made as to which type of dressing is most cost effective. Decisions on which dressing to apply should be based on the local costs of dressings and the preferences of the practitioner or patient.

▶ Dressings applied over ulcers are generally thought to aid healing and improve patient comfort. However, a confusing array of dressings are available, and they contribute significantly to the cost of ulcer care; moreover, their effectiveness has been questioned.[1] Palfreyman et al performed a systematic review and meta-analysis to compare the results of clinical trials that evaluated the use of dressings in the treatment of venous leg ulcers. They excluded trials that included patients with arterial and diabetic ulcers and those that involved topical agents and skin grafting. The authors found insufficient evidence to recommend any type of dressing over another, and found that hydrocolloid dressings offer no healing benefit compared with simple dressings under compression. They concluded that given the expense of many of these dressings and the absence of healing benefit, cost should be an important factor in the choice of dressings.

B. H. Thiers, MD

Reference

1. Palfreyman SJ, Nelson EA, Lochiel R, Michaels JA. Dressings for healing venous leg ulcers. *Cochrane Database Syst Rev.* 2006;3:CD001103.

Long term results of compression therapy alone versus compression plus surgery in chronic venous ulceration (ESCHAR): randomised controlled trial
Gohel MS, Barwell JR, Taylor M, et al (Cheltenham Gen Hosp, Gloucester, England; Derriford Hosp, Plymouth, England; Southmead Hosp, Bristol, England; et al)
BMJ 335:83, 2007

Objective.—To determine whether recurrence of leg ulcers may be prevented by surgical correction of superficial venous reflux in addition to compression.

Design.—Randomised controlled trial.

Setting.—Specialist nurse led leg ulcer clinics in three UK vascular centres.

Participants.—500 patients (500 legs) with open or recently healed leg ulcers and superficial venous reflux.

Interventions.—Compression alone or compression plus saphenous surgery.

Main Outcome Measures.—Primary outcomes were ulcer healing and ulcer recurrence. The secondary outcome was ulcer free time.

Results.—Ulcer healing rates at three years were 89% for the compression group and 93% for the compression plus surgery group (P=0.73, log rank test). Rates of ulcer recurrence at four years were 56% for the compression group and 31% for the compression plus surgery group (P<0.01). For patients with isolated superficial reflux, recurrence rates at four years were

51% for the compression group and 27% for the compress plus surgery group (P<0.01). For patients who had superficial with segmental deep reflux, recurrence rates at three years were 52% for the compression group and 24% for the compression plus surgery group (P=0.04). For patients with superficial and total deep reflux, recurrence rates at three years were 46% for the compression group and 32% for the compression plus surgery group (P=0.33). Patients in the compression plus surgery group experienced a greater proportion of ulcer free time after three years compared with patients in the compression group (78% *v* 71%; P=0.007, Mann-Whitney U test).

Conclusion.—Surgical correction of superficial venous reflux in addition to compression bandaging does not improve ulcer healing but reduces the recurrence of ulcers at four years and results in a greater proportion of ulcer free time.

▶ Chronic venous ulceration is an expensive and common clinical problem that often is associated with superficial venous reflux. The authors sought to delineate the effect of surgery and compression on healing and recurrence rates in patients with chronic venous leg ulceration. Early results had suggested that compression along with superficial venous surgery could in fact reduce recurrence rates.[1] Here, they present long-term data that confirm the previous findings in that surgical correction of superficial venous reflux in addition to compression bandaging did not appear to improve ulcer healing rates but did however reduce the recurrence of ulcers. This supports the argument for widespread provision of color duplex scanning and superficial venous surgery for patients with chronic venous leg ulcers.

B. H. Thiers, MD

Reference

1. Barnwell JR, Davies CE, Deacon J, et al. Comparison of surgery and compression with compression alone in chronic venous ulceration (ESCHAR study): randomised controlled trial. *Lancet.* 2004;363:1854-1859.

Application of topical mitomycin C to the base of shave-removed keloid scars to prevent their recurrence

Bailey JNR, Waite AE, Clayton WJ, et al (Royal Free Hosp, London)
Br J Dermatol 156:682-686, 2007

Background.—Keloid scars are formed by over-activity of fibroblasts producing collagen and they cause significant morbidity both from their appearance and from their symptoms. Existing treatments are often unsatisfactory. Topical mitomycin C is known to inhibit fibroblast proliferation.

Objectives.—To determine whether application of mitomycin C to the base of shave-removed keloids would prevent their recurrence.

Methods.—Ten patients had all or part of their keloid shave-removed. After haemostasis topical mitomycin C 1 mg mL^{-1} was applied for 3 min. This application was repeated after 3 weeks. The keloids were photographed before treatment and the patients were reviewed every 2 months for a total of 6 months when a final photograph of the keloid site was taken. The patients and the Clinical Trials Unit staff scored the outcome on a linear analogue scale of 0–10, where 0 = disappointed and 10 = delighted. The pretreatment and 6-month post-treatment photographs were also assessed by two dermatologists who were not involved in the clinical trial.

Results.—Four of the 10 patients were delighted with the outcome of treatment and only one was disappointed. On average there was an 80% satisfied outcome.

Conclusions.—This new treatment of keloids has been shown to be effective in the majority of patients but further studies are required to confirm this benefit.

▶ Although keloids can be surgically removed, a major problem is recurrence, even when postoperative irradiation and intralesional steroids are used. Topical mitomycin C has been used by otolaryngologists and ophthalmologists to either prevent the scarring or the recurrence of scarring after certain surgical procedures. On the basis of this clinical experience and laboratory studies, the authors applied mitomycin C to the base of wounds created by the shaved excision of keloids. According to them, the results were encouraging; however, a major deficiency of this study is the short-term follow-up (6 months). This is inadequate to assess the frequency of recurrence and the viability of this strategy to prevent scar formation.

P. G. Lang, Jr, MD

The Results of Surgical Excision and Adjuvant Irradiation for Therapy-Resistant Keloids: A Prospective Clinical Outcome Study

van de Kar AL, Kreulen M, van Zuijlen PPM, et al (Academic Med Ctr, Amsterdam; Red Cross Hosp, Beverwijk, The Netherlands)
Plast Reconstr Surg 119:2248-2254, 2007

Background.—There is no consensus on the best way to treat keloids, because adequate studies on this subject are sparse. Surgical excision in combination with radiotherapy is considered the most efficacious treatment available in severe keloids following the International Clinical Recommendations on Scar Management. Unfortunately, the recommendations are mainly based on retrospective studies that do not define recurrence.

Methods.—The authors evaluated the recurrence rate of therapy-resistant keloids treated with excision followed by radiotherapy (1200 cGy in three or four fractions). The minimum follow-up period was 12 months. The therapeutic outcome was judged as recurrence (elevation of the lesion not confined to the original wound area) or nonrecurrence. An evaluation of the outcome of the scars was obtained by using the Patient and Observer Scar Assessment Scale.

Results.—Twenty-one patients with 32 keloids were evaluated. The recurrence rate was 71.9 percent after a mean follow-up period of 19 months.

Conclusions.—This high recurrence rate suggests that radiotherapy might be less efficacious than suggested by other studies. On the basis of the authors' results, surgical excision combined with radiotherapy should be reserved as a last resort in the treatment of therapy-resistant keloids.

▶ Unfortunately, this was a small study. It would have been more interesting if a larger number of keloids had been treated and if there were more comparison groups, eg, surgery alone, surgery plus irradiation, surgery plus intralesional steroids, and surgery plus irradiation and intralesional steroids. Moreover, it would have been most informative if the keloids could have been analyzed in terms of their location. Some previous investigators have extolled the effectiveness of postoperative irradiation in the management of keloids; however, as the authors remark, this could have been due to a number of factors, including: (1) short-term follow-up, (2) a predominance of low-risk locations, and (3) the inclusion of hypertrophic scars. Despite the small number of patients studied, 2 observations can be made: (1) keloids of the ear lobes appear to recur less frequently and (2) despite postoperative irradiation almost three fourths of the keloids recur. These observations parallel those of this reviewer, who has found the benefits of postoperative irradiation to be disappointing.

P. G. Lang, Jr, MD

20 Miscellaneous Topics in Cosmetic and Laser Surgery

Evaluation of the effectiveness of a broad-spectrum sunscreen in the prevention of chloasma in pregnant women

Lakhdar H, Zouhair K, Khadir K, et al (Univ Teaching Hosp Ibn Rochd, Casablanca, Morocco; La Roche Posay Pharmaceutical Labs, Asnières, France)

J Eur Acad Dermatol Venereol 21:738-742, 2007

Background.—Chloasma, or melasma, is a pigmentary disorder that can affect between 50% and 70% of pregnant women. During pregnancy, chloasma does not require any particular treatment beside the use of an effective sunscreen and avoiding the use of any photosensitizing products or inappropriate skin care routine. However, there exist very few studies related to the benefits of sunscreens to prevent this dermatosis.

Objective.—The aim of this study was to assess the role of a broad-spectrum sunscreen in the prevention and treatment of chloasma in pregnant women.

Methods.—We tested the effectiveness and tolerance of a sunscreen composition (SPF 50+, UVA-PF 28) during a 12-month clinical trial on 200 parturients.

Results.—The 'excellent' tolerance of the sunscreen under evaluation was confirmed. Out of 185 patients who completed the study, only five new cases of chloasma were noted, an occurrence of 2.7%, which is much lower than the 53% previously observed in an usual condition study (same investigators, same geographical area and same time frame). In addition, the clinical effectiveness of the evaluated sunscreen was judged 'excellent' by the majority of parturients and by the research dermatologists during all the consultations. It is also worth noting that at 6 months, a clinical improvement was observed in 8 out of 12 volunteers who were affected by a pre-existing chloasma observed during their inclusion visit. Colorimetric measurements showed that, at the end of their pregnancy, the parturients' skin was, on average, significantly lightened (increase of parameter L* in 38% cases) and less pigmented (reduction of parameter b* in 50% cases); thus, resulting in a

411

significantly lighter skin colour (increase of ITA° in 69% cases) compared to their inclusion visit.

Conclusions.—This study clearly demonstrates the effectiveness of the well-tolerated broad-spectrum sunscreen evaluated, in the prevention of the development of chloasma in pregnant women.

▶ Sun protection is an important, although often forgotten, part of the treatment program for chloasma. Lakhdar et al clearly demonstrate the value of a broad-spectrum sunscreen for preventing the development of chloasma in pregnant women. A cursory review of the sunscreen labels of several products disclosed no warnings or cautions against use during pregnancy.

B. H. Thiers, MD

Efficacy and safety of serial glycolic acid peels and a topical regimen in the treatment of recalcitrant melasma
Erbil H, Sezer E, Taştan B, et al (Güllane Military Med Academy, Ankara, Turkey)
J Dermatol 34:25-30, 2007

Melasma is a common acquired disorder of facial hyperpigmentation. In this study we investigated the efficacy and safety of a combined treatment regimen including serial glycolic acid peels, topical azelaic acid cream and adapalene gel in the treatment of recalcitrant melasma. Twenty-eight patients with recalcitrant melasma were enrolled in a prospective, randomized, controlled trial lasting 20 weeks. The patients of the group receiving chemical peels underwent serial glycolic acid peels in combination with topical azelaic acid 20% cream (b.i.d.) and adapalene 0.1% gel (q.i.d., applied at night). The control group received only topical treatment including topical azelaic acid and adapalene. The clinical improvement was assessed with the Melasma Area Severity Index (MASI) at baseline and monthly during the 20-week treatment period. The results showed a prominent decrease in MASI scores at the end of the treatment in both groups, although the results were better in the group receiving chemical peels ($P=0.048$). All patients tolerated the topical agents well with minimal irritation observed in the first few weeks of the therapy. Three patients in the glycolic acid peel group developed a mild-degree postinflammatory hyperpigmentation with total clearance at the end of the treatment period. Therefore, the present study suggests that combined treatment with serial glycolic acid peels, azelaic acid cream and adapalene gel should be considered as an effective and safe therapy in recalcitrant melasma.

▶ Melasma can be a difficult management problem. Topical therapy alone is not always successful in its treatment. In this study, a combination of 20% azelaic acid and 0.1% adapalene gel were used in combination with a series of glycolic acid peels to successfully treat a group of patients with recalcitrant melasma. After analyzing their data, the authors concluded that their results possibly could have been improved had they used a stronger concentration of glycolic acid (50%). This study demonstrates that multiple modalities some-times need to be used to effectively treat this condition.

P. G. Lang, Jr, MD

Cardiac Complications in Deep Chemical Peels
Landau M (Wolfson Med Ctr, Holon, Israel)
Dermatol Surg 33:190-193, 2007

Background.—Deep chemical peels have been used in dermatology for more than a century. The main indications for this procedure include photoaging, perioral wrinkling, acne scars, and precancerous skin lesions. The most important potential complication of deep peels is cardiotoxicity.

Objective.—The objective was to estimate incidence of cardiac complications during full-face deep chemical peel and to suggest the methods to reduce the rate of this potential complication.

Methods.—Clinical data on the patients being treated by full-face deep chemical peel between December 1, 2004, and November 30, 2005, were recorded. Full cardiomonitoring was performed during the peeling procedure. Any arrhythmia or medical intervention was recorded.

Results.—A total of 181 patients have been treated during the study period. All the patients were female; the mean age was 56 years (range, 30–77 years). In 12 patients (6.6%), cardiac arrhythmia has been recorded during the procedure. Cardiac arrhythmia was more common in patients with diabetes, hypertension, and depression. In 4 patients the arrhythmia was self-limited and did not require any intervention. In the other 8 patients, 100 mg of lidocaine was given intravenously to control the arrhythmia.

Conclusion.—The incidence of cardiac complications in appropriately performed deep chemical peeling is lower than previously appreciated.

▶ Phenol is cardiotoxic; consequently, great care must be taken when using this agent for deep chemical peeling. Hydration, the induction of diuresis, and good ventilation decrease the risk of systemic toxicity. In this report, the author studied the frequency of cardiac arrhythmias in patients undergoing deep chemical peeling with phenol and found an incidence of 6.6%. Whether this was directly related to cardiotoxicity or was due to other factors (eg, poor analgesia) is not clear. In some instances, the arrhythmia required treatment with lidocaine. Pretreatment with propranol seemed to help prevent this complication. This study confirms the relative safety of using phenol for deep chemical peels, but it also demonstrates the importance of cardiac monitoring.

P. G. Lang, Jr, MD

Fraxel Skin Resurfacing
Collawn SS (Univ of Alabama, Birmingham)
Ann Plast Surg 58:237-240, 2007

Fractional photothermolysis is a new skin resurfacing laser technology for treating wrinkles, melanocytic pigmentation, scars, and photodamaged skin. Treatment with the Fraxel laser (Reliant Technologies, Inc.) creates microzones of injury in the skin that are surrounded by normal intervening skin that rapidly heals the injured tissue. From June to November of 2005, 70 patients underwent 2 to 6 treatments with the Fraxel laser (Reliant Technologies, Inc.) on the face and/or extremities for abnormal pigmentation, wrinkles, and scars. Treatments were 1 to 3 weeks apart. Clinically, the patient experienced little downtime other than erythema and edema for a few days followed by light skin exfoliation for a few days. After treatment, skin color and texture were more homogeneous with a decrease in the unwanted melanocytic pigmentation. The skin showed a decrease in rhytids. In summary, fractional photothermolysis improved skin color and texture and decreased fine wrinkles and melanocytic pigmentation with minimal downtime for the patient.

▶ There has been an explosion in the development of ablative and nonablative fractional resurfacing devices, which appear to yield results superior to those of prior nonablative devices. One such device is the Fraxel laser. Patients treated with this device heal in 24 to 48 hours and have minimal down time. However, multiple treatments (4 to 6) are required, and maximum improvement may not occur for months after the last treatment. Fraxel was 1 of the earlier devices developed for fractional resurfacing. Since then a number of other devices, including erbium:YAG and CO_2 lasers, have been developed; these may be more effective, require fewer treatments, and may be used on areas other than the face. It will be interesting to follow the evolution of this new technology.

P. G. Lang, Jr, MD

Safety and Efficacy of Poly-L-Lactic Acid in HIV Lipoatrophy and Lipoatrophy of Aging
Hanke CW, Redbord KP (Laser and Skin Surgery Ctr of Indiana, Carmel)
J Drugs Dermatol 6:123-128, 2007

Background.—Poly-L-lactic acid (PLLA) is an injectable filler used for the treatment of facial fat loss secondary to HIV and aging. The US FDA approved PLLA for the treatment of HIV lipoatrophy in August 2004.
Observations.—Sixty-five patients were treated with PLLA; 27 were HIV positive and 38 were HIV negative. The HIV patients had more severe facial lipoatrophy at presentation and improved more given their level of severity. The HIV positive patients required more treatment sessions and more PLLA to reach full correction than the non-HIV patients. Ninety-four percent of all

patients had no complications and the effects of PLLA were similar in both groups. All complications were temporary and resolved over time. Patient satisfaction metrics indicated that all patients were "very satisfied" with their treatment. The HIV lipoatrophy patients indicated marked quality of life improvement.

Conclusions.—PLLA is a safe, efficacious, and satisfying treatment for facial fat loss associated with HIV and aging.

▶ Until recently, there was little to offer patients with lipoatrophy. Although fat transfer sometimes can be successful, with time, the correction often is lost. Moreover, in some patients, there is no fat reservoir from which to harvest material for injection. In recent years, encouraging results have been reported with the use of PLLA. This study confirms the reports of others that it is effective for both HIV-associated lipoatrophy and age-related lipoatrophy and lasts at least 2 years. The major side effect appears to be the development of papules in the skin that resolve with time. This complication can be avoided if (1) the material is adequately diluted; (2) the injections are kept deep; (3) massage is carried out posttreatment; and (4) thin skin is avoided. The primary drawback would appear to be cost since multiple visits and injections are required for adequate correction, especially, in HIV-positive patients.

P. G. Lang, Jr, MD

Long-Lasting and Permanent Fillers: Biomaterial Influence over Host Tissue Response
Nicolau PJ (Assistance Publique Hopitaux de Paris)
Plast Reconstr Surg 119:2271-2286, 2007

Background.—The purpose of this study was to attempt to understand why some injectable fillers produce frequent ill effects and some do not, by reviewing the available agents and analyzing them through the knowledge of biomaterial studies, which show clearly what type of reactions can be expected according to the chemical used.

Methods.—A study of long-lasting and permanent fillers was performed in an attempt to understand the specific reactions induced by each agent. Agents were then compared with manufacturers' allegations and published data on complications.

Results.—All the available products have a potential for complications. However, the difference between the normal healing process and true inflammatory granuloma must be established. For a volume effect, the implant, although deep, should induce the smallest inflammatory reaction, to avoid any long-term side effects. Particulate implants with porous or irregular surfaces are potentially more reactive than spherical, smooth-surface particles. Gels and oils have a potential for fragmentation, and each droplet will start a new inflammatory phase. For a superficial treatment, it seems better to use a "passive" filler, which should have no inflammatory reaction. The problem remains for combined indications: volume and smoothing, deep and superficial. After hyaluronic acid injections in areas previously treated with a nonresorbable agent, severe inflammatory granulomas have appeared, and it is not possible to state whether they are attributable to the new product, even a resorbable one, or to reactivation of the sleeping reaction from the previous implant.

Conclusion.—There is an obvious need for serious, precise, and objective studies on most of the available fillers, which have not been properly scientifically studied on human skin.

▶ Physicians using or anticipating using long-lasting and permanent fillers should read this article. It is a comprehensive review of agents available in this country as well as abroad.

P. G. Lang, Jr, MD

Technique for calcium hydroxylapatite injection for correction of nasolabial fold depressions
Alam M, Yoo SS (Northwestern Univ, Chicago)
J Am Acad Dermatol 56:285-289, 2007

Background.—Injectable calcium hydroxylapatite is a soft-tissue augmentation material that is used off-label for facial augmentation, including repletion of depressed nasolabial folds.

Objective.—We sought to assess the safety of calcium hydroxylapatite injection for correction of nasolabial fold depressions. Specifically, we sought to obtain a quantitative assessment of injection-related adverse events using a reproducible placement technique with long-term follow-up.

Methods.—We conducted an open-label, single-center prospective study using reproducible technique with 1- to 1.5-year follow-up. All patients were treated with infraorbital nerve blocks. Then, parallel linear threading technique using 27-gauge/1.25-in needles was used to place 1 to 2 mL of injectant at the dermal subcutaneous junction into each pair of depressed folds. A triangular array of injectant was deposited under the melonasal junction. At follow-up at 2 to 3 weeks and at 1 to 1.5 years, respectively, patients were asked to report and characterize injection-related redness, swelling, bruising, nodule or granuloma formation, asymmetric correction, textural change, hypersensitivity reactions, degree of correction remaining, and overall satisfaction. In addition, patients who had received other injectable soft-tissue materials were asked to compare these with calcium hydroxylapatite in terms of risk profile and longevity of effect.

Results.—In all, 22 patients were treated and complete follow-up data were obtained from 18. Of the 18 patients, all reported at least mild postinjection redness and swelling, which abated within 1 to 5 days. Bruising was reported by fewer than half, and resolved within 4 to 10 days. Palpable but not visible nodules were reported by 2 of 18 patients; these resolved within 3 months of injection. Asymmetric correction, textural change, granulomas, and hypersensitivity reactions were not reported. In all, 14 of 18 patients re-

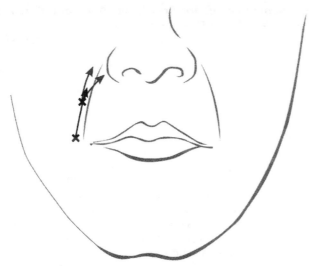

FIGURE 1.—Linear threading technique. Needle is inserted parallel to skin at base of nasolabial fold adjacent to mouth (*lower "x"*), advanced until few millimeters beyond middle of fold, and then withdrawn as injectant is delivered. Process is then repeated twice starting with insertion at midpoint of fold (*upper "x"*). Two upper threads are placed in "V" configuration to support junction of upper fold with nasal ala. (Courtesy of Alam M, Yoo SS. Technique for calcium hydroxylapatite injection for correction of nasolabial fold depressions. *J Am Acad Dermatol*. 2007;56:285-289. Copyright Elsevier, 2007.)

ported that cosmetically significant correction lasted longer than 1 year. Two thirds of injected patients who had received other fillers for nasolabial fold correction preferred calcium hydroxylapatite, with the primary reason being increased longevity of effect.

Limitations.—There was a lack of objective outcomes measures.

Conclusions.—When a consistent, defined injection technique is used, injectable calcium hydroxylapatite appears to be a well-tolerated soft-tissue augmentation material for correction of nasolabial fold depressions. A long duration of effect may make this material particularly desirable for some patients (Fig 1).

▶ When using fillers, injection technique is important to achieve the best possible result. In these authors' experience, a threading technique is optimal (Fig 1). Interestingly, there is little emphasis placed on the depth of placement. Moreover, the majority of follow-up was by phone, with only some patients returning for reexamination 6 to 18 months after treatment.

P. G. Lang, Jr, MD

Cosmetic Permanent Filllers for Soft Tissue Augmentation: A New Contraindication for Interferon Therapies

Fischer J, Metzler G, Schaller M (Eberhard-Karls-Univ Tübingen, Germany)
Arch Dermatol 143:507-510, 2007

Background.—Most of the new fillers used for soft tissue augmentation in aesthetic dermatology are considered well tolerated, but very little data are available on their long-term tolerability, especially in patients receiving immunomodulatory therapy.

Observations.—A 48-year-old woman presented with disfiguring facial edema 10 weeks after she began antiviral therapy with peginterferon alfa-2a and ribavirin for chronic hepatitis C infection. The major affected sites had been treated 10 years before with Artecoll, a permanent filler containing polymethylmethacrylate. A treatment attempt with allopurinol was initiated while antiviral therapy was continued and was successfully completed after 6 months. Despite significant improvement, extended plastic surgery was necessary for facial reconstruction.

Conclusions.—The normal host response to a cosmetic filler is a weak granulomatous reaction. Interferon and other immunostimulatory medications can lead to an exacerbation of this preexisting low-grade chronic inflammation that is quite similar to interferon-triggered sarcoidosis. This potential long-term risk has medicolegal implications for informed consent and for the potential use of both permanent fillers and interferon (Fig 1B).

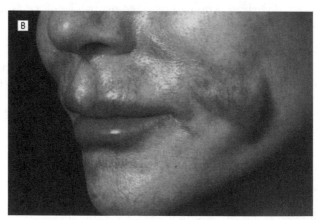

FIGURE 1B.—Swelling of the lips and formation of a cyst along the left nasolabial groove after 15 weeks. (Courtesy of Fischer J, Metzler G, Schaller M. Cosmetic permanent filllers for soft tissue augmentation: A new contraindication for interferon therapies. *Arch Dermatol.* 2007;143:507-510. Copyright 2007, American Medical Association.)

▶ Although only a single case report, the message of this article appears to be that patients who have received permanent fillers (polymethylmethacrylate) should not be treated with interferon, which may enhance a chronic low-grade inflammatory response to the filler, with potentially devastating results (Fig 1B).

P. G. Lang, Jr, MD

Use of oral glycopyrronium bromide in hyperhidrosis
Bajaj V, Langtry JAA (Univ Hosp of North Durham, England; Royal Victoria Infirmary, Newcastle upon Tyne, England)
Br J Dermatol 157:118-121, 2007

Background.—Idiopathic hyperhidrosis may be a disabling condition causing emotional stress and negative impact on a patient's quality of life. Oral anticholinergics are one of the treatments available. There are few published data on the use of the anticholinergic drug glycopyrronium bromide (glycopyrrolate) given orally in the treatment of hyperhidrosis.

Objectives.—To report a retrospective analysis describing the treatment responses, doses and side-effects of oral glycopyrrolate in the treatment of idiopathic hyperhidrosis.

Methods.—Review of case notes in a series of 24 patients, nine with generalized and 15 with localized hyperhidrosis.

Results.—Fifteen of 19 evaluable patients (79%) responded to oral glycopyrrolate. However, treatment was limited by side-effects in around one third of patients.

Conclusions.—A prospective clinical study to compare the efficacy and side-effects of oral anticholinergics is warranted.

▶ Anticholinergic drugs, such as glycopyrrolate, act as competitive antagonists of acetylcholine at the muscarinic receptor. Because muscarinic receptors are present throughout the central and autonomic nervous system as well as sweat ducts, the pharmacologic action of anticholinergic drugs can be appreciated in many organ systems. Bajaj and Langtry found oral glycopyrrolate to be effective in 75% of patients with both generalized and localized hyperhidrosis. However, side effects limited treatment in approximately one third of patients. They suggest a prospective clinical study to assess the efficacy and side effects of oral anticholinergic drugs in the treatment of hyperhidrosis. Unfortunately, the list of viable alternative treatment candidates is quite limited.

B. H. Thiers, MD

Treatment of axillary hyperhidrosis with botulinum toxin type A reconstituted in lidocaine or in normal saline: a randomized, side-by-side, double-blind study

Vadoud-Seyedi J, Simonart T (Erasme Univ, Brussels, Belgium)

Br J Dermatol 156:986-989, 2007

Background.—Botulinum toxin type A represents a safe and effective treatment for primary axillary hyperhidrosis. One of the most troublesome disadvantages associated with this therapy is pain at the injection sites. Reconstitution of botulinum toxin A in a solution of lidocaine could be an easy alternative procedure to reduce the discomfort associated with those injections. However, the current recommendations are that botulinum toxin A should be reconstituted in normal saline.

Objectives.—To compare the efficacy and tolerance profile of saline-diluted botulinum toxin A and lidocaine-diluted botulinum toxin A in patients with axillary hyperhidrosis.

Methods.—In a double-blind, side-by-side, controlled, randomized clinical trial, 29 patients were injected with 100 mouse units of botulinum toxin A (Botox®; Allergan Pharmaceuticals Ireland, Westport, Ireland) reconstituted in lidocaine into one axilla and with the same dosage of the toxin, reconstituted in an equal volume of saline, into the other axilla. The patients were followed up for 8 months. Quantification of sweat production was performed by iodine-starch tests and by the patients' own rating of sweating. The intensity of pain associated with the botulinum toxin intracutaneous injections was self-assessed by the patients and was evaluated using a 100-mm visual analogue scale.

Results.—Botulinum toxin A diluted in normal saline and botulinum toxin A diluted in lidocaine were similarly effective in terms of control of onset of sweat production, duration of effect and subjective percentage of mean decrease in sweating. Both treatments were well tolerated, and there were no lasting or severe adverse effects. However, the mean ± SD pain score during the procedure was significantly lower in the axillae treated with lidocaine-reconstituted botulinum toxin than in the axillae treated with saline-reconstituted botulinum toxin (29.3 ± 20.1 vs. 47.5 ± 24.0; $P = 0.0027$).

Conclusions.—Short- and long-term results show the equal effectiveness of botulinum toxin A reconstituted in saline or in lidocaine. However, because injections of botulinum toxin A reconstituted in lidocaine are associated with significantly reduced pain, lidocaine-reconstituted botulinum toxin A may be preferable for treating axillary hyperhidrosis.

▶ One of the main drawbacks to using Botox for hyperhidrosis is the pain associated with multiple injections. This study demonstrates that reconstituting the toxin with lidocaine decreases pain and does not have an adverse effect on its efficacy or duration of action.

P. G. Lang, Jr, MD

Botulinum toxin type A in the treatment of primary axillary hyperhidrosis: A 52-week multicenter double-blind, randomized, placebo-controlled study of efficacy and safety
Lowe NJ, for the North American Botox in Primary Axillary Hyperhidrosis Clinical Study Group (Cranley Clinic, London; et al)
J Am Acad Dermatol 56:604-611, 2007

Background.—The long-term effects of botulinum toxin type A (BoNTA) on the global impairment associated with severe primary axillary hyperhidrosis have not been comprehensively assessed relative to placebo.

Objective.—To assess the efficacy and safety of 2 dosages of BoNTA compared with placebo in subjects with primary axillary hyperhidrosis.

Methods.—Subjects (N = 322) were randomized to the use of BoNTA (75 U or 50 U/axilla) or placebo in this 52-week, multicenter, double-blind study.

Results.—BoNTA treatment significantly reduced daily activity limitations at 4 weeks after injection. A 2-point improvement on the 4-point Hyperhidrosis Disease Severity Scale (HDSS) was reported in 75% of subjects in the 75-U and 50-U BoNTA groups and in 25% of the placebo group ($P <$ .001). Improvements in HDSS scores were corroborated by gravimetric results. The median duration of effect was 197 days, 205 days, and 96 days in the 75-U, 50-U, and placebo groups, respectively. BoNTA was well tolerated.

Limitations.—The effect of total surface area involvement on treatment efficacy was not evaluated.

Conclusion.—BoNTA treatment effectively reduces the symptoms of primary axillary hyperhidrosis and is well tolerated.

▶ This double-blind, randomized, placebo-controlled study demonstrates the efficacy of BoNTA for the treatment of axillary hyperhidrosis. The response generally lasts for 6 to 7 months.

P. G. Lang, Jr, MD

Skin Cooling for Botulinum Toxin A Injection in Patients With Focal Axillary Hyperhidrosis: A Prospective, Randomized, Controlled Study
Bechara FG, Sand M, Altmeyer P, et al (Ruhr-Univ Bochum, Germany; Univ of California-Los Angeles)
Ann Plast Surg 58:299-302, 2007

Background.—Botulinum toxin A (BTX-A) injections are a commonly used and effective therapy for patients with focal axillary hyperhidrosis. However, injections are often painful. Therefore, we studied whether skin cooling decreases pain during injection.

Methods.—Thirty-one patients (n = 31) with focal axillary hyperhidrosis were enrolled in the present study. Patients were treated with 50 MU BTX-A (Botox; Allergan, Irvine, CA) in each axilla. One group (n = 21) received a skin cooling using a cold-air system (SmartCool; Cynosure, Westford, MA) versus no cooling on the other side. In the second group (n = 10), patients were cooled with the same cold air blower on one axilla and ice cubes on the other. For evaluation of the effect of cooling in both groups, relative pain scores using a visual analog scale (VAS) were recorded.

Results.—In the first group, the air-cooled-side pain scores ranged from 0 to 4 (average: 2.5) versus 5 to 10 (average: 7.4) on the noncooled side. The air-cooled side showed a 66.2% higher reduction in pain score. In the second group, no significant difference was seen between air and ice cooling (average pain score 2.0 versus 2.4; $P > 0.05$).

Conclusion.—Skin cooling decreases pain during injection of BTX-A in patients with focal axillary hyperhidrosis, with ice and air cooling showing the same efficacy.

▶ This is another study that addresses the pain associated with BTX-A injections and strategies to minimize it. In this instance cooling of the skin was used and found to provide analgesia. Air cooling and application of ice cubes were equally effective.

P. G. Lang, Jr, MD

Tumescent Suction Curettage in the Treatment of Axillary Hyperhidrosis: Experience in 63 Patients
Böni R (Whitehouse Ctr for Liposuction, Zurich, Switzerland)
Dermatology 213:215-217, 2006

Background.—Axillary hyperhidrosis is a common and most distressing problem, which can be addressed by a variety of treatment modalities.

Objective.—To assess the value of tumescent suction curettage in the treatment of axillary hyperhidrosis.

Methods.—63 patients (39 female, 25 male; mean age 30.3 ± 7.6 years) with axillary hyperhidrosis were enrolled in the study. All patients were treated in an outpatient setting with tumescent suction curettage of the axillary cavity, using two entry sites. The results were evaluated with the iodine-starch test after 4 weeks and after 6 months. Two years after the procedure, patient satisfaction was evaluated as 'satisfied', 'partially satisfied' or 'dissatisfied'.

Results.—None of the patients had early postoperative complications of infection or seroma. All patients had a marked reduction of hyperhidrosis after 4 weeks, confirmed by the iodine-starch test. After 6 months, 15 patients had high sweat rates and asked for repeat surgery. Two years after the procedure, 49 patients were satisfied, 11 patients were partially satisfied and 3 patients were dissatisfied.

Conclusion.—Tumescent suction curettage is a safe and effective treatment of axillary hyperhidrosis resulting in a high level of patient satisfaction. Some patients will need repeat surgery. Suction curettage, however, should not be used as the first line of treatment in axillary hyperhidrosis.

▶ Tumescent suction curettage has been reported to be effective for the treatment of axillary hyperhidrosis. In this series, a significant number of patients required a second procedure for adequate reduction of sweating. Were these findings operator dependent, or was the technique less effective than we have been led to believe?

P. G. Lang, Jr, MD

Repeat liposuction-curettage treatment of axillary hyperhidrosis is safe and effective
Bechara FG, Sand M, Tomi NS, et al (Ruhr-Univ Bochum, Germany; Augusta Kranken Anstalt Academic Teaching Hosp, Bochum, Germany)
Br J Dermatol 157:739-743, 2007

Background.—Liposuction-curettage (LC) is an effective surgical therapy option for axillary hyperhidrosis, with less scarring compared with radical excision of axillary skin. Although this method has proven to be effective, the treatment of nonresponders to minimally invasive surgery has not been previously defined. Whether these patients benefit from a second surgical procedure has not been evaluated so far.

Objectives.—To investigate efficacy and side-effects of a second LC with an aggressive rasping cannula in patients with insufficient prior surgery.

Methods.—Nineteen nonresponders to prior LC (13 female and six male) underwent a second LC with a rasping cannula. Gravimetry was performed before and 8 months after surgery. Side-effects, patient satisfaction, the surgeons' intraoperative evaluation and the Vancouver Scar Scale (VSS) before and after surgery were documented.

Results.—Sweat rates showed a reduction of 69% in 17 (89%) patients. Two patients (11%) did not respond to surgery. Eighty-four per cent of all patients were completely satisfied or satisfied with postoperative results. No severe side-effects were observed. The surgeon reported slightly increased difficulties during dissection of dermis from subcutaneous fat in three patients. Assessment of scars showed an excellent aesthetic outcome (mean VSS 0.79 before vs. 1.1 after surgery).

Conclusions.—LC using an aggressive cannula is an effective therapy option for patients with insufficient response to prior LC surgery, with a low risk of side-effects.

▶ As noted in Böni's study,[1] a significant number of patients with axillary hyperhidrosis will not achieve an acceptable decrease in sweating following liposuction-curettage. This study by Bechara et al would suggest that, at least in part, this could relate to the type of cannula used. The use of a sharp, rasplike cannula appears to be more effective but carries with it the risk of skin necrosis. However, in experienced hands, it can help achieve a significant decrease in sweating in patients who previously failed liposuction-curettage without an increase in complications.

P. G. Lang, Jr, MD

Reference

1. Böni R. Tumescent suction curettage in the treatment of axillary hyperhidrosis: experience in 63 patients. *Dermatology.* 2006;213:215-217.

The Effect of Thoracoscopic Sympathectomy on Quality of Life and Symptom Management of Hyperhidrosis
Boley TM, Belangee KN, Markwell S, et al (Southern Illinois Univ, Springfield)
J Am Coll Surg 204:435-438, 2007

Background.—Success with thoracoscopic sympathectomy (TS) for hyperhidrosis is 93% to 100%. We wished to determine if hyperhidrosis patients who do not undergo TS have decreased quality of life (QOL).

Study Design.—Data collection was retrospective, with telephone calls to hyperhidrosis patients who qualified for sympathectomy. Data collection included assessing sweating severity; overall QOL; social, professional, and cosmetic satisfaction; and comfort with daily activities.

Results.—Between 1998 and 2005, 60 patients met the criteria for sympathectomy. Twenty-two patients who qualified but did not undergo operations (no TS) and 26 TS patients were contacted. Change in symptoms on a 10-point scale for hands was: no TS, -0.30 and TS, -6.25, $p < 0.0001$, and QOL, on a 1-to-5 scale, increased (no TS, 0.27 and TS, 1.65, $p = 0.0003$). Satisfaction was very good/excellent socially for 9 of 22 no TS patients and 23 of 26 TS patients ($p = 0.002$); professionally for 12 of 22 no TS patients and 23 of 26 TS patients ($p = 0.021$); and cosmetically for 10 of 22 no TS patients and 23 of 26 TS patients ($p = 0.004$). Patients were very satisfied with shaking hands (9 of 22 no TS patients and 24 of 26 TS patients, $p = 0.0003$); writing (9 of 11 no TS patients and 25 of 26 TS patients, $p = 0.0001$); eating (11 of 22 no TS patients and 25 of 25 TS patients, $p = 0.0008$). TS patients had more sweating on the abdomen (no TS patients, 0.0 and TS patients, 1.75, $p = 0.0001$), on the groin (no TS patients, 0.00 and TS patients, 2.9, $p = 0.0009$), and on the back (no TS patients, 0.48 and TS patients, 4.96, $p = 0.0001$). QOL was very good/excellent at followup for 13 of 22 no TS patients and 23 of 26 TS patients ($p = 0.04$).

Conclusions.—TS controls palmar hyperhidrosis, and, despite compensatory sweating, patients having the procedure are very satisfied. Patients who did not have surgery have decreased satisfaction, comfort, and QOL, and increased symptoms.

▶ TS is usually reserved for those patients who have failed other forms of therapy. This study demonstrates that this surgical procedure is effective for controlling palmar and axillary hyperhidrosis but is accompanied by compensatory hyperhidrosis elsewhere. Despite this, it is claimed that these patients are quite satisfied and feel their QOL has been improved.

P. G. Lang, Jr, MD

Prospective Study of Infantile Hemangiomas: Demographic, Prenatal, and Perinatal Characteristics

Haggstrom AN, and The Hemangioma Investigator Group (Univ Dermatology Associates, Washington, DC; et al)
J Pediatr 150:291-294, 2007

Objectives.—To characterize demographic, prenatal, and perinatal features of patients with infantile hemangiomas and to determine the importance of these factors in predicting rates of complication and treatment.

Study Design.—We conducted a prospective study at 7 U.S. pediatric dermatology clinics. A consecutive sample of 1058 children, aged 12 years and younger, with infantile hemangiomas was enrolled between September 2002 and October 2003. A standardized questionnaire was used to collect demographic, prenatal, perinatal, and hemangioma-specific data. National Vital Statistic System Data (NVSS) was used to compare demographic variables and relevant rates of prenatal events.

Results.—In comparison with the 2002 United States National Vital Statistics System birth data, we found that infants with hemangiomas were more likely to be female, white non-Hispanic, premature ($P < .0001$) and the product of a multiple gestation (10.6% versus 3.1%; $P < .001$). Maternal age was significantly higher ($P < .0001$), and placenta previa (3.1%) and pre-eclampsia (11.8%) were more common.

Conclusions.—Infants with hemangiomas are more likely to be female, white non-Hispanic, premature, and products of multiple gestations. Prenatal associations include older maternal age, placenta previa, and preeclampsia. No demographic, prenatal, and perinatal factors predicted higher rates of complications or need for treatment.

▶ This report and a report by the same group of authors, Chamlin et al,[1] were based on findings in 1096 infants with hemangiomas prospectively followed at 7 sites in the United States and 1 in Barcelona, Spain (although the 38 infants enrolled in the Barcelona site were not included in the first report as United States National Vital Statistics System birth data was used for comparison). The authors confirm that infants with hemangiomas are more likely to be female, non-Hispanic white, premature, and the product of a multiple gestation. In addition they found that maternal age was significantly higher and placenta previa and preeclampsia were more common than in pregnancies resulting in children without hemangiomas. At least some of these findings could suggest a relationship of hemangiomas to placental abnormalities. Ulcerated hemangiomas were most commonly noted on the lower lip, neck, and anogenital region. Ulceration was most likely to occur in segmental hemangiomas with both superficial and deep components, although it must be remembered that localized lesions, which are far more common, may also develop ulceration. Most ulcerations were superficial, and bleeding, when it occurred, was most often mild or moderate. These studies are important because of the standardized review of the prenatal and perinatal history of a large number of infants with hemangiomas and because the authors were able to evaluate and observe these infants prospectively.

S. Raimer, MD

Reference

1. Chamlin SL, Haggstrom AN, Drolet BA, et al. Multicenter prospective study of ulcerated hemangiomas. *J Pediatr*. 2007;151:684-689.

Multicenter Prospective Study of Ulcerated Hemangiomas
Chamlin SL, Haggstrom AN, Drolet BA, et al (Northwestern Univ, Chicago; Indiana Univ, Indianapolis; Med College of Wisconsin, Milwaukee; et al)
J Pediatr 151:684-689, 2007

Objective.—To identify clinical features of infants with ulcerated infantile hemangiomas.

Study Design.—Cross-sectional analysis was conducted within a prospective cohort study of children with infantile hemangiomas. Children younger than 12 years of age were recruited. Demographic and prenatal/perinatal information was collected. Hemangioma size, location, subtype, course, complications, and treatments were recorded.

Results.—One thousand ninety-six patients were enrolled, and 173 (15.8%) patients experienced ulceration. Ulceration occurred in 192 (9.8%) of 1096 total hemangiomas. Hemangiomas with ulcerations were more likely large, mixed clinical type, segmental morphologic type, and located on the lower lip, neck, or anogenital region. Ulceration occurred at a median age of 4 months, most often during the proliferative phase. Children with ulcerated hemangiomas were more likely to present to a pediatric dermatologist at a younger age and to require treatment. Bleeding occurred in 41% of ulcerated lesions but was rarely of clinical significance. Infection occurred in 16%.

Conclusions.—Ulceration occurs in nearly 16% of patients with infantile hemangiomas, most often by 4 months of age, during the proliferative phase. Location, size, and clinical and morphologic type are associated with an increased risk for development of ulceration.

▶ This report and a report by the same group of authors, Haggstrom et al,[1] were based on findings in 1096 infants with hemangiomas prospectively followed at 7 sites in the United States and 1 in Barcelona, Spain (although the 38 infants enrolled in the Barcelona site were not included in the first report as United States National Vital Statistics System birth data was used for comparison). The authors confirm that infants with hemangiomas are more likely to be female, non-Hispanic white, premature, and the product of a multiple gestation. In addition they found that maternal age was significantly higher and placenta previa and preeclampsia were more common than in pregnancies resulting in children without hemangiomas. At least some of these findings could suggest a relationship of hemangiomas to placental abnormalities. Ulcerated hemangiomas were most commonly noted on the lower lip, neck, and anogenital region. Ulceration was most likely to occur in segmental hemangiomas with both superficial and deep components, although it must be remembered that localized lesions, which are far more common, may also develop ulceration. Most ulcerations were superficial, and bleeding, when it occurred, was most often mild or moderate. These studies are important because of the standardized review of the prenatal and perinatal history of a large number of infants with hemangiomas and because the authors were able to evaluate and observe these infants prospectively.

S. Raimer, MD

Reference

1. Hemangioma Investigator Group, Haggstrom AN, Drolet BA, Baselga E, et al. Prospective study of infantile hemangiomas: demographic, prenatal, and perinatal characteristics. *J Pediatr*. 2007;150:291-294.

No Evidence for Maternal–Fetal Microchimerism in Infantile Hemangioma: A Molecular Genetic Investigation
Pittman KM, Losken HW, Kleinman ME, et al (Duke Univ Med Ctr, Durham, NC; Univ of North Carolina Shcool of Medicine, Chapel Hill; New York Univ; et al)
J Invest Dermatol 126:2533-2538, 2006

In this study, using the placental origin theory as a basis, we set out to explore whether hemangioma endothelial cells (HEC) were maternal in origin. We rigorously addressed this hypothesis using several molecular genetic techniques. Fluorescent *in situ* hybridization on surgical specimens of proliferating hemangiomas ($n=8$) demonstrated no XX-labeled HEC from resected tumors of male infants. This analysis was followed by PCR genotyping of HEC ($n=11$) using microsatellite markers where cellular components were genotyped and compared to genomic DNA of corresponding mother-child pairs. In the seven informative mother-child pairs, HEC matched the genotype of the child and not the maternal genotype. Concerned that HEC represented a mixed population of cells, we subsequently enriched for cells using the placental-specific endothelial cell (EC) marker, FcγRII. Three informative mother-child pairs exhibited only the genotype of the child in our enriched cell population. Using sequence analysis, we identified an informative single nucleotide polymorphism in an exon of the placental-EC-specific protein, GLUT1. When comparing GLUT1 complementary DNA (cDNA) with mother-child DNA, the genotype of the cDNA matched the constitutional DNA of the child. Our results indicate that hemangiomas are not microchimeric in origin. This study provides further insight into the origin of a tumor whose pathogenesis remains elusive.

▶ A strong immunohistochemical correlation has been demonstrated between placental vasculature and the endothelial cells of hemangiomas. The authors of this article found through molecular genetic analysis that the endothelial cells of hemangiomas appear to be of fetal rather than maternal origin. In addition to the hypothesis that hemangiomas may originate from microembolization of placental cells of fetal origin, the authors also postulate that they could arise from mutation of endothelial cells residing in situ or from stimulation of an endothelial precursor cell in the fetus. Determining that maternal-fetal microchimerism does not appear to occur in hemangiomas is an important step in elucidating their origin.

S. Raimer, MD

Extensive venous/lymphatic malformations causing life-threatening haematological complications
Mazereeuw-Hautier J, Syed S, Leisner RI, et al (Great Ormond Street Hosp for Children NHS Trust, London)
Br J Dermatol 157:558-562, 2007

Background.—Large venous/lymphatic slow-flow malformations (SFM) can be associated with a coagulopathy resulting in thrombosis and haemorrhage. Such potentially life-threatening complications of SFM have been reported only rarely.

Objectives.—To better define the clinical characteristics of haematological complications associated with SFM, to highlight the importance of recognition and to discuss the management of these difficult-to-treat patients.

Patients and Methods.—A cohort of six children who presented with massive SFM associated with serious haematological complications was seen between January 1980 and June 2005 in the Department of Paediatric Dermatology, Great Ormond Street Hospital for Children, London, U.K. (tertiary referral centre for vascular anomalies). Clinical and haematological characteristics were recorded.

Results.—Patients were aged 1–20 years. All suffered with recurrent episodes of pain, localized skin necrosis and bleeding. All had intravascular coagulopathy and life-threatening complications. These included brain haemorrhage, massive bleeding from the uterus and colon, large and extensive thromboses of the deep vessels in the abdomen and pelvis and severe haemoptysis. One patient died suddenly at the age of 20 years from pulmonary thromboembolism and thrombosis within the deep vessels of the vascular malformation. The youngest patient underwent a leg amputation to remove the huge vascular malformation due to the major risk of complications and lack of limb function. Three of the patients underwent anticoagulation treatment and showed improvement in their coagulopathy.

Conclusions.—It is essential that patients with extensive SFM have their coagulation screened regularly to detect intravascular coagulopathy. This may progress to disseminated vascular coagulopathy and a serious risk of thrombosis and haemorrhage. Such patients require early anticoagulation in an attempt to prevent these secondary complications.

▶ The authors report a series of 6 children with extensive large, venous/lymphatic SFMs and complications that developed in these patients. Children with large venous/lymphatic malformations frequently develop localized intravascular coagulopathy that may progress to disseminated intravascular coagulation and can result in life-threatening hemorrhage. This condition must be differentiated from Kasabach-Merritt syndrome, which is characterized by profound thrombocytopenia complicating an aggressive infantile vascular tumor. The cause and treatment of the 2 conditions are completely different. Coagulation studies should be performed at birth on children with extensive large, venous/lymphatic SFMs and then monitored every few months. Anticoagulation therapy should be initiated if abnormalities develop.

S. Raimer, MD

Topical imiquimod in the treatment of infantile hemangiomas: A retrospective study
Ho NTC, Lansang P, Pope E, et al (Univ of Toronto)
J Am Acad Dermatol 56:63-68, 2007

Background.—Active nonintervention remains the mainstay of therapy for most uncomplicated infantile hemangiomas (IH) because of their expected involution. Topical imiquimod, with its ability to induce the production of interferon, tumor necrosis factor-alpha, and the antiangiogenesis factor tissue inhibitor of matrix metalloproteinase, has been recently reported to be efficacious in the treatment of IH.

Objective.—We sought to evaluate the efficacy of imiquimod 5% cream in the treatment of noncomplicated IH and possible side effects.

Methods.—A retrospective chart review analysis was performed in 18 children (16 girls and 2 boys) with a median age of 18 weeks (range: 4-256 weeks). A total of 22 hemangiomas (14 located on head, 3 on genitalia, 2 on trunk, and 3 on extremities) were treated with imiquimod 5% cream. Imiquimod was applied 3 times weekly in 10 patients and 5 times weekly in 8 patients for a mean duration of 17 weeks (7-46 weeks).

Results.—All superficial IH improved, and remission was achieved in 4 hemangiomas. There was little improvement in mixed IH with no or minimal change in all deep hemangiomas. One case with ulcerated hemangioma substantially improved with accelerated ulcer healing and hemangioma size reduction. No systemic complication was observed in any of our patients, with irritation and crusting being the most common reactive effects.

Limitations.—The small-sample, retrospective study limits the interpretation of results.

Conclusion.—Imiquimod 5% cream may be most effective in superficial IH. There was no significant correlation between response and early onset of treatment for any IH in our small sample study. Pharmacokinetic analysis

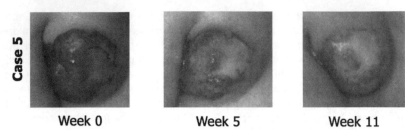

Week 0　　　　　**Week 5**　　　　　**Week 11**

FIGURE 1.—Before and after treatment. Case 5, ulcerated infantile hemangioma, demonstrated accelerating healing and great tolerance. (Courtesy of Ho NTC, Lansang P, Pope E, et al. Topical imiquimod in the treatment of infantile hemangiomas: a retrospective study. *J Am Acad Dermatol.* 2007;56:63-68. Copyright Elsevier, 2007.)

and placebo-controlled study should follow to ascertain the safety and efficacy of imiquimod 5% cream in the pediatric age group (Fig 1).

▶ In this study, complete remission of hemangiomas occurred in only 4 of the 22 lesions treated. From the photographs it appears that imiquimod caused ulceration of lesions and that the lesions resolved with scarring (Fig 1, Case 5). Only the superficial or the superficial component of mixed superficial and deep hemangiomas responded to treatment. This type of hemangioma would be expected to resolve spontaneously without scarring. Such lesions also frequently respond to high-potency topical corticosteroids, which should not cause ulceration or scarring. Imiquimod would seem contraindicated for application to hemangiomas in cosmetically sensitive areas such as the face.

S. Raimer, MD

Redarkening of Port-Wine Stains 10 Years after Pulsed-Dye–Laser Treatment
Huikeshoven M, Koster PHL, de Borgie CAJM, et al (Univ of Amsterdam)
N Engl J Med 356:1235-1240, 2007

Background.—Although pulsed-dye–laser therapy is currently the gold standard for the treatment of port-wine stains, few objective data are available on its long-term efficacy. Using objective color measurements, we performed a 10-year follow-up of a previously conducted prospective clinical study of the treatment of port-wine stains with a pulsed-dye laser.

Methods.—We invited the patients to undergo repeated color measurements performed by the same procedures as in the previous study. The results at long-term follow-up were compared with color measurements obtained before treatment and after completion of an average of five laser treatments of the complete port-wine stain. A questionnaire was used to investigate patients' satisfaction with the treatment and their perception of long-term changes in the stain.

Results.—Of the 89 patients from whom color measurements were obtained in the previous study, 51 were included in this study. The patients had received a median of seven additional treatment sessions since the last color measurement, which had been made after an average of five treatments. The median length of follow-up was 9.5 years. On average, the stain when measured at follow-up was significantly darker than it was when measured after the last of the initial five laser treatments (P=0.001), but it was still significantly lighter than it was when measured before treatment (P<0.001). Fifty-nine percent of patients were satisfied with the overall treatment result. Six percent of patients reported that the stain had become lighter since their last treatment, 59% that it was unchanged, and 35% that it had become darker.

Conclusions.—Using objective color measurements, we observed significant redarkening of port-wine stains at long-term follow-up after pulsed-dye–laser therapy. Patients should be informed about the possibility of redarkening before beginning treatment.

▶ It is usually not possible to completely resolve extensive port-wine stains (PWS); it would be hoped that any lightening achieved would be permanent. Unfortunately, this study, albeit small, suggests that redarkening of PWS is common even though they often remain lighter than they were before treatment. These studies were all performed with the first generation of pulsed-dye lasers (PDL). It is not known what effect longer wavelengths and pulse durations, along with cooling devices that allow treatment with higher fluences, might have on the permanency of lightening of PWS.

P. G. Lang, Jr, MD

Subject Index

A

Author Index